Ophthalmology Review

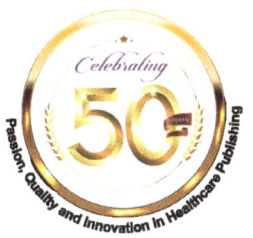

Ophthalmology Review

3rd Edition

Editor-in-chief
Myron Yanoff MD
Chair Emeritus, Department of Ophthalmology
Professor, Department of Ophthalmology and Pathology
Drexel University College of Medicine
Philadelphia, Pennsylvania, USA

Editors

Uriel Schechter OD
Instructor, Drexel University College of Medicine
American Optometric Association
Philadelphia, Pennsylvania, USA

Vincent B Lam MD
Assistant Professor
Drexel University College of Medicine
Philadelphia, Pennsylvania, USA

Kelly A Williamson MD
Assistant Professor, Department of Ophthalmology
Drexel University College of Medicine
Philadelphia, Pennsylvania, USA

Weiye Li MD PhD
Professor, Department of Ophthalmology
Drexel University College of Medicine
Philadelphia, Pennsylvania, USA

An Vo MD
Assistant Professor
Department of Ophthalmology
Drexel University College of Medicine
Philadelphia, Pennsylvania, USA

Nancy Crawford MD
Assistant Clinical Professor
Pennsylvania College of Osteopathic Medicine
Program Director
Department of Ophthalmology
Drexel University College of Medicine
Philadelphia, Pennsylvania, USA

Stephanie J Weiss DO
Clinical Instructor
Department of Ophthalmology
Weill Cornell Medical College
New York, USA

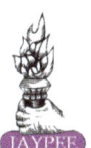

JAYPEE BROTHERS MEDICAL PUBLISHERS
The Health Sciences Publisher
New Delhi | London | Panama

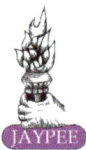 **Jaypee Brothers Medical Publishers (P) Ltd**

Headquarters
Jaypee Brothers Medical Publishers (P) Ltd
4838/24, Ansari Road, Daryaganj
New Delhi 110 002, India
Phone: +91-11-43574357
Fax: +91-11-43574314
Email: jaypee@jaypeebrothers.com

Overseas Offices

J.P. Medical Ltd
83 Victoria Street, London
SW1H 0HW (UK)
Phone: +44 20 3170 8910
Fax: +44 (0)20 3008 6180
Email: info@jpmedpub.com

Jaypee-Highlights Medical Publishers Inc
City of Knowledge, Bld. 235, 2nd Floor
Clayton, Panama City, Panama
Phone: +1 507-301-0496
Fax: +1 507-301-0499
Email: cservice@jphmedical.com

Jaypee Brothers Medical Publishers (P) Ltd
Bhotahity, Kathmandu, Nepal
Phone: +977-9741283608
Email: kathmandu@jaypeebrothers.com

Website: www.jaypeebrothers.com
Website: www.jaypeedigital.com

© 2019, Jaypee Brothers Medical Publishers

The views and opinions expressed in this book are solely those of the original contributor(s)/author(s) and do not necessarily represent those of editor(s) of the book.

All rights reserved. No part of this publication may be reproduced, stored or transmitted in any form or by any means, electronic, mechanical, photocopying, recording or otherwise, without the prior permission in writing of the publishers.

All brand names and product names used in this book are trade names, service marks, trademarks or registered trademarks of their respective owners. The publisher is not associated with any product or vendor mentioned in this book.

Medical knowledge and practice change constantly. This book is designed to provide accurate, authoritative information about the subject matter in question. However, readers are advised to check the most current information available on procedures included and check information from the manufacturer of each product to be administered, to verify the recommended dose, formula, method and duration of administration, adverse effects and contraindications. It is the responsibility of the practitioner to take all appropriate safety precautions. Neither the publisher nor the author(s)/editor(s) assume any liability for any injury and/or damage to persons or property arising from or related to use of material in this book.

This book is sold on the understanding that the publisher is not engaged in providing professional medical services. If such advice or services are required, the services of a competent medical professional should be sought.

Every effort has been made where necessary to contact holders of copyright to obtain permission to reproduce copyright material. If any have been inadvertently overlooked, the publisher will be pleased to make the necessary arrangements at the first opportunity. The **CD/DVD-ROM** (if any) provided in the sealed envelope with this book is complimentary and free of cost. **Not meant for sale.**

Inquiries for bulk sales may be solicited at: jaypee@jaypeebrothers.com

Ophthalmology Review

First Edition: 2000
Second Edition: 2012
Third Edition: **2019**
ISBN: 978-93-5270-610-5

Contributors

Clifford Goodrich MD
Ophthalmology Resident, PGY-4
Drexel University College of Medicine
Philadelphia, Pennsylvania, USA

Nicole Pumariega MD MS
Drexel University College of Medicine
Hahnemann University Hospital
Philadelphia, Pennsylvania, USA

Nida Khan MD
Department of Ophthalmology
Drexel University College of Medicine
Philadelphia, Pennsylvania, USA

Prashanth Iyer MD
Department of Ophthalmology
Drexel College of Medicine
Philadelphia, Pennsylvania, USA

Robert T Spector MD FACS
Medical Doctor
Professor, Department of Ophthalmology and Pediatrics
St Christopher's Hospital for Children
Drexel University College of Medicine
Philadelphia, Pennsylvania, USA

Ryan McGuire MD
Chief Resident, Department of Ophthalmology
Hahnemann University Hospital
Drexel University College of Medicine
Philadelphia, Pennsylvania, USA

Stephanie J Weiss DO
Clinical Instructor, Department of Ophthalmology
Weill Cornell Medical College
New York, USA

Preface to the Third Edition

The third edition of *Ophthalmology Review* has been updated with new knowledge and additional information covering all ophthalmic subspecialties. In this edition, the answers section has been further expanded to provide answers with complete explanations. New illustrations and images are also included throughout wherever needed both in the question and in the answer sections.

The book is intended to review the essentials of clinical and basic ophthalmic sciences and ophthalmic surgery. It not only provides an excellent review of ophthalmology but also quite useful as a study guide for those taking primary or recertification examinations in ophthalmology and optometry. Practicing ophthalmologists and optometrists should also find it useful as a general review.

We hope that students, residents, and practicing clinicians will use this book to explore the considerable knowledge in the ophthalmic literature that we have distilled into an easy-to-read format.

Myron Yanoff

Preface to the First Edition

Ophthalmology Review contains a series of questions covering all ophthalmic subspecialties. Answers are keyed to page numbers in the textbook *Ophthalmology*, edited by Myron Yanoff and Jay S Duker, and published by Mosby International Ltd in 1998. In some sections the *incorrect* response is sought, in others the *correct* response. The instructions for each section are given at the beginning of that section.

Ophthalmology Review is intended as a re-examination of the fundamentals of basic and clinical ophthalmic sciences and ophthalmic surgery. It is especially useful for those taking primary or recertification examinations in ophthalmology and optometry. Practicing ophthalmologists and optometrists will also find it helpful for a general review. We hope that students, residents, and practitioners will use *Ophthalmology Review* to revisit and explore the considerable knowledge available in the ophthalmic literature.

Myron Yanoff
Gary R Diamond

Acknowledgments

I am grateful to the whole team of M/s Jaypee Brothers Medical Publishers (P) Ltd, Shri Jitendar P Vij (Group Chairman), Mr Ankit Vij (Managing Director), Mr MS Mani (Group President), Ms Chetna Malhotra Vohra (Associate Director–Content Strategy), Ms Pooja Bhandari (Production Head), Ms Kritika Dua (Senior Development Editor), Mr Rajesh Sharma (Production Coordinator), Ms Seema Dogra (Cover Visualizer), Mr Akshay Thakur (Typesetter), Ms Ritika Ahuja (Proofreader), and Mr Radhey Shyam (Graphic Designer) for all their support extended to us in this project and make it a success. Without their cooperation, I could not have completed this project.

Contents

1. **Optics and Refraction** — 1
   Uriel Schechter, Clifford Goodrich

2. **Genetics and Ocular Embryology** — 13
   Kelly A Williamson

3. **Uveitis and Other Intraocular Inflammations** — 20
   Kelly A Williamson

4. **Cornea and External Disease** — 49
   An Vo

5. **Refractive Surgery** — 82
   An Vo

6. **Lens** — 93
   Myron Yanoff, Nicole Pumariega

7. **Orbit and Oculoplastics** — 123
   Vincent B Lam, Ryan McGuire, Nida Khan

8. **Retina and Vitreous** — 149
   Weiye Li, Stephanie J Weiss

9. **Glaucoma** — 207
   Nancy Crawford, Prashanth Iyer

10. **Intraocular Tumors** — 229
    Myron Yanoff, Nicole Pumariega

11. **Neuro-ophthalmology** — 257
    Stephanie J Weiss, Robert T Spector

12. **Strabismus** — 287
    Stephanie J Weiss, Robert T Spector

CHAPTER 1

Optics and Refraction

Uriel Schechter, Clifford Goodrich

QUESTIONS

Identify the incorrect answer for all questions (unless instructed otherwise).

1. **Visible light:**
   A. Wavelengths represent about 1% of the electromagnetic spectrum.
   B. Has wavelengths about the size of bacteria.
   C. Has shorter wavelengths than ultraviolet light.
   D. Has shorter wavelengths than radiowaves.
   E. Has wavelengths about 400–700 nm.

2. **Earth's atmosphere:**
   A. Absorbs potentially harmful ultraviolet and infrared radiation.
   B. Contains oxygen, carbon dioxide, and water vapor as protective substances.
   C. Is held in place by gravity.
   D. Contains water vapor from the oceans.
   E. Contains ozone formed by the reaction between diatomic oxygen and ultraviolet radiation.

3. **Rhodopsin:**
   A. Functions as a light-powered transmembrane ion pump in many single-celled organisms.
   B. Is present in anaerobic bacteria.
   C. Undergoes cis-trans isomerization shortly after light stimulation.
   D. Responds best to light at 605 nm.
   E. Is the precursor to human cone color pigments.

4. **Potential acuity measurement:**
   A. May use interferometry.
   B. Requires clear lens areas.
   C. Requires the patient's understanding of the testing goals.
   D. Tends to overestimate visual acuity when the media are very dense.
   E. Tends to overestimate acuity in patients who have macular edema.

5. Epithelial edema-induced halos:
A. Occur when the cornea acts as a diffraction grating.
B. Are white when white-light objects are viewed.
C. Can be seen by patients who have contact lens overwear.
D. Are colored when white objects are viewed.
E. Are usually seen around bright lights at night.

6. Polarized light:
A. Is totally reflected when incident on a surface at the Brewster angle.
B. Is partial under most circumstances.
C. Is vertical in most human surroundings.
D. From the corneal surface may affect calculations of corneal shape.
E. Oscillates in a single plane.

7. The ozone layer:
A. Is found high in the atmosphere.
B. Is depleted by halogenated organic molecules.
C. Reacts with the solar winds to form the aurora borealis.
D. Can be formed during lightning strikes.
E. Filters out most harmful ultraviolet light rays.

8. Ultraviolet light:
A. Constitutes 25% of the energy output of the sun.
B. Contains ultraviolet (UV)-A, -B, and -C.
C. Causes greater damage in older individuals.
D. Is filtered from the retina by the crystalline lens.
E. Obeys Planck's equation: The energy content of radiation is 1240/wavelength (nm).

9. Ultraviolet (UV) light:
A. Is divided into UV-A, UV-B, and UV-C, with UV-A being the most harmful to the superficial layers of the skin.
B. Can be harmful on a partly cloudy day.
C. Is essential to vitamin D creation.
D. Induces age spots, skin dryness, and wrinkling.
E. Can cause basal and squamous cell carcinomas.

10. Damage to the eye from ultraviolet light:
A. Is dependent on intensity and duration of exposure.
B. May result in conjunctival tumors.
C. Usually causes superficial punctate keratopathy about 2–3 hours after exposure.
D. May produce spheroidal degeneration after long exposure.
E. May produce pterygium after long exposure.

11. The crystalline lens:
A. Is susceptible to cataract formation by ultraviolet (UV) light exposure.
B. Is susceptible to cataract formation by infrared light exposure.
C. Contains enzymes that are affected by exposure to UV-C light.

D. Is susceptible to presbyopia at a younger age at lower latitudes.
E. Responds to UV light by the creation of free radicals and molecular bond breakage.

12. All sunglasses:
A. Protect against light damage to the eye.
B. Improve contrast sensitivity.
C. Improve dark adaptation.
D. Reduce glare sensitivity.
E. Vary in how much ultraviolet (UV) light they block from entering through the pupil.

13. Photochromic lenses:
A. Darken when they contact UV light.
B. Take longer to darken than lighten.
C. Are excellent UV absorbers when dark.
D. May be of glass or plastic.
E. Absorb about 80% of incident light when maximally darkened.

14. Ultraviolet-absorbing lenses:
A. Include almost all dark lenses.
B. Include clear plastic allyl diglycol carbonate (CR-39) lenses.
C. Include polycarbonate lenses.
D. Cannot be fabricated from glass materials.
E. Of CR-39 are more effective than those made of CR+39.

15. Identify the incorrect statement.
A. A photon of blue light carries more energy than a photon of red light.
B. A photon's energy is proportional to its frequency.
C. Stimulated emission produces incoherent light.
D. Spontaneous emission is a random process.
E. Stimulated emission is not a random process.

16. Identify the incorrect statement.
A. Gas lasers are the most frequently used ophthalmic lasers.
B. Population inversion is caused by lights external to the cavity or by an electric discharge.
C. Once achieved, population inversion needs not to be maintained.
D. Most high-energy states decay in a few nanoseconds by spontaneous emission.
E. Population inversion occurs when electrons in high-energy states outnumber those in low-energy states.

17. Identify the incorrect statement.
A. Pulsed lasers deliver more energy overtime than continuous lasers.
B. "Laser" is an acronym for "light amplification by stimulated emission of radiation".
C. Continuous lasers allow more control over energy than pulsed lasers.
D. Excimer and neodymium-doped yttrium aluminum garnet (Nd:YAG) lasers are pulsed.

E. Excimer lasers emit a beam of light with a wavelength of less than 200 nm.

18. Identify the incorrect statement.
    A. The number of available laser wavelengths can be increased by harmonic generation and use of organic dyes.
    B. The argon ion produces wavelengths of blue-green and green wavelengths.
    C. Xanthophyll pigment is abundant in the human macula and highly absorbs green light.
    D. Lasers may use gases, liquids, or solids as exciting materials.
    E. Krypton red lasers operating at 647 nm are commonly available.

19. Identify the incorrect statement.
    A. Powerful lasers that are useful as weapons are commonly available.
    B. Laser photocoagulation involves tissue light absorption which generates heat.
    C. Laser photodisruption is a mechanical process that creates a small, but high-energy shock wave at its focus.
    D. Laser photoablation breaks chemical bonds essentially vaporizing tissue.
    E. The laser-specific wavelength determines which light-tissue interaction occurs.

20. Identify the incorrect statement.
    A. In retinal photocoagulation, laser light is absorbed by the pigment in the retinal pigment epithelium and choroid.
    B. In photocoagulation, the energy is uniformly distributed across the whole diameter of the aiming beam.
    C. A tenfold increase in exposure time roughly doubles laser lesion diameter.
    D. Assuming constant laser power and duration, a smaller spot size is more likely to cause complications than a larger spot size.
    E. Doubling power doubles the lesion size.

21. Identify the incorrect statement.
    A. As a rule, contact lenses that invert the fundus view roughly double the spot size.
    B. Whenever laser spot size is changed, power must be adjusted to maintain an equal burn intensity.
    C. Contact lenses giving direct fundus view (e.g. Goldmann three-mirror lens) do not change spot size.
    D. Smaller spot sizes are rarely necessary outside the posterior pole.
    E. Shorter duration burns are less likely to disrupt Bruch's membrane than longer duration burns, given the same power and size.

22. Identify the incorrect statement.
    A. The retina thins in the periphery, so less power is necessary in that area.

B. Treatment of the peripheral retina is often painful for the patient.
C. A noncircular aiming beam has lower power density than a circular type.
D. The laser beam is rarely parfocal with the slit-lamp's viewing optics.
E. Treatment of the posterior pole requires brief exposure times.

23. **Identify the incorrect statement.**
    A. The neodymium-doped yttrium aluminum garnet laser is a photo-disruptor.
    B. High-energy requirements of the Nd:YAG demand a pulsed energy system.
    C. Q-switching describes the method of changing a laser's frequency.
    D. Mode locking produces the shortest and most powerful pulses.
    E. Most clinical photodisruptors are Q-switched.

24. **The neodymium-doped yttrium aluminum garnet laser:**
    A. Produces visible red light.
    B. Rarely coincides with the aiming beam.
    C. Produces a cone of light.
    D. Is used in capsulectomy by focusing in the anterior vitreous and moving forward.
    E. Is more likely to damage silicone intraocular lenses optically than acrylic ones.

25. **Identify the incorrect statement.**
    A. The total chromatic aberration of the human eye is approximately 3 diopters.
    B. Maximum eye sensitivity occurs at about 560 nm.
    C. Retinal photoreceptors point toward the second nodal point of the eye.
    D. The cornea-aqueous interface is the site of the greatest change in refractive index within the eye.
    E. Depth of focus increases, as pupillary diameter decreases.

26. **Identify the incorrect statement.**
    A. The Snellen formula assumes that each element in a 20/20 (6/6) target subtends 5 minutes of arc.
    B. The high contrast of a Snellen acuity chart does not represent the contrast of everyday targets.
    C. The Bailey–Lovie acuity chart uses 10 letters of similar difficulty with 5 per line.
    D. The Bailey–Lovie acuity chart uses a uniform change in angular size for each line.
    E. The Snellen acuity chart does not have an orderly progression of target size changes from line to line.

27. **Identify the incorrect statement.**
    A. Contrast is the difference in luminance of objects against a background.

B. Contrast sensitivity decreases with age.
C. Contrast sensitivity decreases with decreased luminance.
D. Pupil size of 1 mm gives the maximal modulation transfer function for high spatial frequencies.
E. Visual acuity of 20/20 (6/6) is equivalent to 30 cycles per degree.

28. **Identify the incorrect statement.**
    A. Vernier acuity testing involves cortical processing, and allowing a subject to detect targets that are smaller than the diffraction limit of the eye.
    B. Retinal photoreceptors are triggered by a minimum of 3 quanta of visible light.
    C. Professional tennis players cannot visually follow the ball to the racquet with accuracy.
    D. Babe Ruth was only able to see 20/200 (6/60) out of his left eye, but was able to see 20/15 (6/4.5) out of his right eye.
    E. More than three retinal ganglion cells are connected to each foveal cone.

29. **Identify the incorrect statement.**
    A. Myopia has a racial predilection.
    B. Prolonged near work may cause increased myopia.
    C. The majority of myopes have refractive errors exceeding 2 diopters.
    D. Approximately, 1–3% of the population has pathologic myopia.
    E. The majority of a typical medical school class is likely to be myopic.

30. **Identify the incorrect statement.**
    A. About half of all infants less than 2 years of age have more than 1 diopter of astigmatism.
    B. About 2% of adults have astigmatism more than 3 diopters.
    C. Most neonatal astigmatism persists into adulthood.
    D. Neonatal astigmatism changes at different ages in different populations around the world.
    E. Neonatal astigmatism may permit the infant with uncorrected myopia to have a better acuity by using accommodation.

31. **Identify the incorrect statement.**
    A. Presbyopia occurs earlier in persons who live closer to the equator because of ambient temperature effect.
    B. Presbyopes purchase two-third of spectacles in developed countries.
    C. The mean axial length of a full-term neonate measures 16–18 mm.
    D. Suturing together a monkey's eyelids leads to axial myopia.
    E. By age of 3 years, a human eye is about 20 mm in diameter.

32. **A Jackson's cross cylinder test:**
    A. Involves the principle of placing the circle of least confusion on the retina.
    B. Cannot determine the power of the astigmatic correction.
    C. Verifies the axis and power of the correcting cylindrical lens.

D. Uses a lens in which the principal powers are equal and opposite in sign.
   E. Has markings (red dots) on each end of the minus axis.

33. **A red–green duochrome test:**
   A. Is used for binocular balance.
   B. Makes use of the eye's chromatic aberration.
   C. Uses a pair of colored slides at 500 nm (green) and 670 nm (red).
   D. Should be performed prior to performing the Jackson's cross cylinder test.
   E. Is sensitive to 0.25 diopter.

34. **A stenopeic slit:**
   A. Acts as a line of pinholes.
   B. Can be used to screen for astigmatism.
   C. Is most useful in patients who have better than 20/40 (6/12) visual acuity.
   D. Is found in most trial lens sets.
   E. Is useful in patients who have scarred corneas.

35. **Identify the incorrect statement.**
   A. The optical center of a lens is the point where the prismatic displacement is zero.
   B. A low-Abbe number implies greater chromatic aberration by the lens.
   C. Polycarbonate lenses must be able to withstand the impact of dropping 16 g steel balls from the height of 10 feet.
   D. No IR lenses absorb infrared radiation without significantly decreasing transmission of visible light.
   E. Polycarbonate lenses are usually the material of choice for children's glasses.

36. **Identify the incorrect statement.**
   A. Pantoscopic tilt describes the positioning of a bifocal toward the nasal aspect of a prescription lens.
   B. Antireflective coatings are generally single layer of material equal in thickness to 0.25 of the wavelength of yellow light
   C. Antireflective coatings cannot be applied to glass lenses.
   D. Antiscratch properties can be added to lenses by heat treatment or dipping.
   E. Weak minus lenses are particularly susceptible to the creation of double imaging when viewed by others.

37. **Identify the incorrect statement.**
   A. Most patients are intolerant of a vertical prism imbalance of more than 0.5 diopter.
   B. Bicentral (slab-off) grinding is an inexpensive way of correcting induced vertical prism.
   C. A 3% size difference between the eyes is often sufficient for the creation of asthenopia.

D. A few laboratories can furnish iseikonic ("size") lenses.
E. A light shined through a 1 prism diopter lens deflects a ray of light 1 cm at a target distance of 1 meter.

38. **Identify the incorrect statement.**
    A. Flat top segments cause minimal image jump.
    B. Round top segments cause maximal image jump.
    C. In myopes, flat top segments minimize image displacement.
    D. In hyperopes, base-up prisms minimize image displacement.
    E. Franklin segments cause no image jump.

39. **Progressive addition lenses:**
    A. Are unable to use laboratory-applied coatings.
    B. Are available in glass and plastic.
    C. Are right and left eye specific.
    D. May disturb peripheral visual space.
    E. Require the patient to learn head turning.

40. **Identify the incorrect statement.**
    A. Hydrogel contact lenses have names ending in "filcon".
    B. Nonhydrogel contact lenses have names ending in "focon".
    C. Lenses with less than 10% water content are considered "low-water content" lenses by the US Food and Drug Administration.
    D. The Dk of contact lenses refers to the oxygen permeability of the lens.
    E. Central oxygen transmissibility of a contact lens depends on lens thickness.

41. **Soft contact lenses fitted for extended wear:**
    A. Contain essentially the same materials as soft lenses fitted for daily wear.
    B. Are associated with a 10–15 times greater incidence of microbial keratitis than daily wear lenses.
    C. May not contain the proper Dk/t necessary to maintain a healthy cornea.
    D. Are fit less frequently than rigid gas-permeable lenses for extended wear.
    E. Are approved by the US Food and Drug Administration for up to 7 days' wear.

42. **Soft contact lenses that:**
    A. Fit too steeply will show minimal movement upon blinking.
    B. Fit too flatly will show excessive movement upon blinking.
    C. Are dry will exhibit poor keratometric mires.
    D. Fit too flatly may cause patient discomfort upon blinking.
    E. Fit steeply will decenter easily.

43. **Corneal fluorescein staining with contact lens wear may be due to:**
    A. Mechanical trauma.
    B. Metabolic interference.

C. Exposure keratitis.
D. Chemical toxicity.
E. Excessive lens permeability.

44. Corneal edema associated with contact lens wear:
   A. Appears as a central circular whitish gray opacity in patients wearing rigid gas-permeable lenses.
   B. Appears as posterior stroma striae or endothelial folds in patients wearing soft lenses.
   C. Usually occurs to some extent, patients who wear extended wear soft lenses.
   D. When appearing as stromal striae is usually oriented horizontally.
   E. Is usually caused by hypoxia.

45. Corneal microcysts:
   A. On slit-lamp examination distribute light similarly to the background.
   B. Are caused by disrupted cell growth resulting from hypoxia.
   C. May work through the corneal surface to cause fluorescein staining.
   D. Present after contact lenses are discontinued may increase for a few weeks.
   E. Are accumulations of dead cellular material.

46. Superior limbic keratoconjunctivitis:
   A. Is caused most often by extended wear of soft contact lenses in those who wear contact lenses.
   B. Is located in the posterior stroma.
   C. Is often quite painful.
   D. May be seen in individuals who do not wear contact lenses.
   E. Is usually not associated with epithelial defects.

47. Giant papillary conjunctivitis in contact lens wearers:
   A. Can be caused by mechanical irritation of the conjunctiva by the lens.
   B. Can be caused by an autoimmune reaction to the patient's mucoproteins on the lens.
   C. Includes papillae with a diameter of more than 0.5 mm.
   D. Consists of papillae containing lymphocytes and plasma cells.
   E. Does not significantly respond to mast cell stabilizers.

48. Identify the incorrect statement.
   A. A myope who wears contact lenses must accommodate more than one who wears glasses.
   B. A myope must converge more through glasses than contact lenses.
   C. A hyperope must converge less through glasses than contact lenses.
   D. Contact lenses induce a prismatic effect on convergence.
   E. A hyperope who wears contact lenses must accommodate less than one who wears glasses.

49. During retinoscopy:
   A. At neutralization, the far point of the patient's eye is focused at the peephole of the retinoscope.

B. A typical working distance is 75 cm.
C. The far point of the uncorrected hyperope is behind the patient's retina.
D. The closer to neutrality, the faster the reflex movement.
E. The closer to neutrality, the brighter the reflex movement.

50. Identify the incorrect statement regarding keratometry.
A. It assumes that the cornea is spherical or toric.
B. Placido disc topography is primarily a qualitative assessment of the cornea.
C. It measures only the anterior corneal power.
D. It works well enough to permit accurate contact lens fittings.
E. It compensates for the negative posterior corneal power by using a lower corneal refractive index.

51. A lensometer:
A. Measures the focal length of the lens.
B. Consists of a movable target, a powerful fixed lens, and a telescopic eyepiece.
C. Maintains proportion among the power of the unknown lens, the target, and the fixed field lens.
D. Can be used with progressive multifocal lenses.
E. Has changed little in design since automation.

52. Indirect ophthalmoscope:
A. Provides a real and inverted aerial image of the patient's illuminated fundus.
B. When used with stronger lenses, it provides a larger field of retinal view.
C. In examination of an emmetropic eye with a 20 diopter lens, it provides 2× magnification.
D. Produces magnified images of small changes in retinal topography.
E. Brings the patient's and the examiner's pupils into conjugate relationship.

ANSWERS

1. C. Visible light has longer wavelengths than ultraviolet light.
2. B. The earth's atmosphere contains ozone, carbon monoxide, and water vapor as protective substances.
3. D. Rhodopsin responds best to light at 495 nm, but also responds to almost all visible light.
4. D. When the media are very dense, interferometry may not be possible to find two clear areas to form an interference pattern on the retina.
5. B. Haloes produced by epithelial edema are colored when white-light objects are viewed.
6. C. Polarization of light is horizontal in most human surroundings.
7. C. The ozone layer has no role in the creating the aurora borealis.

Optics and Refraction

8. A. Ultraviolet light constitutes about 10% of the energy emitted by the sun.
9. A. Damage to the superficial layers of the skin often referred to as "sunburn", is caused mostly by ultraviolet (UV)-B.
10. C. Ultraviolet light damage to the eye usually causes superficial punctate keratopathy about 8–12 hours after exposure.
11. C. The crystalline lens enzymes are affected by exposure to ultraviolet (UV)-A and B light.
12. A. Sunglasses ironically may increase the chance of light damage to the eye because the pupil dilates behind dark glasses and may actually allow more ultraviolet (UV) radiation to enter the eye.
13. B. Photochromic lenses take longer to lighten than darken.
14. D. Ultraviolet-absorbing lenses can be fabricated from glass materials.
15. C. Stimulated emission produces coherent light.
16. C. Once achieved, population inversion needs to be maintained.
17. A. Continuous lasers deliver more energy overtime than pulsed lasers. The energy of pulsed lasers is concentrated into very brief time periods.
18. C. Xanthophyll pigment is a common pigment in the macula; however, it does not absorb green light well.
19. A. Regardless of their use in science fiction, lasers are not death rays.
20. B. In most photocoagulators, the energy is concentrated in the center of the beam.
21. E. Keeping power and size constant, a shorter duration burn delivers more power rapidly to the tissue, increasing the chance to disrupt Bruch's membrane.
22. C. A noncircular aiming beam has a higher power density than a circular type.
23. C. Q-switching is a method of producing shorter duration burns. Frequency doubling describes a method of changing a laser's frequency.
24. A. Produces invisible infrared light.
25. D. The air-tear interface is the site of the greatest change in refractive index within the eye.
26. A. The Snellen formula assumes that each element in a 20/20 (6/6) target subtends 1 minutes of arc. The entire letter subtends 5 minutes of arc.
27. D. Pupil size of 2.0–2.8 mm gives the maximal modulation transfer function for high spatial frequencies.
28. B. Retinal photoreceptors can be triggered by a minimum of 1 quanta of visible light.
29. C. The vast majority of myopes have refractive errors of 2 diopters or less.
30. C. Most neonatal astigmatism has disappeared by adulthood.
31. E. By age of 3 years, a human eye is about 23 mm in diameter. The eye at birth is about 18 mm in diameter.
32. B. The Jackson's cross cylinder test determines the correct axis and power of the correcting lens by producing larger or smaller circles of least confusion.

33. A. The red–green duochrome test is used to refine the final sphere by making use of the chromatic aberration of the eye.
34. C. The stenopeic slit is most useful to screen for a high degree of astigmatism in patients who have poor vision.
35. C. Polycarbonate lenses must survive the impact of a 16 g steel ball traveling at a velocity of 16.4 ft/s, and dropped from a height of 4.2 feet (127 cm).
36. A. Pantoscopic tilt refers to the tilting of the bottom of the lenses toward the patient eyes. The average patient's glasses have a pantoscopic tilt of 7–12°.
37. B. Bicentral (slab-off) grinding can correct induced vertical prism but it is an expensive recourse.
38. D. In hyperopes, base down prisms minimize image displacement.
39. A. Laboratory-applied coatings can be used, but may make engraved markings difficult to find.
40. C. Lenses with less than 50% of water content are considered "low-water content" lenses by the US Food and Drug Administration.
41. D. Only a small percentage of patients are fitted for rigid gas-permeable lenses for extended wear; most are fitted with soft contact lenses.
42. E. Soft contact lenses that fit flat may decenter easily. Soft contact lenses that fit steep usually will not decenter.
43. E. Excessive lens permeability protects against corneal damage.
44. D. Corneal edema associated with contact lens wear appears as posterior stromal striae usually oriented vertically.
45. A. Corneal microcysts on slit-lamp examination display reversed illumination, i.e. the distribution of light within the microcysts is opposite to that of the background.
46. B. Superior limbic keratoconjunctivitis secondary to contact lenses is located in the superior cornea.
47. C. Giant papillary conjunctivitis in contact lens wearers includes papillae with a diameter of 0.4–0.9 mm. Normal micropapillae have a diameter of less than 0.3 mm.
48. D. Contact lenses because they remain centered on the eye, do not induce a prismatic effect on convergence.
49. B. During retinoscopy, a typical working distance is 66 cm (25").
50. B. Placido disc topography is a quantitative assessment. A keratoscope is an older hand-held device which uses a Placido disc for qualitative assessments.
51. A. The lensometer does not measure the focal length of the lens, but measures the vertex power which is the reciprocal of the distance between the back surface of the lens and its secondary focal point, this distance being the "back focal length".
52. C. The indirect ophthalmoscope in examination of an emmetropic eye with a 20 diopter lens provides 3× magnification; whereas, a 30-diopter lens provides 2× magnification.

CHAPTER 2

Genetics and Ocular Embryology

Kelly A Williamson

QUESTIONS

Identify the incorrect answer for all questions.

1. **Introns are:**
   A. Deoxyribonucleic acid (DNA) sequences that do not have a specific function.
   B. Not transcribed into ribonucleic acid (RNA) by RNA polymerase.
   C. Not translated into polypeptides and proteins.
   D. Also known as "intervening sequences".
   E. Spliced from heteronuclear RNA.

2. **The DNA molecule:**
   A. Is a double-stranded helix in humans.
   B. Is structured such that adenine always bonds with cytosine and guanine always bonds with thiamine.
   C. Is transcribed into RNA by RNA polymerase.
   D. Possesses four nucleotide bases held together by hydrogen bonds.
   E. Possesses a sugar–phosphate backbone.

3. **Meiotic cell division:**
   A. Results in four haploid cells.
   B. Incorporates crossing over before the first cell division.
   C. Occurs only in gamete cell lines.
   D. Requires the enzyme DNA polymerase.
   E. Results in diploid cells that are exact replicas of the original cell.

4. **If two traits are on separate chromosomes:**
   A. They respect the law of independent assortment.
   B. The resultant gamete has a 50% chance of inheriting alleles from each locus.
   C. They segregate, as if they were located far apart on the same chromosome.
   D. Recombination will rarely occur between the two loci.
   E. They obey Mendel's first law, the principle of segregation.

5. Identify the incorrect response.
A. Point mutations are the most common mutation encountered in human genetics.
B. Missense mutations are caused by insertion of DNA blocks.
C. Point mutations may decrease the level of polypeptide production.
D. A mutated gene may lead to production of a protein product that works poorly.
E. Point mutations involve the substitution of a single base pair.

6. Trinucleotide repeats are:
A. Associated with the phenomenon of "anticipation".
B. The cause of myotonic dystrophy and Huntington's disease.
C. The underlying reason why children with myotonic dystrophy are often affected later in life than their parents or grandparents.
D. A type of insertion mutation.
E. Less common than point mutations.

7. DNA-based diagnosis:
A. Uses genetic linkage analysis.
B. Assists in genetic counseling.
C. Does not permit early disease recognition.
D. Identifies individuals at risk for an inherited condition.
E. Identifies specific changes in DNA sequences.

8. Linkage analysis:
A. May be used to diagnose any genetically inherited disorder.
B. Requires physical gene isolation.
C. Does not require gene sequencing.
D. Requires DNA from multiple family members.
E. May result in misdiagnosis because of recombination between genetic markers used for testing and the disease-causing mutation.

9. Direct mutation analysis:
A. Does not rely on DNA sequencing.
B. Does not rely on segregation of genetic markers.
C. Does not require multiple family members' DNA samples.
D. Is not subject to potential errors caused by rare recombinant events.
E. Relies on isolating and sequencing the gene responsible for the disease.

10. Autosomal dominant traits:
A. Result in clinical expression of the gene in heterozygotes.
B. Affect both sexes equally.
C. Have a "vertical" pattern of transmission in pedigree drawings.
D. Usually demonstrate expression of the gene in at least three successive generations.
E. Can result in male-to-male transmission of the gene with both sexes showing the typical phenotype.

Genetics and Ocular Embryology

11. **Autosomal recessive traits:**
    A. Must be inherited from only one parent who is a carrier in order for an offspring to be affected.
    B. Affect both sexes equally.
    C. Are often traits involving enzymes.
    D. Are associated with consanguineous parental relationships.

12. **X-linked recessive traits:**
    A. Affect men more frequently than women.
    B. Are transmitted to half of the sons of affected men.
    C. May affect the obligate maternal carrier.
    D. Are transmitted to all the daughters of affected men; these daughters are carriers.
    E. Are transmitted to half the daughters of maternal carriers; these daughters are carriers.

13. **Examples of autosomal dominant anterior stromal corneal dystrophies are:**
    A. Macular dystrophy.
    B. Granular dystrophy.
    C. Lattice dystrophy.
    D. Avellino (combined granular-lattice) dystrophy.
    E. Reis–Bucklers dystrophy.

14. **The autosomal dominant anterior stromal corneal dystrophies:**
    A. Have all been mapped to a common locus on chromosome 5q31.
    B. Have been associated with several different mutations.
    C. Have been associated with different genes on different chromosomes.
    D. Are caused by variations in the structure of keratoepithelin.
    E. Have varying clinical and pathologic features.

15. **Mutations in the *PAX6* gene:**
    A. Are responsible for aniridia, Peters' anomaly, and Meesmann's dystrophy.
    B. Result in mutation of one copy of the gene.
    C. Alter the paired-box sequence, an important regulatory element.
    D. Regulate lens crystalline proteins.
    E. Exhibit extensive phenotypic variability.

16. **Rieger's syndrome:**
    A. May include corectopia.
    B. Is often caused by a gene on chromosome 4q25.
    C. Is genetically heterogeneous.
    D. Is associated with glaucoma in 10% of affected individuals.
    E. Is caused by genes that code for transcription factors induced in early eye development.

17. **Congenital cataracts:**
    A. Are familial in one-third of cases.
    B. May be caused by abnormalities in lens crystalline proteins.

C. Termed "Cerulean" are diffusely blue.
D. Termed "Coppock" involve the embryonic lens.
E. Are associated with abnormalities in beta-crystalline genes.

18. Retinitis pigmentosa may be:
A. Inherited as a digenetic trait.
B. Caused by genes with systemic effect.
C. Caused by many genes.
D. Caused by rhodopsin gene mutation.
E. Caused by a null mutation in autosomal dominant cases.

19. Stargardt disease:
A. Is usually caused by a point deletion.
B. Causes dark-appearing choroid on fluorescein angiography.
C. Is inherited as an autosomal recessive trait.
D. May have loss of central visual acuity as a teenager.
E. Is caused by a defect in a retina-specific adenosine triphosphate-binding transporter gene.

20. X-linked juvenile retinoschisis:
A. Is inherited as an X-linked trait.
B. Does not manifest in heterozygous female carriers.
C. Is caused by nonsense mutations in all cases.
D. Involves retinal splitting caused by Müller cell dysfunction.
E. Is caused by creation of an inactive protein product.

21. Gyrate atrophy:
A. Results in circular areas of chorioretinal atrophy.
B. Is caused by the overproduction of a specific enzyme, ornithine aminotransferase.
C. Is caused by hyperornithinemia.
D. Is an autosomal recessive trait.
E. May be reversed by a diet that is low in arginine.

22. Defective red–green color vision:
A. Involves genes arranged in head-to-head tandem array.
B. Affects 2–6% of men.
C. Involves red and green pigment genes that are 98% identical.
D. In extreme forms causes blue cone monochromacy.
E. Usually involves a single amino acid change.

23. Retinoblastoma:
A. Is caused by a gene located on chromosome 13q14.
B. Is often inherited as an autosomal dominant trait.
C. Requires mutations of both copies of the product of the retinoblastoma gene.
D. Does not occur in 25% of those inheriting a mutant gene copy.
E. Involves a gene product vital to cell cycle regulation.

Genetics and Ocular Embryology

24. **Mitochondrial DNA:**
    A. Mutations cause Leber's optic neuropathy.
    B. Is derived from maternal egg cell cytoplasm and divides by simple fission.
    C. Is not present in sperm.
    D. Mutations may segregate to daughter mitochondria in unequal amounts.
    E. Is not transmitted by the father.

25. **The following structures are all derived from neuroectoderm, *except*:**
    A. Iris pigment epithelium.
    B. Iris sphincter.
    C. Optic nerve axons and glia.
    D. Neurosensory retina.
    E. Trabecular meshwork.

26. **The following are all derived from cranial neural crest cells, *except*:**
    A. Corneal stroma and endothelium.
    B. Iris pigment epithelium.
    C. Uveal melanocytes.
    D. Crystalline lens.
    E. Sclera.

27. **Hyaloid artery:**
    A. Is a branch of the ventral ophthalmic artery.
    B. Forms an anastomosis with the tunica vasculosa lentis.
    C. Begins to regress in the third trimester of gestation.
    D. Is not patent by the 7th gestational month.
    E. May persist on the disc as a Bergmeister's papilla.

28. **Identify the incorrect response.**
    A. The primary vitreous is associated with the hyaloid artery.
    B. The secondary vitreous is avascular and surrounds the primary vitreous.
    C. The hyaloid artery travels in the canal of Cloquet.
    D. The tertiary vitreous connects the retina to the secondary vitreous.
    E. The lens zonules develop from tertiary vitreous.

29. **The crystalline lens:**
    A. Is induced by the optic vesicle.
    B. Is derived from surface ectoderm.
    C. Contains an anterior upright Y suture and posterior inverted Y suture.
    D. Is derived from tissue that initially forms a plate-shaped disc.
    E. Changes shape from ellipsoidal to spherical as embryogenesis proceeds.

30. **A congenital finding depicted below:**
    A. Results from incomplete cleavage of the embryonic fissure at 5–8 weeks of gestation.

B. If typical is inferotemporal in location.
C. If typical is usually bilateral.
D. Of the iris alone may be isolated.
E. Of the retinal pigment epithelium may lead to failure of development of other ocular layers.

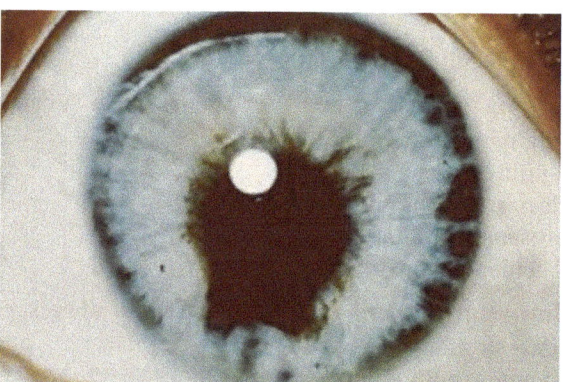

Fig. 2.1: Inferior iris coloboma.

ANSWERS

1. B. Introns are transcribed into the initial RNA product (hnRNA = heteronuclear RNA) and are later spliced out prior to translation of RNA into polypeptides.
2. B. In DNA molecules, adenine always binds with thiamine, while cytosine always binds with guanine.
3. E. As a consequence of crossing over and recombination events that occur during the pairing of homozygous chromosomes prior to the first division, the four haploid cells are not identical.
4. D. If two traits are on separate chromosomes, recombination events occur 50% of the time.
5. B. Missense mutations are DNA point mutations that result in a change in the amino acid sequence of the polypeptide chain.
6. C. Trinucleotide repeats result in more severe changes in the activity of a protein product. They are found in patients with certain neurodegenerative disorders such as Huntington disease, Fragile X syndrome, and myotonic dystrophy. This is the underlying reason why the children with these disorders are often affected earlier in life than their parents or grandparents.
7. C. DNA-based diagnosis permits early recognition of a medical condition, so that interventions are made to prevent or reverse the disease process.
8. B. Linkage analysis does not require physical isolation and sequencing of the abnormal gene.

9. A. Direct mutation analysis techniques are based on the DNA sequence of a gene to identify the specific base-pair change that is responsible for the disease.
10. E. Every generation has an affected member.
11. A. Autosomal recessive traits must be inherited from both parents who are carriers in order for an offspring to be affected.
12. B. X-linked recessive traits are not transmitted to the sons of affected males.
13. A. Macular corneal dystrophy is inherited in the autosomal recessive manner due to a mutation in the *CHST6* gene on chromosome 16. All of the other dystrophies listed are due to mutations of the *TGFB1* gene at the 5q31 locus.
14. C. All autosomal dominant (AD) anterior stromal dystrophies are mapped to the same gene located on the same chromosome.
15. A. Meesmann's dystrophy is not associated with a mutation in the *PAX6* gene; it is associated with mutations in the *KRT12* and *KRT3* genes.
16. D. Approximately, 50% of Rieger's syndrome patients develop glaucoma.
17. C. Cerulean cataracts demonstrate bluish and white peripheral opacification in concentric layers.
18. E. Retinitis pigmentosa may be caused by a Missense mutation in the autosomal dominant forms and by a null mutation in the autosomal recessive forms.
19. A. Stargardt's disease is usually caused by Missense mutations. Both copies of the responsible gene have to be inactivated for the disease to manifest.
20. C. Multiple cases of the X-linked juvenile retinoschisis were studied. Mutation analysis demonstrated nonsense, frameshift, splice acceptor, and Missense mutations.
21. B. A Missense mutation results in the deficiency of a specific enzyme, ornithine aminotransferase.
22. A. Genes are arranged in the head-to-tail tandem array.
23. D. Approximately, 10% of individuals, who inherit a mutant copy of the gene, do not sustain a second mutation and do not develop retinoblastoma due to incomplete penetrance.
24. C. Sperm contains mitochondria, but does not transmit it to the fertilized egg.
25. E. Trabecular meshwork is derived from the cranial neural crest cells.
26. D. Lens is derived from the surface ectoderm.
27. A. The hyaloid artery is a branch of the dorsal ophthalmic artery.
28. D. The canal of Cloquet is formed in the area of condensation between the primary and secondary vitreous.
29. E. The crystalline lens changes shape from spherical to ellipsoidal, as embryogenesis proceeds.
30. B. Iris colobomas are typically inferonasal in location.

CHAPTER 3

Uveitis and Other Intraocular Inflammations

Kelly A Williamson

QUESTIONS

Identify the incorrect answer for all questions (unless instructed otherwise).

1. **B cells:**
   A. Require the presence of a compatible antigen-presenting cell to recognize a specific antigen.
   B. Produce antibodies.
   C. Are a form of leukocyte.
   D. Mature in the bone marrow of mammals.
   E. Are derived from bone marrow stem cells.

2. **T cells:**
   A. Express surface markers such as CD4 or CD8.
   B. May be "helper" or cytotoxic cells.
   C. May be "natural killer" cells.
   D. Usually express T-cell antigen receptors alpha or beta.
   E. Are "educated" in the thymus.

3. **Identify the incorrect statement.**
   A. Neutrophils are the hallmark of acute inflammation.
   B. Eosinophils release the "major basic protein" which is toxic to worms.
   C. Eosinophils seem to dampen the immune response.
   D. Mast cells release histamine.
   E. Basophils confer—immunity to parasites.

4. **Tolerance to self:**
   A. May be mediated by clonal deletion or negative selection.
   B. May be mediated by clonal energy.
   C. Is maintained by requiring a T cell to receive three signals before responding to an antigen.
   D. Is thought to be due to a block in transcription of the interleukin-2 gene.
   E. May be mediated by programmed cell death, called apoptosis.

Uveitis and Other Intraocular Inflammations

5. Human leukocyte antigens associated with ocular diseases include:
- A. Anterior uveitis: HLA-B27.
- B. Behcet's syndrome: HLA-B52.
- C. Birdshot retinochoroidopathy: HLA-A29.
- D. Intermediate uveitis: HLA-B8, HLA-DR2.
- E. Vogt-Koyanagi-Harada syndrome: HLADR4.

6. Identify the incorrect statement.
- A. Type I hypersensitivity reactions are the result of an immunoglobulin E response to an antigen.
- B. Type II hypersensitivity reactions are the result of an antibody's binding to a cell surface antigen.
- C. Type III hypersensitivity reactions are the result of immune complex formation and complement activation.
- D. Type IV hypersensitivity reactions are regulated by T-cells.
- E. Type II hypersensitivity reactions are mediated by mast cells.

7. Which of the following is the correct pairing of a hypersensitivity reaction and the ocular disease that causes it?
- A. Type I: Allergic conjunctivitis.
- B. Type II: Ocular pemphigus.
- C. Type III: Sympathetic uveitis.
- D. Type IV: Tuberculous uveitis.
- E. Type V: Myasthenia gravis.

8. Immune privilege of the eye is dependent on:
- A. Tight blood-ocular barriers.
- B. Selective iris B-cell deficiency.
- C. Lack of an intraocular lymphatic system.
- D. Immunosuppressive intraocular environment.
- E. Intact blood-retinal barrier.

9. The ciliary processes:
- A. Contain an inner nonpigmented epithelial layer and an outer pigmented epithelial layer.
- B. Contain two epithelial cell layers arranged apex to apex.
- C. Contain aqueous-secreting nonpigmented epithelium.
- D. Are attached to the lens zonules.
- E. Are derived from neuroectoderm.

10. Cyclosporine:
- A. Is produced by fungi.
- B. Has a more specific immunosuppressive effect than corticosteroids or cytotoxic agents.
- C. Is a cytotoxic drug.
- D. Inhibits T-cell recruitment.
- E. Is effective in posterior and intermediate uveitis.

11. **Elevated intraocular pressure (IOP) may be associated with uveitis because of:**
    A. Trabeculitis.
    B. Formation of peripheral anterior synechiae.
    C. Formation of posterior synechiae.
    D. Corticosteroid-induced IOP elevation.
    E. Iris stromal edema.

12. **Granulomatous uveitis is associated with:**
    A. Large, poorly defined keratic precipitates.
    B. Koeppe nodules of iris at the papillary border.
    C. Darkly pigmented keratic precipitates.
    D. Bullous iris nodules within the stroma.
    E. Hypopyon.

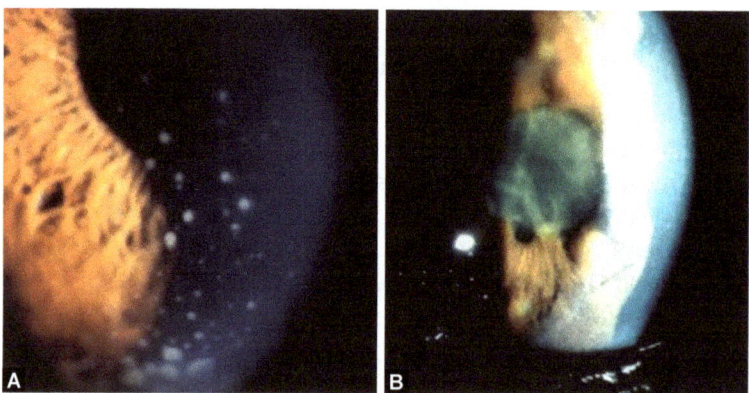

Figs 3.1A and B: (A) Mutton-fat keratic precipitates on the cornea just to the right of the light reflex; (B) Flare and posterior synechiae in granulomatous uveitis.

13. **Early immunosuppressive therapy is strongly recommended by the International Uveitis Study Group for:**
    A. Intermediate uveitis in children.
    B. Behcet's syndrome.
    C. Vogt-Koyanagi-Harada disease.
    D. Sympathetic uveitis.
    E. Rheumatoid sclerouveitis.

14. **Anterior uveitis:**
    A. May be induced by a virus.
    B. Is always unilateral.
    C. May have strong ethnic associations.
    D. May not be associated with pain or erythema.
    E. May be associated with high or low intraocular pressure.

15. **All the following are associated with bilateral anterior uveitis, *except*:**
    A. Spondyloarthritis.
    B. Behcet's syndrome.

C. Juvenile rheumatoid arthritis.
D. Sarcoidosis.
E. Inflammatory bowel disease.

16. The HLA-B27 histocompatibility complex marker:
    A. Is present in 6–8% of the US Caucasian population.
    B. Predisposes to ankylosing spondylitis and Reiter's syndrome.
    C. Is present in 50% of individuals who have sudden-onset anterior uveitis.
    D. Predisposes to simultaneous bilateral uveitis.
    E. Is associated with anterior uveitis that tends to resolve completely in 2–3 weeks.

17. Uveitis in association with inflammatory bowel disease:
    A. May begin insidiously.
    B. Is usually bilateral.
    C. Rarely has a posterior component.
    D. Is more common in women than in men.
    E. Is more likely associated with Crohn's disease than with ulcerative colitis.

18. A 6-year-old Caucasian female presents to an ophthalmologist for failing a routine vision screen at school. She has not noticed vision problems prior to the screening. She has complained to her parents regarding intermittent pain in several joints. Her visual acuity is 20/200 in the right eye and 20/50 in the left eye. Intraocular pressures (IOPs) are 20 OD and 18 OS. Anterior segment examination is significant for cortical and posterior subcapsular cataracts in the right eye more than in the left. There is a small area of band keratopathy visible on the right temporal cornea. Anterior segment examination is significant for +1–2 cell and flare in the right eye and trace cell and flare in the left eye. Uveitis in association with this condition:
    A. Occurs predominantly in girls.
    B. Involves a few (four or fewer) joints.
    C. Is usually of insidious onset.
    D. First appears with pain and erythema.
    E. Is usually associated with a positive test for antinuclear antibodies and a negative test for rheumatoid factor.

19. A 38-year-old Caucasian female with anterior uveitis was found to have white blood cells on the urinalysis screen in the absence of infection. Uveitis associated with this systemic condition:
    A. Is of sudden onset.
    B. Is bilateral.
    C. Is more common in adolescent girls and women.
    D. Usually is found in systemically ill patients.
    E. Responds well to topical corticosteroids alone.

20. Kawasaki disease (mucocutaneous lymph node syndrome):
   A. Is the form of vasculitis most likely to involve the eye.
   B. Is a disease of teenagers.
   C. Is associated with conjunctival erythema and bilateral sudden-onset anterior uveitis.
   D. May affect the coronary arteries.
   E. Is treated with high-dose intravenous immunoglobulin.

21. After hiking in a wooded area, a 19-year-old college student develops a low-grade fever, large rash on his trunk, and conjunctivitis. In the systemic condition described in this patient:
   A. Spread is by an arthropod vector, the *Ixodes* tick.
   B. The rash has an annular expanding margin of at least 5 cm.
   C. The most common ocular involvement is bilateral uveitis.
   D. Vitreous organization known as "spider web" uveitis may occur.
   E. Serologic testing has many false-positive results.

22. Phakoanaphylactic endophthalmitis:
   A. Often involves the retina.
   B. Usually develops days to weeks after lens capsule disruption.
   C. May occur within 24 hours of lens extraction in a patient sensitized to lens protein.
   D. Is usually granulomatous and zonal.
   E. Is usually less painful than typical acute infectious endophthalmitis.

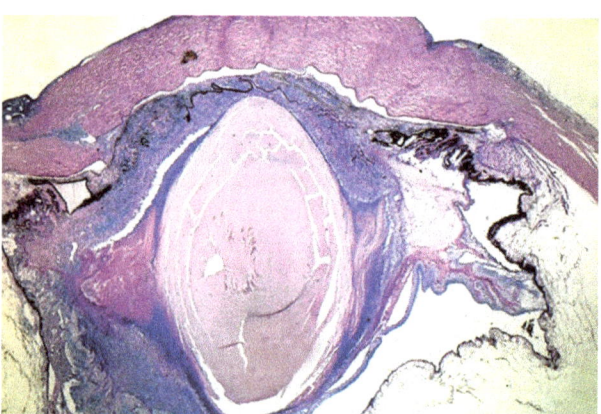

Fig. 3.2: Zonular granuloma around the lens nucleus in Phakoanaphylactic endophthalmitis.

23. Organisms commonly associated with late-onset postoperative endophthalmitis include:
   A. *Staphylococcus epidermidis*.
   B. *Propionibacterium acnes*.
   C. *Candida parapsilosis*.
   D. *Staphylococcus aureus*.
   E. Fungi.

24. **Herpetic iridocyclitis caused by herpes simplex or herpes zoster:**
    A. May be associated with hyphema.
    B. Is usually nongranulomatous.
    C. Is never associated with vasculitis.
    D. May be associated with atrophy of the iris pigment epithelium.
    E. May be associated with severely elevated intraocular pressure.

25. **Varicella-zoster virus iridocyclitis:**
    A. Is more frequently granulomatous than the iridocyclitis seen with herpes simplex.
    B. Is less frequently associated with sector iris atrophy than is herpes simplex.
    C. Is often associated with a skin rash in the trigeminal distribution.
    D. Is less likely to be associated with corneal anesthesia than is herpes simplex.
    E. Has a bimodal age distribution.

26. **Syphilitic uveitis:**
    A. May be granulomatous or nongranulomatous.
    B. In human immunodeficiency virus (HIV)-positive individuals may include posterior pole lesions at the level of the retinal pigment epithelium.
    C. May be associated with marginal infiltrates of the anterior corneal stroma.
    D. Has decreased significantly in the past years.
    E. May first appear as acute uveitis.

27. **False-positive nontreponemal serologic findings may occur in:**
    A. Human immunodeficiency virus (HIV)-positive individuals.
    B. Patients with leprosy.
    C. Patients of advanced age.
    D. Patients who have neurosyphilis.
    E. Pregnancy.

28. **Identify the incorrect statement.**
    A. Primary syphilis is characterized by a chancre anywhere on the skin or a mucous membrane.
    B. Primary syphilis is often associated with a maculopapular rash.
    C. Secondary syphilis has the highest systemic treponemal load.
    D. Central nervous system infection can be documented in nearly 25% of patients who have early syphilis (primary, secondary, or early latent phases).
    E. Tertiary syphilis occurs in about one-third of untreated patients.

29. **Treatment of syphilis may be considered adequate when:**
    A. Signs and symptoms improve.
    B. Seroconversion occurs.

C. Nontreponemal tests show low titers.
D. A four-fold to eight-fold decrease in nontreponemal titers occurs.
E. Corneal ghost vessels disappear.

30. Tuberculous uveitis:
   A. Is usually granulomatous.
   B. May occur without systemic evidence of disease.
   C. May be associated with acid-fast bacilli in the anterior chamber.
   D. Is commonly isolated to the choroid.
   E. Is becoming more common.

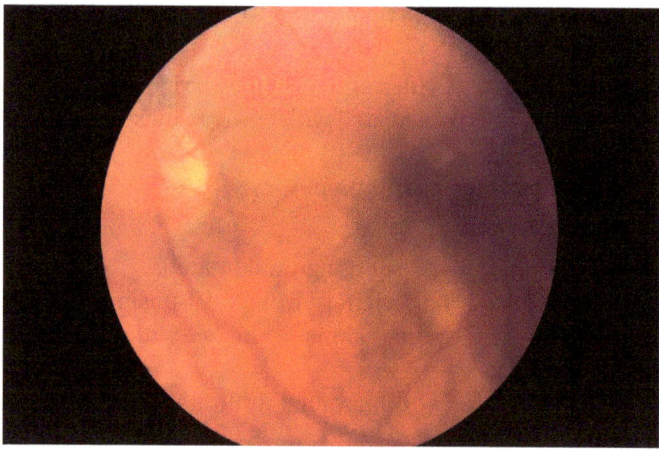

Fig. 3.3: Tuberculous choroiditis.

31. Treatment of tuberculous uveitis:
   A. Is justified in patients who have a positive purified protein derivative but no other evidence of tuberculosis.
   B. Usually requires at least two drugs.
   C. By corticosteroids is usually avoided.
   D. Early in the disease course usually has a good prognosis.
   E. Depends on the individual's immune status.

32. Leprous uveitis:
   A. Is usually an acute granulomatous iridocyclitis.
   B. Is associated with iris pearls.
   C. Is usually treated with a multiple-drug regimen.
   D. Occurs in about 7% of patients who have leprosy.
   E. Is usually caused by direct bacterial ocular spread.

33. Brucellosis uveitis:
   A. Is the most common eye manifestation of *Brucella*.
   B. Is always granulomatous.
   C. May occur in the anterior, intermediate, and posterior forms.
   D. May cause choroiditis.
   E. May be associated with retrobulbar neuritis.

Uveitis and Other Intraocular Inflammations

34. Fuchs' heterochromic iridocyclitis:
A. Occurs with equal frequency in men and women.
B. May appear at any age.
C. Has been theorized to be associated with rubella virus.
D. Has minimal inflammatory symptoms.
E. Is usually bilateral.

35. Eyes that have active Fuchs' heterochromic iridocyclitis:
A. Usually have diffuse stellate keratic precipitates.
B. Often have iris stromal atrophy.
C. Usually develop posterior synechiae and pupillary block glaucoma.
D. Manifest elevated intraocular pressure in 25–60% of cases.
E. Develop cataracts in 80% of cases.

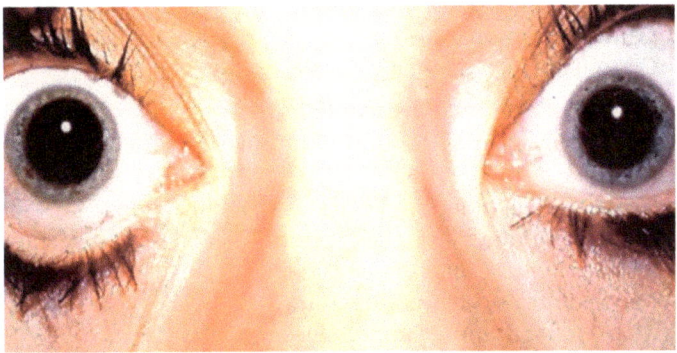

Fig. 3.4: Iris heterochromia of left iris in Fuchs' heterochromic iridocyclitis.

36. Treatment of Fuchs' heterochromic iridocyclitis:
A. By topical corticosteroids usually produces rapid and complete resolution.
B. Associated cataracts extraction may be performed safely during periods of active inflammation.
C. By nonsteroidal anti-inflammatory agents does not alter the disease course.
D. Associated glaucoma by filtration surgery has a poor prognosis.
E. Aggressive treatment of intraocular inflammation is not indicated.

37. Glaucomatocyclitic crises (Posner–Schlossman syndrome):
A. Are seen in males in 80% of cases.
B. Are rarely seen in older adults.
C. Occur in white eyes.
D. Are associated with marked anterior chamber flare but few cells.
E. Usually occur unilaterally.

38. Pars planitis:
A. Usually occurs in young patients (age 5–40 years).
B. Comprises 85–90% of all intermediate uveitis cases.
C. Is usually seen in girls and women.

D. Is usually (in 80% of cases) bilateral.
E. By definition is intermediate uveitis in the absence of an associated infection or systemic disease.

39. **Intermediate uveitis has been associated with:**
    A. Lyme disease.
    B. Familial tendency.
    C. T-cell lymphoma virus.
    D. Multiple sclerosis.
    E. HLA-B27 histocompatibility antigen.

40. **Intermediate uveitis is frequently associated with:**
    A. Posterior synechiae.
    B. Inferior "snowbank" on the inferior pars plana and peripheral retina.
    C. Corneal band keratopathy.
    D. Cataract formation.
    E. Cystoid macular edema.

41. **Treatment of intermediate uveitis:**
    A. Is generally reserved for those who have visual acuity less than 20/40 (6/12).
    B. Should not include depot corticosteroid injections.
    C. Includes cryotherapy or laser photocoagulation of the "snowbank" if steroids do not improve visual acuity.
    D. May require pars plana vitrectomy.
    E. May require immunosuppressive treatment.

42. **The course of intermediate uveitis:**
    A. Usually involves at least 3 years of inflammation.
    B. Tends to "burnout" after 5–15 years.
    C. Is consistent with good visual acuity if macular edema does not occur.
    D. Is one of exacerbation and remission in most patients.
    E. Associated with T-cell lymphoma virus that is not usually consistent with good visual acuity.

43. **A 28-year-old patient with history of *Pneumocystis carinii* pneumonia, complains of blurred vision and floaters in the left eye. His visual acuity (VA) is 20/20 OD and 20/400 OS. Anterior chamber examination shows trace cell and flare in the left eye. Dilated retinal examination is significant for an area of retinal infarction intermixed with hemorrhages extending from temporal periphery to the posterior pole. Upon further work-up, the patients CD4 count was found to be 43 cells/mm^3. This type of retinitis:**
    A. Is the most common ocular infection in patients who have acquired immunodeficiency syndrome (AIDS).
    B. Results in blindness if untreated.
    C. Rarely occurs, except in immunocompromised patients.
    D. May occur concomitantly with viral esophagitis.
    E. Incidence decreases as the CD4 circulating lymphocyte count declines.

44. **Cytomegalovirus retinitis:**
    A. Spreads from retinal cell to retinal cell.
    B. Is associated with less vitritis since the introduction of highly active antiretroviral therapy.
    C. Lesions are typically multifocal.
    D. Is associated with retinal detachment in 25–50% of cases.
    E. May appear with retinal vascular sheathing.

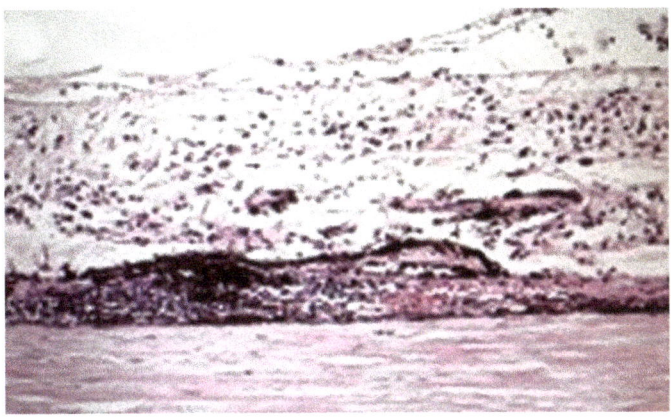

Fig. 3.5: Retinal disorganization with congenital cytomegalovirus (CMV) retinitis.

45. **Treatment of cytomegalovirus retinitis with ganciclovir:**
    A. Often involves intravenous therapy.
    B. Is initially effective in 90–100% of recently diagnosed cases.
    C. Exhibits a clinical effect in 2–3 weeks.
    D. Rarely causes neutropenia.
    E. If given as an intravitreal injection or implant, does not provide coverage of systemic cytomegalovirus (CMV) infection.

46. **Congenital cytomegalovirus retinitis:**
    A. Is often associated with systemic manifestations such as fever, thrombocytopenia, anemia, and hepatosplenomegaly.
    B. Can result in hyper- and hypopigmented retinal lesions after resolution of active inflammation.
    C. Rarely results in retinal detachment.
    D. Can result in optic atrophy and cataract in some patients.
    E. Is the most common cause of congenital viral infection.

47. **More recent treatment approaches to cytomegalovirus retinitis include:**
    A. Oral ganciclovir.
    B. Intravenous cidofovir.
    C. Ganciclovir intravitreal implant.
    D. Intravitreal foscarnet injection.
    E. Foscarnet intravitreal implant.

48. Retinitis caused by varicella-zoster virus:
A. Is seen only in adults who are immunocompromised.
B. Has been termed as acute retinal necrosis syndrome.
C. Can cause an outer retinal infection in patients who have advanced acquired immunodeficiency syndrome.
D. Occurs equally among men and women.
E. Has certain human leukocyte antigen (HLA) histocompatibility groups as a predisposing factor.

49. Congenital herpes simplex virus (HSV) retinitis:
A. Is rarely documented.
B. Is usually monocular.
C. Occurs in children of mothers who have a history of HSV-2 genital disease during the 2nd trimester of pregnancy.
D. Is uncommonly associated with HSV keratitis.
E. Is associated with HSV encephalitis.

50. Acute retinal necrosis syndrome:
A. Starts in the posterior retina.
B. Progresses to retinal detachment in 4–8 weeks in 75% of patients.
C. Involves 80% of second eyes within 3 months of disease onset in the first eye.
D. Responds better to treatment than progressive outer retinal necrosis.
E. May appear with severe ocular pain.

51. Viral retinitis may be caused by:
A. Western equine encephalomyelitis virus.
B. Measles virus.
C. Influenza A virus.
D. Rubella virus.
E. Epstein-Barr virus.

52. Whipple's disease:
A. May begin in the eye with corneal infiltrates.
B. Is usually diagnosed by colonic biopsy.
C. Affecting the brain causes gradual dementia, supranuclear ophthalmoplegia, and ocular myoclonic movements.
D. Is associated with periodic acid-Schiff-positive material in many organs.
E. Is caused by rod-like bacteria.

53. Treatment of Whipple's disease:
A. Can improve dementia.
B. Involves oral penicillin.
C. Is lifelong in some cases because recurrences are common.
D. Reverses vitreous opacities.
E. Improves the bowel biopsy findings.

Uveitis and Other Intraocular Inflammations

54. *Histoplasma capsulatum:*
    A. Has not been definitely identified histopathologically in eyes of patients who have ocular histoplasmosis syndrome.
    B. Endophthalmitis rarely occurs in immunocompromised individuals.
    C. Endophthalmitis is usually associated with active pulmonary disease.
    D. Complement fixation titers are elevated (>1:32) in disseminated disease.
    E. Is transmitted with wind-blown soil and pigeon droppings.

55. The ocular histoplasmosis syndrome:
    A. Is most frequently found in the Mississippi and Ohio river valleys, where histoplasmosis is endemic.
    B. Can result in poor visual acuity if the macula is involved.
    C. Is not associated with anterior segment inflammation.
    D. Is often associated with vitritis.
    E. May be associated with equatorial linear streak lesions.

56. Treatment of choroidal neovascularization in patients who have ocular histoplasmosis syndrome:
    A. May include laser photocoagulation, photodynamic therapy (PDT) with verteporfin, and the off-label use of intravitreal antivascular endothelial growth factor (VEGF) agents.
    B. Is associated with recurrence in 25% of patients.
    C. Is more effective if krypton red laser is used.
    D. By laser is controversial if the neovascularization is subfoveal.
    E. May include surgical removal of a subfoveal net if present.

57. *Candida albicans* endophthalmitis:
    A. Is usually seen in immunocompromised patients.
    B. Typically appears with white, fluffy chorioretinal lesions with overlying vitritis.
    C. Is usually treated with intravenous and intravitreal antifungals.
    D. Treatment can lead to nephrotoxicity.
    E. Is rarely associated with septicemia.

58. Toxoplasmosis:
    A. Is the most common infectious retinitis.
    B. Infection is not of concern for the majority of pregnant women, as most already have antibodies to *Toxoplasma gondii*.
    C. Is associated with the ingestion of raw meat.
    D. Is disseminated by feline feces.
    E. Is disseminated by an obligate intracellular parasite.

59. Toxoplasmosis retinitis:
    A. Is usually active in 1 eye at a time.
    B. Is always associated with vitritis.
    C. Spares retinal nerve fiber layer.
    D. May be disseminated in immunocompromised patients.
    E. Often induces anterior segment inflammation.

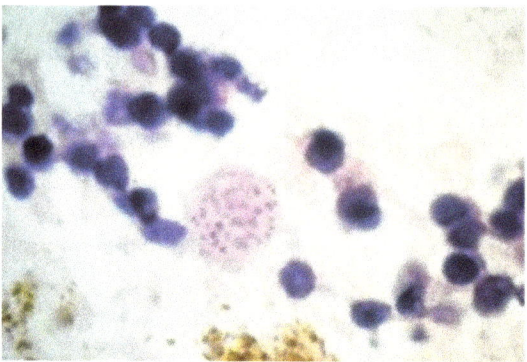

Fig. 3.6: Toxoplasma cyst within the retinal tissue.

60. **Congenital toxoplasmosis may first appear as:**
    A. Microcephaly.
    B. Pneumonitis.
    C. Thrombocytopenia.
    D. Cataracts.
    E. Microphthalmia.

61. **Treatment of toxoplasmic retinitis should be considered for:**
    A. A lesion causing vitritis sufficient to result in a two-line drop in visual acuity.
    B. Persistence of a lesion for more than 1 month.
    C. A lesion near the optic nerve.
    D. A lesion greater than 1 disc diameter in size.
    E. An eye with one single active lesion.

62. **Identify the incorrect statement.**
    A. Folic acid antagonists kill only metabolically active trophozoites.
    B. Clindamycin has poor ocular penetration.
    C. Clindamycin eliminates encysted *Toxoplasma* bradyzoites.
    D. Systemic corticosteroids can be initiated as long as there is appropriate concomitant antimicrobial coverage.
    E. Use of depot steroid injections in patients who have active toxoplasmic retinitis is discouraged.

63. **Identify the incorrect statement.**
    A. Pyrimethamine is safe for use in pregnant women.
    B. Treatment of active congenital toxoplasmosis should be continued for at least 1 year in newborns with the disease.
    C. Any active toxoplasmic lesion should be treated in an immunocompromised host.
    D. Pyrimethamine is often contraindicated for use in an immunocompromised host.
    E. Zidovudine action is often antagonistic to that of pyrimethamine.

64. *Toxocara canis*:
A. Can infect wolves and foxes as well as dogs.
B. Usually depends on puppies for transmission to other hosts.
C. Is a flatworm similar to *Ascaris* organisms.
D. Larvae cannot complete their life cycle in humans.
E. May infect as many as 80% in endemic areas.

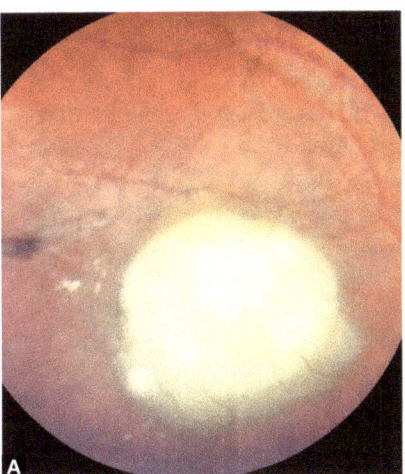 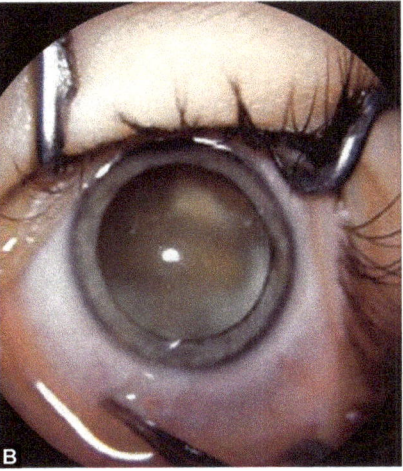

Figs. 3.7A and B: *Toxocara canis* granuloma. (A) Posterior pole involvement; and (B) Leukokoria.

65. Visceral larva migrans:
A. Generally occurs in children at about 2 years of age.
B. May leave encysted larvae in the brain, liver, and lungs.
C. Is usually associated with eosinophilia.
D. Does not usually present with systemic symptoms.
E. Cannot be diagnosed by checking stools for ova and parasites.

66. Ocular *Toxocara* lesions may appear as:
A. Hemorrhagic retinitis.
B. A dense, white retinal granuloma in the posterior pole or periphery.
C. Endophthalmitis.
D. Tiny mobile larvae in the lens or subretinal space.
E. Neuroretinitis.

67. Compared with patients who have *Toxocara* retinitis, patients who have retinoblastoma are:
A. Less likely to have a cataract.
B. More likely to have calcification in the mass.
C. More likely to have vitreoretinal traction around the mass.
D. More likely to have overlying clear vitreous.
E. Usually younger.

68. Compared with patients who have *Toxocara* retinitis, patients who have Coats' disease are:
   A. More likely to have surrounding exudative retinal detachment.
   B. Less likely to have granuloma formation.
   C. More likely to be boys.
   D. More likely to have unilateral disease.
   E. More likely to demonstrate abnormal retinal vasculature.

69. Cysticercosis:
   A. Is caused by larvae of adult *Taenia* tapeworms.
   B. Is usually identified in patients who have visceral organ findings.
   C. Is common in Mexico and Central America.
   D. May involve any part of the visual system.
   E. Is transmitted by eating raw pork.

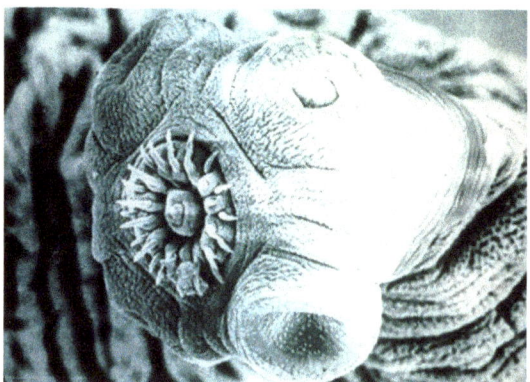

Fig. 3.8: Electron micrograph of the organism causing cysticercosis.

70. Onchocerciasis:
   A. Is endemic in equatorial Africa.
   B. Is transmitted by the blackfly.
   C. May cause blinding chorioretinitis.
   D. Microfilariae can be noted floating in the anterior chamber.
   E. Microfilariae can usually be identified clinically in the conjunctiva of affected patients.

71. Ocular onchocerciasis may cause:
   A. Sclerosing keratitis.
   B. Profound vitritis.
   C. Chorioretinitis.
   D. Optic nerve atrophy.
   E. Posterior synechiae.

72. Acute posterior multifocal placoid pigment epitheliopathy:
   A. Is usually unilateral.
   B. Affects the choriocapillaris, retinal pigment epithelium, and outer retinal segments.

64. *Toxocara canis*:
A. Can infect wolves and foxes as well as dogs.
B. Usually depends on puppies for transmission to other hosts.
C. Is a flatworm similar to *Ascaris* organisms.
D. Larvae cannot complete their life cycle in humans.
E. May infect as many as 80% in endemic areas.

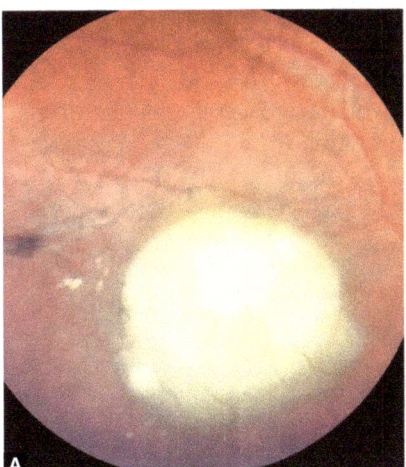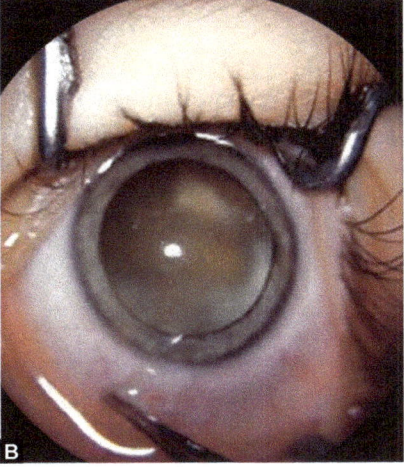

Figs. 3.7A and B: *Toxocara canis* granuloma. (A) Posterior pole involvement; and (B) Leukokoria.

65. Visceral larva migrans:
A. Generally occurs in children at about 2 years of age.
B. May leave encysted larvae in the brain, liver, and lungs.
C. Is usually associated with eosinophilia.
D. Does not usually present with systemic symptoms.
E. Cannot be diagnosed by checking stools for ova and parasites.

66. Ocular *Toxocara* lesions may appear as:
A. Hemorrhagic retinitis.
B. A dense, white retinal granuloma in the posterior pole or periphery.
C. Endophthalmitis.
D. Tiny mobile larvae in the lens or subretinal space.
E. Neuroretinitis.

67. Compared with patients who have *Toxocara* retinitis, patients who have retinoblastoma are:
A. Less likely to have a cataract.
B. More likely to have calcification in the mass.
C. More likely to have vitreoretinal traction around the mass.
D. More likely to have overlying clear vitreous.
E. Usually younger.

68. **Compared with patients who have *Toxocara* retinitis, patients who have Coats' disease are:**
    A. More likely to have surrounding exudative retinal detachment.
    B. Less likely to have granuloma formation.
    C. More likely to be boys.
    D. More likely to have unilateral disease.
    E. More likely to demonstrate abnormal retinal vasculature.

69. **Cysticercosis:**
    A. Is caused by larvae of adult *Taenia* tapeworms.
    B. Is usually identified in patients who have visceral organ findings.
    C. Is common in Mexico and Central America.
    D. May involve any part of the visual system.
    E. Is transmitted by eating raw pork.

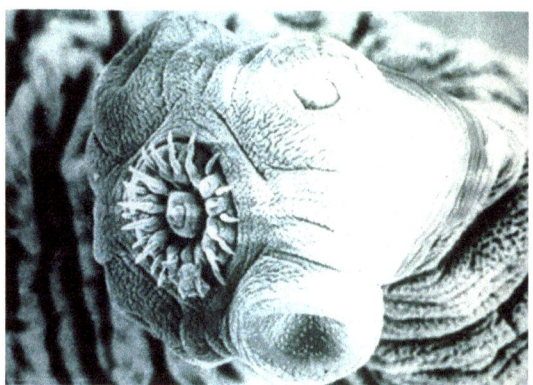

Fig. 3.8: Electron micrograph of the organism causing cysticercosis.

70. **Onchocerciasis:**
    A. Is endemic in equatorial Africa.
    B. Is transmitted by the blackfly.
    C. May cause blinding chorioretinitis.
    D. Microfilariae can be noted floating in the anterior chamber.
    E. Microfilariae can usually be identified clinically in the conjunctiva of affected patients.

71. **Ocular onchocerciasis may cause:**
    A. Sclerosing keratitis.
    B. Profound vitritis.
    C. Chorioretinitis.
    D. Optic nerve atrophy.
    E. Posterior synechiae.

72. **Acute posterior multifocal placoid pigment epitheliopathy:**
    A. Is usually unilateral.
    B. Affects the choriocapillaris, retinal pigment epithelium, and outer retinal segments.

C. May be preceded by a viral syndrome.
D. Affects men and women equally.
E. Shows a typical pattern of early blockage and late staining of lesions on fluorescein angiography.

73. **Acute posterior multifocal placoid pigment epitheliopathy:**
    A. Is usually self-limited.
    B. Has been documented to be associated with adenovirus 5.
    C. May result in pigment epithelial mottling.
    D. Usually results in normal visual acuity after the condition resolves.
    E. Commonly results in choroidal neovascular membranes.

74. **Multiple evanescent white dot syndrome:**
    A. Is usually unilateral.
    B. Primarily affects healthy women between ages 20 years and 60 years.
    C. Exhibits multiple white dots at the level of the retinal pigment epithelium.
    D. Usually results in loss of visual acuity.
    E. Often exhibits typical changes in macular photoreceptor of inner/outer segment junction appearance on spectral domain optical coherence tomography (SDOCT).

75. **Serpiginous choroiditis:**
    A. Affects men and women equally from the 2nd to 6th decades of life.
    B. Presents with loss of visual acuity.
    C. Demonstrates early hyperfluorescence and late hypofluorescence of active lesions on fluorescein angiography.
    D. Has a progressive, stepwise course.
    E. Results in final visual acuity of 20/200 to counting fingers in up to 38% of patients in the affected eye.

76. **Birdshot retinochoroidopathy:**
    A. Is usually found in patients who are positive for HLA-A29.
    B. Typically affects men between the 2nd and 6th decades of life.
    C. Is associated with vitritis and disc edema.
    D. Is associated with cystoid macular edema.
    E. Exhibits depressed rod and cone function on electroretinography.

77. **Sarcoidosis:**
    A. Occurs in family clusters.
    B. Presents with noncaseating granulomas without evidence of infection.
    C. Is found 10–20 times more frequently in blacks than in Caucasians in the United States.
    D. Affects the eye rarely.
    E. Usually affects both eyes.

78. **Ocular sarcoidosis-associated:**
    A. Retinitis is rare but is related to central nervous system sarcoidosis.
    B. Posterior uveitis typically first appears with periphlebitis.

C. Vitritis can mimic intermediate uveitis with "snowbank" overlying the peripheral retina and pars plana.
D. Choroiditis is associated with profound vitritis.
E. Vasculitis may be associated with "candle wax" retinal exudates.

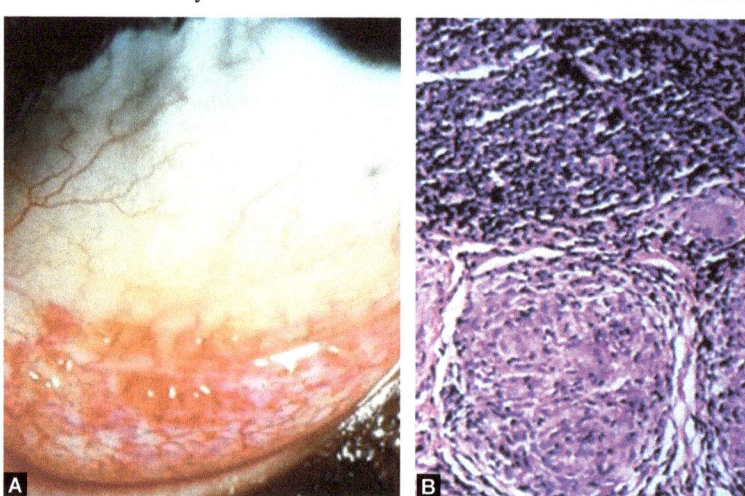

Figs. 3.9A and B: Conjunctival granulomas in ocular sarcoidosis. (A) Clinical appearance of granulomas; and (B) Histology of zonal granulomas.

79. **The diagnosis of sarcoidosis:**
    A. Is assisted by finding elevated serum angiotensin-converting enzyme (ACE).
    B. Is suggested by gallium scanning showing bilateral hilar adenopathy in affected patients.
    C. Is supported by a decreased helper/suppressor T-cell ratio.
    D. By conjunctival biopsy yields better results when granulomas are sampled.
    E. Cannot be definitively made based on the appearance of skin lesions alone.

80. **Early-onset sarcoidosis in children younger than 4 years:**
    A. Has a distinct clinical picture of rash, polyarthritis, and granulomatous uveitis.
    B. Commonly includes pulmonary disease.
    C. Is often a systemic disease with cardiac abnormalities and hepatosplenomegaly.
    D. Tends to have a chronic course.
    E. May be confused with juvenile rheumatoid arthritis.

81. **Behcet's syndrome:**
    A. Is more common in women.
    B. Results in more severe ocular disease in men than in women.
    C. Is associated with HLA-B51.

D. Is associated with ocular involvement in 70% of cases.
E. Involves both eyes in 70–80% of cases.

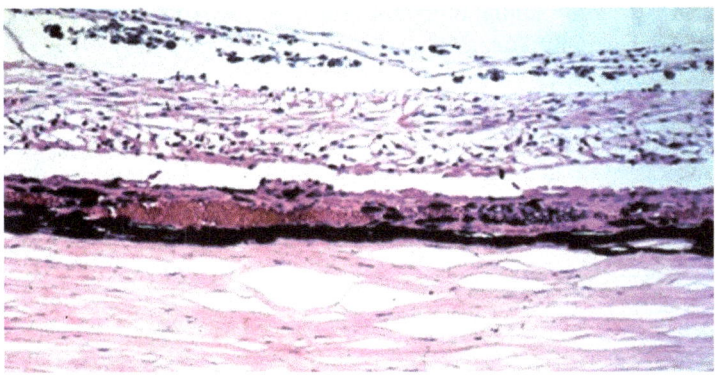

Fig. 3.10: Retinal involvement in the Behcet's disease. Retina is completely disorganized secondary to retinal vasculitis.

82. **Behcet's syndrome involving the eye:**
    A. Is associated with the hypopyon uveitis in one-third of patients.
    B. Is associated with a hypopyon that may change location with change in head position.
    C. Is rarely associated with optic disc edema.
    D. May lead to ischemic retinal changes caused by vascular thromboses.
    E. Is commonly associated with retinal vasculitis.

83. **Systemic manifestations of Behcet's syndrome include:**
    A. Recurrent oral mucosal aphthous ulcers.
    B. Erythema nodosum lesions of the face, arm, and legs.
    C. Arthritis and gastrointestinal ulcers.
    D. Hearing loss.
    E. Painful "punched-out" genital lesions.

84. **Treatment of Behcet's syndrome:**
    A. May include the use of systemic steroids.
    B. Includes cytotoxic agents in children.
    C. With cyclosporine may cause nephrotoxicity.
    D. In Japan avoids the use of cyclophosphamide.
    E. With cyclophosphamide controls inflammation better than with corticosteroids.

85. **Vogt-Koyanagi-Harada syndrome:**
    A. Is more common in lightly pigmented races.
    B. Is more common in women.
    C. Is usually linked to HLA-DR4 and HLA-Dw53.
    D. Is of unknown cause.
    E. Causes bilateral uveitis.

86. **Features of Vogt-Koyanagi-Harada syndrome include:**
    A. Cerebrospinal fluid pleocytosis.
    B. Low cerebrospinal fluid glucose.
    C. Sensorineural hearing loss.
    D. Vitiligo.
    E. Alopecia.

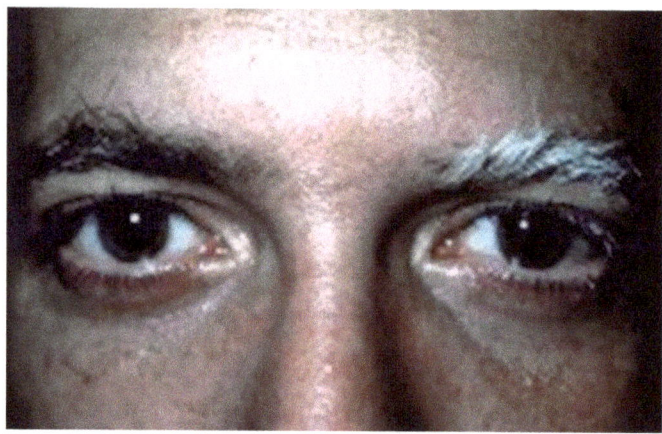

Fig. 3.11: Poliosis of the left eye in a patient with the Vogt-Koyanagi-Harada (VKH) syndrome.

87. **Retinal detachment in patients who have Vogt-Koyanagi-Harada syndrome:**
    A. Shows elevated retinal folds radiating from the macula.
    B. Is bullous in severe cases.
    C. May exhibit a cloverleaf pattern in the posterior fundus.
    D. Is rhegmatogenous.
    E. Often resolves after treatment with oral corticosteroids.

88. **The pathologic complex of Vogt-Koyanagi-Harada syndrome:**
    A. Is very similar to that of sympathetic uveitis.
    B. May exhibit Dalen-Fuchs nodules.
    C. Exhibits inflammation that appears directed toward choroidal melanocytes.
    D. Exhibits sparing of the choriocapillaris by lymphocytes.
    E. May exhibit subretinal neovascularization in chronic cases.

89. **Sympathetic ophthalmia:**
    A. Requires presence of a perforating scleral wound.
    B. Is associated with a cell-mediated immune response to retinal antigen.
    C. May be associated with papillitis.
    D. May cause macular scarring.
    E. Is most common in young adults between the ages of 20 years and 40 years.

Uveitis and Other Intraocular Inflammations

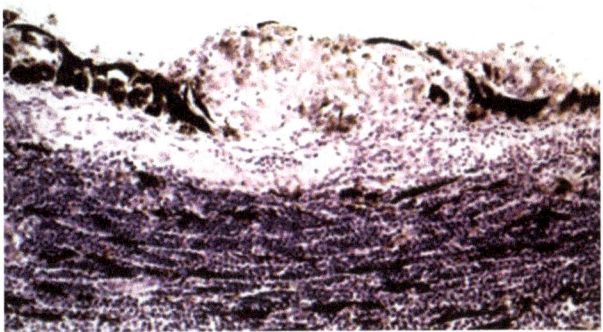

Fig. 3.12: Subretinal pigment epithelial Dalen-Fuchs nodules in an eye with sympathetic ophthalmia.

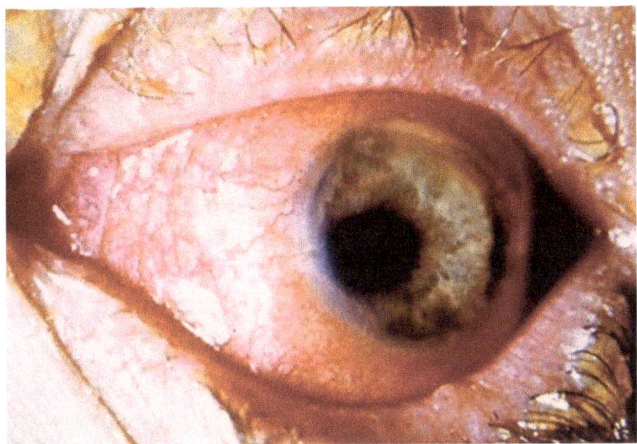

Fig. 3.13: Significant conjunctival infection in an eye with sympathetic ophthalmia.

90. **Identify the incorrect statement.**
    A. Sympathetic uveitis can usually be distinguished histopathologically from Vogt-Koyanagi-Harada syndrome.
    B. In sympathetic uveitis the choroid is uniformly infiltrated with mononuclear and epithelial cells.
    C. Sympathetic uveitis may be associated with spinal fluid pleocytosis, tinnitus, and dysacusis.
    D. Enucleation should be performed within 2 weeks of the penetrating injury in order to decrease the risk of sympathetic uveitis in the noninjured eye.
    E. Sympathetic uveitis may rarely develop in the noninjured eye after the injured eye has been removed.

91. **Identify the incorrect statement.**
    A. Endophthalmitis after cataract extraction is usually caused by the patient's lid or conjunctival flora.

B. Endophthalmitis after cataract extraction is usually caused by *Staphylococcus epidermidis, Staphylococcus aureus,* or *Streptococcus pneumoniae.*
C. Endophthalmitis related to filtering blebs is usually caused by a *Streptococcus* species or *Haemophilus influenzae.*
D. Most patients with endophthalmitis related to filtering blebs have a negative Seidel's test at the site of the bleb.
E. Endophthalmitis related to filtering blebs is more common in patients who have inferior filtering blebs.

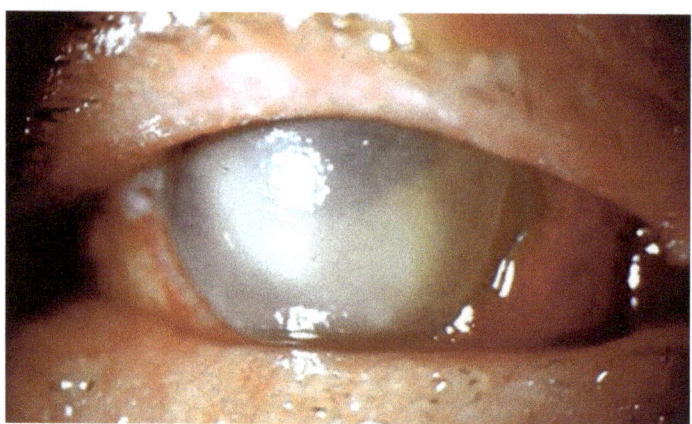

Fig. 3.14: An eye with endophthalmitis.

92. **Acute infectious endophthalmitis after cataract surgery:**
    A. May be painless.
    B. Is usually associated with decreased visual acuity.
    C. Is associated with edematous lids.
    D. Usually includes hypopyon.
    E. May be associated with a normal red reflex.

93. **Endogenous infectious endophthalmitis:**
    A. Is associated with less inflammation and pain than is exogenous endophthalmitis.
    B. May cause vitritis with white, fluffy exudates.
    C. Involves both eyes in 75% of cases.
    D. Most frequently appears with floaters and decreased visual acuity.
    E. Frequently, it is associated with a nonocular infectious focus.

94. **Aqueous and vitreous samples from patients with suspected infectious endophthalmitis:**
    A. Should be placed on thioglycollate broth and an anaerobic medium.
    B. Should be sent for Gram and Giemsa staining.
    C. Should include a minimum of 1.0 mL of liquid vitreous.
    D. Show positive cultures in about 65% of cases.
    E. Should be placed on blood and chocolate agar.

Uveitis and Other Intraocular Inflammations

95. In the treatment of infectious endophthalmitis:
  A. Gentamicin or amikacin is the intravitreal agent of choice for gram-negative coverage.
  B. Intravitreal amikacin is a common cause of macular infarction.
  C. Ceftazidime is a reasonable choice for intravitreal coverage for gram-negative bacteria.
  D. The addition of intravitreal dexamethasone has been associated with good visual outcomes.
  E. Vancomycin is the intravitreal agent of choice for gram-positive bacterial coverage.

96. The Endophthalmitis Vitrectomy Study concluded that in eyes with endophthalmitis found within 6 weeks of cataract surgery:
  A. Vitrectomy yielded better final visual acuity in eyes having initial acuity of hand motions or better.
  B. Vitrectomy yielded better final visual acuity in eyes having initial acuity of light perception only.
  C. Vitrectomy yielded no better culture results than vitreous tap alone.
  D. Retinal detachment is difficult to treat after vitrectomy for endophthalmitis treatment.
  E. The outcome of the endophthalmitis should not be assumed to be similar to that of endophthalmitis developing after procedures other than cataract surgery.

97. The Endophthalmitis Vitrectomy Study found the risk factors at initial ocular examination that are predictive of decreased final acuity to be:
  A. Acuity of light perception only.
  B. Perforated posterior lens capsule.
  C. Rubeosis.
  D. Absent red reflex.
  E. Pain.

98. Progressive outer retinal necrosis in a patient who has acquired immunodeficiency syndrome (AIDS):
  A. Usually progresses to full-thickness retinal necrosis in a few days.
  B. Spares the perivascular retina in the initial stages of disease.
  C. Involves the second eye in weeks to months.
  D. Rarely drops visual acuity to light perception only.
  E. May begin in the posterior pole.

99. Toxoplasmic retinochoroiditis in patients who have AIDS:
  A. Is bilateral and multifocal.
  B. Is usually associated with pre-existing chorioretinal scarring.
  C. Is commonly associated with vitritis, although the vitritis may be less severe than in immunocompetent patients.
  D. Is associated with intracranial toxoplasmosis in 25% of patients.
  E. Is more common in South America than in the United States.

100. Infectious multifocal choroiditis in patients who have AIDS:
A. Occurs in 10% of terminally ill patients.
B. May be caused by *Pneumocystis carinii* or *Cryptococcus* or *Mycobacterium* organisms.
C. Has a specific clinical picture for each organism.
D. May be found in asymptomatic patients.
E. Does not cause lesions that coalesce with time.

101. Molluscum contagiosum in patients who have AIDS:
A. Tends to be multiple sited and bilateral.
B. Spreads to the head and neck areas.
C. Is caused by a deoxyribonucleic acid (DNA) virus.
D. Results in a papillary conjunctivitis.
E. Is not associated with dermal necrosis.

102. Kaposi's sarcoma:
A. Is endemic in Kenya and Nigeria where it accounts for 20% of all malignancies.
B. Occurs commonly in men infected with human immunodeficiency virus (HIV).
C. Associated with HIV rarely disseminates to the visceral organs.
D. Is a vascular lesion that may be flat or elevated.
E. Is the most common ocular neoplasm found in individuals infected with HIV.

103. Non-Hodgkin's lymphoma associated with AIDS:
A. More commonly has extranodal involvement than non-AIDS-related lymphoma.
B. Is likely to be a high-grade B-cell malignancy.
C. When intraocular exhibits peripapillary hemorrhage and subretinal infiltrates.
D. When intracranial is typically periventricular in location.
E. Is commonly intraocular.

104. Non-Hodgkin's lymphoma involving the eye:
A. May be primary or secondary to systemic lymphoma.
B. Is usually a B-cell lymphoma.
C. When secondary is usually vitreal.
D. Has increased in incidence in recent years.
E. Usually presents as anterior uveitis.

105. Primary intraocular lymphoma:
A. Usually appears as panuveitis.
B. Is usually unilateral.
C. May cause mound-like elevations of the retinal pigment epithelium by lymphoma cells.
D. May cause secondary glaucoma.
E. Demands lumbar puncture as part of the systemic work-up.

106. **Secondary ocular lymphomas in patients who have systemic lymphoma:**
    A. Occurs predominantly in women.
    B. Are typically unilateral.
    C. Appear most commonly as choroidal masses.
    D. Often extend through the sclera into the orbit.
    E. Show little tissue necrosis on histopathologic examination.

ANSWERS

1. A. B cells are able to recognize antigens that have not been presented or processed by other cells.
2. C. Natural killer cells represent a separate group of lymphocytes that lack both immunoglobulins (as in B cells) and antigen receptors [i.e. T-cell receptor (TCR), as in T-cells].
3. E. Basophils and eosinophils are the cells involved in allergic reactions. Eosinophils confer immunity to the parasitic worms.
4. C. Tolerance to self is maintained by requiring T-cells to receive two signals before responding to an antigen. Clonal deletion and anergy are the two mechanisms of control of one's autoreactivity. T cells receive two signals, binding of an antigen to the T-cell receptor (TCR) and binding of a costimulatory molecule on the antigen presenting cell (APC). Clonal anergy is a process of T-cell inactivation, instead of elimination that occurs when an antigen binds a TCR without the presence of a costimulatory molecule.
5. B. Behcet's syndrome is associated with HLA-B51.
6. E. Type II hypersensitivity reactions represent an antibody-binding response. Antibody binds to a cell surface antigen or tissue resulting in the damage of the involved cell or tissue that presented that antibody. Examples of type II hypersensitivity reactions are hemolytic anemia and ocular cicatricial pemphigoid. Mast cells mediate type I hypersensitivity reactions.
7. C. Sympathetic uveitis is an example of a type IV (T-cell mediated) hypersensitivity reaction. Scleritis is an example of a type III (immune complex-mediated) hypersensitivity reaction.
8. B. ACAID is an anterior chamber-associated immune deviation. Antigens cannot escape from the anterior chamber, thus not eliciting a normal host immune response.
9. A. The ciliary processes contain an inner pigmented epithelial layer and an outer nonpigmented epithelial layer.
10. C. Cyclosporine is a cytostatic drug which suppresses the immune response.
11. E. Iris stromal edema is not a factor in the uveitis-related intraocular pressure (IOP) elevation.

12. C. Keratic precipitates (KPs) represent inflammatory cells on the corneal endothelium. In a setting of acute uveitis, KPs are lightly pigmented. They turn darker and shrink with time.
13. A. The value of early immunosuppressive therapy in children is questionable.
14. B. Anterior uveitis may be unilateral or bilateral. Herpes simplex virus (HSV)- and herpes zoster virus (HZV)-related uveitis may present with elevated intraocular pressure. Vogt-Koyanagi-Harada (VKH) Behcet's have strong ethnic predispositions. Uveitis with insidious onset or chronic smoldering uveitis may not be associated with pain and redness.
15. A. Anterior uveitis associated with spondyloarthritis is typically acute in onset, unilateral, recurrent, and self-limited.
16. D. Anterior uveitis associated with HLA-B27 is usually unilateral.
17. C. Uveitis associated with inflammatory bowel disease commonly has a posterior component.
18. D. Juvenile rheumatoid arthritis (JRA)-related uveitis is typically asymptomatic, insidious, and frequently detected during a routine screening of visual acuity.
19. E. Interstitial nephritis with uveitis responds well to high-dose oral corticosteroids.
20. B. Kawasaki disease is a disease of children.
21. C. Conjunctivitis is the most common ocular presentation of Lyme disease. An annular rash of at least 5 cm with central clearing, low-grade fever, and flu-like symptoms are typically present as well.
22. A. Phakoanaphylactic endophthalmitis usually presents with an abrupt-onset ocular inflammation, mutton-fat keratic precipitates, a hypopyon, and posterior synechiae. There is no retinal, choroidal, or optic nerve involvement.
23. D. *Staphylococcus aureus* is an organism involved in the acute form of endophthalmitis.
24. C. Herpes viruses can cause blepharitis, conjunctivitis, scleritis, keratitis, anterior uveitis, vitritis, retinitis, and retinal vasculitis.
25. B. Inflammation associated with varicella-zoster virus (VZV) is more severe than that caused by herpes simplex virus (HSV). Iritis is granulomatous in presentation. VZV infection can result in sectoral iris atrophy due to the occlusive vasculitis.
26. D. There has been an increase in the incidence of syphilitic uveitis in the past years due to bacterial resistance, socioeconomic factors, and human immunodeficiency virus (HIV).
27. D. Patients with neurosyphilis have positive treponemal and nontreponemal tests which have to be confirmed by checking cerebrospinal fluid (CSF)-VDRL levels. In tertiary or latent syphilis, nontreponemal tests are negative, but the treponemal tests are positive.

Uveitis and Other Intraocular Inflammations

28. B. Secondary syphilis is associated with a maculopapular rash.
29. E. Upon resolution of acute interstitial keratitis, deep ghost vessels remain within the cornea.
30. D. The most common presentation of the tuberculous uveitis is anterior uveitis and choroiditis or chorioretinitis.
31. C. Low-dose corticosteroids may be administered to control inflammation under close follow-up of an ophthalmologist.
32. A. Chronic bilateral anterior uveitis is more common than acute iridocyclitis in the cases of leprous uveitis.
33. B. Brucellosis uveitis can present with unilateral or bilateral, granulomatous or nongranulomatous inflammation.
34. E. Unilateral anterior uveitis is a typical presentation of Fuchs' heterochromic iridocyclitis.
35. C. About 20–30% of patients with Fuchs' heterochromic iridocyclitis develop small peripheral anterior synechiae which do not coalesce to produce angle closure glaucoma.
36. A. Eyes with Fuchs' heterochromic iridocyclitis respond poorly to topical corticosteroids and their use probably does not change the course of the disease.
37. D. Anterior uveitis in the glaucomatocyclitic crises is significant for a marked cellular response.
38. C. Pars planitis does not have any apparent gender predilection.
39. E. Intermediate uveitis is associated with HLA-DR15, similar to multiple sclerosis.
40. A. Posterior synechiae are uncommon in intermediate uveitis. If they do develop, they are broader-based and are more difficult to break.
41. B. Treatment of intermediate uveitis may include posterior sub-Tenon's injections of triamcinolone (40 mg/mL) or methylprednisolone acetate depot preparation (80 mg/mL).
42. E. Intermediate uveitis associated with T-cell lymphoma responds well to oral and topical corticosteroids. Long-term disease course and visual outcomes have not been reported.
43. E. This vignette describes a case of cytomegalovirus (CMV) retinitis in an immunocompromised patient. The risk and the incidence of CMV retinitis rise as CD4 count decreases, especially to the levels below 50 cells/mm^3.
44. B. As immune system recovers, strengthened host response causes an increase level of vitritis.
45. D. Treatment of CMV retinitis with ganciclovir causes neutropenia in 30–40% of patients.
46. C. Retinal detachment occurs in up to one-third of children with congenital CMV retinitis.
47. E. There is no foscarnet intravitreal implant available for use.
48. A. Varicella-zoster virus can cause retinitis in either immunocompetent or immunocompromised individuals.
49. B. Ocular findings of congenital HSV retinitis are usually bilateral.

50. A. Acute retinal necrosis starts in the periphery and becomes confluent within a week.
51. A. Western equine encephalomyelitis virus does not cause viral retinitis. In addition to those listed, viral retinitis can be caused by West Nile virus, rift valley fever virus, human T-cell lymphotropic virus type 1, dengue fever, and Chikungunya fever.
52. B. Diagnosis of Whipple's disease is made by duodenal biopsy. Biopsy specimens show periodic acid-Schiff (PAS)-positive bacilli in macrophages. PAS-positive cells may also be found in the anterior chamber, vitreous, brain, lungs, tonsils, and synovial fluid.
53. B. Treatment of Whipple's disease typically includes systemic trimethoprim-sulfamethoxazole. Patients with sulfa allergies can be treated with ceftriaxone, tetracycline, or chloramphenicol.
54. A. Despite the fact that no serologic confirmation of histoplasmosis infection has been reported in patients with ocular histoplasmosis syndrome (OHS), *Histoplasma capsulatum* organisms have been identified within choroidal granulomas of OHS patients.
55. D. Lack of vitritis is typical of OHS.
56. C. The Macular Photocoagulation Study (MPS) group found that krypton red and argon blue lasers are equally effective in the treatment of choroidal neovascular membranes caused by OHS.
57. E. Septicemia requiring long-term antibiotic therapy via indwelling vascular catheters is a risk factor for *Candida albicans* endogenous endophthalmitis.
58. B. About 70–80% of pregnant women in the United States are thought to lack antibodies to *Toxoplasma gondii*, placing them at risk for infection.
59. C. Toxoplasmosis retinitis involves the retinal nerve fiber layer in most cases.
60. D. Congenital toxoplasmosis does not initially present with cataracts.
61. E. Multiple active lesions due to toxoplasmosis uveitis are a relative indication for treatment.
62. B. Clindamycin exhibits excellent ocular penetration. It kills bradyzoites (an encysted form of *Toxoplasma capsulatum*) and acts synergistically with pyrimethamine and sulfonamides.
63. A. Pyrimethamine causes bone marrow suppression and is teratogenic.
64. C. *Toxocara canis* is a roundworm, similar to *Ascaris lumbricoides*.
65. D. Visceral larva migrans results in typical clinical manifestations including irritability, fever, pulmonary and dermatologic findings.
66. A. In addition to the other listed options, ocular *Toxocara* lesions may appear as radial peripheral retinal folds.
67. C. Retinoblastoma lesions do not cause retinal traction.
68. D. Unilateral disease is more common than bilateral disease in both ocular toxocariasis and Coats disease.
69. B. Cysticercosis may be present in any tissue or organ. It can be identified only in patients with ocular and cerebral findings.

70. E. Onchocerciasis can present in the anterior segment as live microfilariae in the cornea, uveitis, limbitis, and microfilariae swimming in the anterior chamber.
71. B. Ocular onchocerciasis infection leads to chorioretinitis. Vitritis is not a typical feature of this disease.
72. A. Acute posterior multifocal placoid pigment epitheliopathy (APMPPE) affects both eyes in the majority of cases. Patients may initially present with a headache, meningismus, hearing loss, and visual disturbances.
73. E. Acute posterior multifocal placoid pigment epitheliopathy lesions resolve over a 2-6 weeks period of time. Patients are left with residual retinal pigment epithelium (RPE) mottling. Choroidal neovascular membranes are rare.
74. D. Multiple evanescent white dot syndrome (MEWDS) lesions resolve over a 2-6 weeks period of time. Visual acuity returns to baseline. Recurrences are uncommon. Visual prognosis is good even with recurrences.
75. C. Serpiginous choroiditis demonstrates early hypofluorescence and late hyperfluorescence of active lesions on the intravenous angiography.
76. B. Birdshot retinochoroidopathy affects healthy patients, mostly females, between the ages of 30 and 60 years.
77. D. Ocular involvement of sarcoidosis is common. It occurs in up to 50% of patients.
78. D. With choroidal lesions, the eye is remarkably quiet. It may mimic other diseases such as pneumocystis choroiditis that present with sub-retinal pigment epithelium (Sub-RPE) choroidal granulomas.
79. C. Bronchoalveolar lavage sample analysis helps with the diagnosis. Lymphocytosis of at least 10% is a sign of alveolitis. Increased helper/suppressor T-cell ratio is almost suggestive of sarcoidosis.
80. B. Children younger than 4 years presenting with sarcoidosis are more likely to have cutaneous disease and arthritis and less likely to have pulmonary disease.
81. A. Behcet's syndrome is more common in men overall. The "complete" type of Behcet's disease (with four major diagnostic criteria present) is more common in men, while "incomplete" Behcet's disease (with three major criteria or ocular involvement with one other major criterion present) is equally common in both sexes.
82. C. Bechet's syndrome is frequently associated with optic disc edema.
83. D. Hearing loss is not one of the features of Behcet's syndrome.
84. D. Treatment of Behcet's disease with tacrolimus and cyclophosphamide has been shown to be successful in Japan.
85. A. Vogt-Koyanagi-Harada (VKH) syndrome is more common in the pigmented races including Asians, Hispanics, Native Americans, and Asian Indians.

86. B. Samples of cerebrospinal fluid (CSF) fluid in the VKH syndrome demonstrate lymphocytic pleocytosis in the setting of normal glucose levels in about 80% of patients that persists for up to 8 weeks.
87. D. Vogt-Koyanagi-Harada patients develop exudative retinal detachments.
88. D. In the VKH syndrome, granulomas are found at the level of the choriocapillaris. Sparing of the choriocapillaris is characteristic of sympathetic ophthalmia.
89. E. Sympathetic ophthalmia (sympathetic uveitis) was historically thought to be more common in children under the age of 10 years (due to ocular injuries) and adults over the age of 60 years (due to surgical interventions). Incidence in children in recent series has decreased due to a decline in the incidence in pediatric ocular trauma.
90. A. Histopathologically, there is no difference between sympathetic uveitis and VKH syndrome. Clinical presentation and history of penetrating ocular injury (or not) are used to differentiate the two entities.
91. D. Most patients with endophthalmitis related to filtering blebs have leaky filtering blebs (demonstrated with a positive Seidel's test).
92. A. Acute infectious endophthalmitis is painful.
93. C. Endogenous infectious endophthalmitis involves both eyes in 25% of cases.
94. C. Fluid samples from patients with suspected endophthalmitis should include a minimum of 0.2 mL of liquid vitreous.
95. B. Intravitreal gentamicin is a common cause of macular infarction.
96. A. The endophthalmitis vitrectomy study (EVS) concluded that vitrectomy yielded better final visual acuity in eyes having initial acuity of light perception (LP) or worse.
97. E. Pain was not a predictor of decreased final acuity.
98. D. Within weeks, vision deteriorates rapidly to light perception or no light perception level.
99. B. Patients with acquired immunodeficiency syndrome (AIDS) may develop primary infection with toxoplasmosis.
100. C. Infectious multifocal choroiditis in patients with AIDS is nonspecific.
101. D. Molluscum contagiosum in patients who have AIDS may result in follicular conjunctivitis.
102. C. Kaposi's sarcoma associated with human immunodeficiency virus (HIV) may disseminate aggressively to various organs including lung, liver, and gastrointestinal (GI) tract.
103. E. Non-Hodgkin's lymphoma associated with AIDS rarely involves eyes.
104. E. Posterior uveitis is the most common presentation.
105. B. Primary intraocular lymphoma is usually bilateral.
106. A. Secondary intraocular lymphoma in patients who have systemic lymphoma occurs predominantly in men.

CHAPTER 4

Cornea and External Disease

An Vo

QUESTIONS

Identify the correct answer for all questions (unless instructed otherwise).

1. **A choristoma is a tumor composed of:**
   A. Cartilage and ectodermal tissue.
   B. Fat and endodermal tissue.
   C. Tissue not normally found in the area of involvement.
   D. Tissue normally found in the area of involvement.
   E. Tissue from each of the three germ layers.

2. **Goldenhar's syndrome contains all the following, *except*:**
   A. Preauricular skin tags.
   B. Blind-ended preauricular fistulas.
   C. Bilateral limbal dermoids.
   D. Hypoplasia of the facial bones.
   E. Polydactylism.

3. **Secondary conjunctival localized amyloidosis may occur in all the following, *except*:**
   A. Stromal corneal dystrophies.
   B. Trachoma.
   C. Trichiasis.
   D. Epithelial corneal dystrophies.
   E. Chronic keratitis.

4. **The most common cause of acute bacterial conjunctivitis worldwide is:**
   A. *Staphylococcus aureus.*
   B. *Streptococcus pneumoniae.*
   C. *Corynebacterium diphtheriae.*
   D. *Staphylococcus albus.*
   E. *Haemophilus influenzae.*

5. The most common cause of chronic bacterial conjunctivitis especially angular blepharoconjunctivitis is:
   A. *Proteus mirabilis.*
   B. *Moraxella lacunata.*
   C. *Escherichia coli.*
   D. *Klebsiella pneumoniae.*
   E. *Serratia marcescens.*

6. Viral conjunctivitis:
   A. Cannot be differentiated from bacterial conjunctivitis without culture.
   B. Usually appears as a bilateral conjunctivitis.
   C. Typically has a purulent discharge.
   D. Unlike bacterial conjunctivitis is almost never accompanied by preauricular lymphadenopathy.
   E. Can usually be diagnosed clinically.

7. Pharyngoconjunctival fever is characterized by all the following, *except*:
   A. It is caused by adenovirus serotypes 3, 4, and 7.
   B. It is the most common ocular adenoviral infection.
   C. It has a short incubation period (<5 days).
   D. It causes a predominantly follicular reaction.
   E. It has an associated preauricular lymphadenopathy in about 90% of cases.

8. Epidemic keratoconjunctivitis is characterized by all the following *except*:
   A. It is associated with membrane formation in about one-third of cases.
   B. Corneal involvement occurs in most cases.
   C. It causes a mixed follicular and papillary reaction.
   D. It is caused by adenovirus serotypes 3, 4, and 7.
   E. It causes a more severe form of conjunctivitis than does pharyngoconjunctival fever.

9. Chlamydial infections cause all the following, *except*:
   A. Trachoma.
   B. Chronic follicular conjunctivitis.
   C. Adult inclusion conjunctivitis.
   D. Middle to deep stromal corneal infiltrates.
   E. Neonatal conjunctivitis.

10. All the following contribute to the cause of neonatal conjunctivitis, *except*:
    A. Inadequate treatment of maternal infection during pregnancy.
    B. Organisms harbored in the mother's birth canal.
    C. 0.10% buffered silver nitrate ocular prophylaxis.
    D. Susceptibility of the infant's eye to infection.
    E. Ocular trauma during delivery.

Cornea and External Disease

11. Allergic conjunctivitis is characterized by all the following, *except*:
   A. Not occurring as part of a generalized allergic reaction.
   B. Type I allergic response.
   C. Mediation by immunoglobulin E.
   D. Bilateral itchy, burning, hyperemic eyes.
   E. Often a family history of atopy.

12. Which of the following statements is true regarding the condition depicted in this figure?

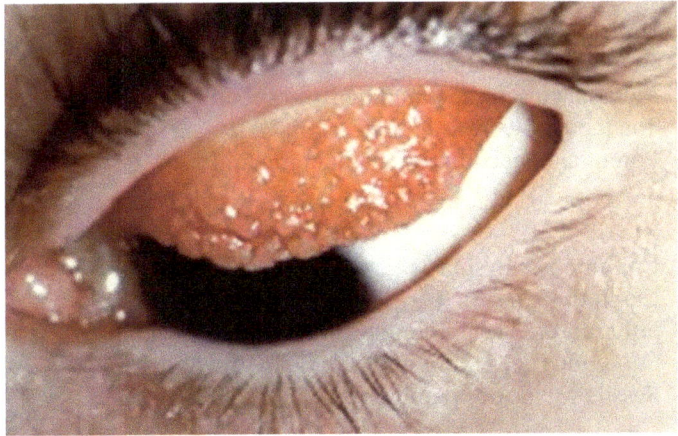

   A. It tends to be unilateral.
   B. It most commonly occurs in the fall and winter.
   C. It usually occurs in young boys (<10 years).
   D. Generally is not self-limiting in children and needs aggressive therapy to cause a remission.
   E. It occurs in palpebral, limbal, and mixed forms.

13. Giant papillary conjunctivitis is seen in all the following, *except*:
   A. Soft contact lens wearers.
   B. Acrylic lens implants.
   C. Hard contact lens wearers.
   D. Ocular prostheses.
   E. Protruding ocular sutures.

14. On examination, a 72-year-old woman has subepithelial conjunctival fibrosis, symblepharon, and fibrotic conjunctival bands. The most likely diagnosis is:
   A. Ligneous conjunctivitis.
   B. Cicatricial pemphigoid.
   C. Toxic follicular conjunctivitis.
   D. Microbiallergic conjunctivitis.
   E. Vernal conjunctivitis.

15. Erythema multiforme major (Stevens–Johnson syndrome) is characterized by all of the following, *except*:

A. It usually occurs in the fifth and sixth decades of life.
B. It can cause an acute, bilateral, mucopurulent conjunctivitis, chemosis, and conjunctival vesicles.
C. Its most severe variant is toxic epidermal necrolysis.
D. Systemic toxicity includes fever, malaise, headache, and fluid imbalance.
E. It may be precipitated by bacteria and sulfonamides.

16. **Primary acquired melanosis is characterized by all the following, *except*:**
    A. Unilaterality.
    B. Brown pigmentation.
    C. Melanocytes in the junctional and subepithelial locations.
    D. The tendency toward progression.
    E. Potential to become a malignant melanoma.

17. **All the following characterize a conjunctival intraepithelial neoplasm, *except*:**
    A. Conjunctival dysplasia.
    B. Carcinoma in situ.
    C. Squamous cell carcinoma with minimal invasion.
    D. Squamous cell carcinoma with deep invasion.
    E. Sessile squamous papilloma.

18. **The corneal epithelium contains all the following, *except*:**
    A. Langerhans cells.
    B. Wing epithelial cells.
    C. Basal epithelial cells.
    D. Dendritic melanocytic nevus cells.
    E. Superficial epithelial cells.

19. **All the following occur within the first few hours after small corneal epithelial injury, *except*:**
    A. Cell spreading.
    B. Cell migration.
    C. Disappearance of anchoring hemidesmosomes.
    D. Cell proliferation.
    E. Contraction of actin fibers.

20. **Recurrent erosion may occur in which of the following conditions:**
    A. Post-traumatic corneal abrasion.
    B. Map-dot-fingerprint (Cogan's microcystic) dystrophy.
    C. Reis-Bückler's dystrophy.
    D. Meesmann's dystrophy.
    E. All of the above.
    F. None of the above.

21. **Typically, the onset of symptoms of recurrent erosion:**
    A. Occurs in midafternoon.
    B. Occurs on awakening in the morning.

C. Is worse in the evening.
D. Is variable throughout the course of the day.
E. Does not seem to occur during the sleeping hours.

22. Treatment of recurrent erosion includes all the following, *except*:
    A. Sharp instrument debridement when large, loose sheets of devitalized cells are present.
    B. Ocular surface lubricants.
    C. Topical hypertonic solutions.
    D. Extended-wear bandage, soft contact lenses.
    E. Anterior stromal micropunctures.

23. The corneal endothelium shows all the following characteristics, *except*:
    A. A monolayer of cells.
    B. Lateral interdigitations of adjacent cells with both gap and tight junctions.
    C. Being devoid of surface villi on the aqueous side.
    D. On specular microscopy, presence of light, well-defined cell borders and dark centers.
    E. Continuous secretion of Descemet's membrane throughout life.

24. Fluid regulation by corneal endothelium is enhanced by all the following, *except*:
    A. Hexagonal arrangement of individual cells.
    B. The barrier portion of the endothelium which is permeable to the extent that it allows enough ion flux to establish the osmotic gradient.
    C. Ca^+ channel enhancer function.
    D. Membrane-bound Na^+/K^+-ATPase sites.
    E. Intracellular carbonic anhydrase pathway.

25. Fuchs' dystrophy:
    A. Is the most common corneal dystrophy to require keratoplasty.
    B. Shows peripheral cornea guttata of Descemet's membrane.
    C. Has as its primary defect an epithelial abnormality.
    D. Is most common in men.
    E. Is not associated with glaucoma.

26. Which of the following symptoms are associated with Fuchs' dystrophy?
    A. Blurred vision.
    B. Recurrent erosions.
    C. Glare.
    D. Pain.
    E. All of the above.

27. Congenital hereditary endothelial dystrophy has all the following attributes, *except*:
    A. Autosomal dominant inheritance pattern.
    B. Onset usually at 3 months in a term infant.

C. Autosomal recessive inheritance pattern.
D. Accumulation of functionally abnormal and structurally exaggerated posterior non-banded Descemet's membrane.
E. Bilateral, symmetric, edematous, and cloudy corneas.

28. **Posterior polymorphous dystrophy has all the following attributes, *except*:**
    A. An autosomal dominant inheritance pattern.
    B. Vesicular, curvilinear, and placoid abnormalities on specular microscopy.
    C. Epithelial-like transformation of corneal endothelium.
    D. An association with glaucoma.
    E. An autosomal recessive inheritance pattern.

29. **Megalocornea:**
    A. Shows a corneal horizontal size more than or equal to 11.5 mm after 2 years of age.
    B. May be autosomal recessive.
    C. May be X-linked recessive.
    D. Shows a decreased endothelial density on specular microscopy.
    E. Often shows a lens dislocated into the vitreous.

30. **All of the following characteristics are associated with Axenfeld-Rieger syndrome, *except*:**
    A. About 50% of the cases are associated with glaucoma.
    B. Results from retention of surface ectodermal tissue.
    C. Iris atrophy, corectopia and polycoria are present.
    D. Dental abnormalities can be present.
    E. Defects in the *PAX2* gene on chromosome 4q25.

31. **Peters' anomaly:**
    A. Does not involve Descemet's membrane.
    B. Does not involve Bowman's membrane.
    C. Is a paracentral, midcorneal stromal defect.
    D. May occur as part of fetal alcohol syndrome.
    E. Is associated with dental and vertebral anomalies.

32. **A 2-year-old child has painful recurrent corneal erosions. Testing shows abnormalities of chromosome 5q. The most likely diagnosis is:**
    A. Superficial granular dystrophy.
    B. Fuchs' combined dystrophy.
    C. Meesmann's dystrophy.
    D. Gelatinous drop-like dystrophy.
    E. Reis-Bückler's dystrophy.

33. **Recurrent corneal erosions are a dominant feature of all of the following, *except*:**
    A. Reis-Bückler's dystrophy.
    B. Honeycomb (Thiel-Behnke dystrophy).
    C. Superficial granular dystrophy.

D. Lattice dystrophy.
E. Macular dystrophy.

34. **Lattice type I (Biber-Haab-Dimmer) dystrophy:**
    A. Is associated with familial amyloidosis.
    B. Shows dichroic, Congo red-positive material in the stroma.
    C. Is associated with development of linear, often branching, stromal opacities in the fifth and sixth decades.
    D. Involves stromal opacities that are most dense just anterior to Descemet's membrane.
    E. Shows abnormalities of chromosome 11p.

35. **A 48-year-old patient presents with mildly decreased vision. Examination shows discrete corneal stromal opacities. The stroma between the opacities is clear. The most likely diagnosis is:**
    A. Granular (Groenouw type I) corneal dystrophy.
    B. Macular corneal dystrophy.
    C. Lattice dystrophy type III.
    D. Gelatinous drop-like dystrophy.
    E. Central cloudy dystrophy.

36. **A 36-year-old patient has decreased vision. Examination demonstrates anterior corneal stromal discrete opacities and posterior stromal linear, often branching, opacities. The most likely diagnosis is:**
    A. Granular (Groenouw type I) corneal dystrophy.
    B. Central cloudy dystrophy.
    C. Lattice dystrophy type III.
    D. Avellino dystrophy.
    E. Posterior amorphous dystrophy.

37. **All the following corneal dystrophies have been mapped to chromosome 5q, *except*:**
    A. Granular (Groenouw type I) corneal dystrophy.
    B. Reis-Bückler's dystrophy.
    C. Lattice dystrophy type II (Meretoja).
    D. Avellino dystrophy.
    E. Lattice dystrophy type I.

38. **All the following statements about the attributes of macular corneal dystrophies are true, *except*:**
    A. These dystrophies show an autosomal recessive pattern.
    B. In type I, typical sulfated keratan sulfate is not present in the cornea or serum.
    C. In type II, antigenic sulfated keratin sulfate is present in the cornea and serum.
    D. Discrete corneal stromal opacities are shown; the stroma between the opacities is cloudy.
    E. Penetrating keratoplasty frequently is followed by recurrence in the graft.

39. On clinical examination, all the following may be seen in the condition depicted by the slit-lamp photo, *except*:

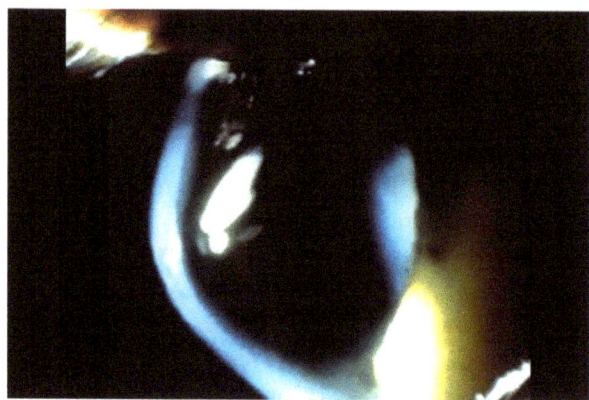

Fig. 4.2: Slit-lamp image.

   A. Corneal epithelium iron deposition in a ring form (Fleischer ring).
   B. Ruptures in Bowman's membrane leading to acute keratoconus.
   C. Protrusion of the lower lid on downgaze (Munson's sign).
   D. Presence of keratometry >47.2 diopters, steepening of the inferior cornea >1.2 diopters (compared with the superior cornea), and skewing of the radial axis of astigmatism more than 21°.
   E. Thinning of the corneal apex.

40. A pterygium is similar to a pinguecula in all the following ways, *except*:
   A. It has an association with ultraviolet light.
   B. It demonstrates elastotic degeneration of the conjunctival substantia propria.
   C. It starts in the region of the limbus.
   D. It shows fibrovascular invasion of Bowman's membrane.
   E. It is a degenerative (as opposed to dysplastic) process.

41. Histologically, arcus senilis shows:
   A. Stromal deposition of lipid.
   B. Peripheral Descemet's membrane deposition of lipid.
   C. Peripheral Bowman's membrane deposition of lipid.
   D. All of the above.
   E. None of the above.

42. Terrien's marginal corneal degeneration:
   A. Occurs most frequently in women in the third to fourth decades.
   B. Has a fairly steep central edge and sloping peripheral edge.
   C. Is unrelated to pellucid marginal corneal degeneration.
   D. Contains a lipid deposit along its peripheral edge.
   E. Involves pain as a prominent symptom.

43. Calcific band keratopathy typically develops in all the following, *except*:

A. Chronic topical epinephrine therapy for glaucoma.
   B. Uveitis.
   C. Juvenile rheumatoid arthritis.
   D. Hyperparathyroidism.
   E. Vitamin D toxicity.

44. A 78-year-old patient shows white-to-gray and light-blue superficial corneal stromal nodules elevating the corneal epithelium. All the following have a likely predisposing association, *except*:
   A. Male gender.
   B. Phlyctenular keratitis.
   C. Vernal keratitis.
   D. Trachoma.
   E. Thygeson's superficial punctate keratitis.

45. Amyloid corneal stromal deposition can be seen in all the following, *except*:
   A. Lattice dystrophy type II (Meretoja).
   B. Gelatinous drop-like dystrophy.
   C. Granular (Groenouw type I) corneal dystrophy.
   D. Climatic proteoglycan stromal keratopathy.
   E. Lattice dystrophy type I.

46. General principles of therapy for noninfectious keratitis include all the following, *except*:
   A. Determining the specific cause.
   B. Using a broad-spectrum antibiotic.
   C. Promoting epithelial healing.
   D. Limiting ulceration and stromal loss.
   E. Supporting repair.

47. All the following are typical of Thygeson's superficial pupctate keratopathy, *except*:
   A. Long duration of exacerbations and remissions.
   B. In some patients an increase in HLA-Dw3 and HLA-DR3 expression.
   C. Central cornea opacities that are small, round, or oval and granular, white-gray, intraepithelial, and dot-like and are often accompanied by subepithelial opacities.
   D. Usual absence of conjunctival inflammation.
   E. Suggestion of male preponderance.

48. A 41-year-old patient has a history of bilateral recurrent inflammation of the superior limbus and conjunctiva. Involvement of the superior tarsal and bulbar conjunctiva is noted. The probable diagnosis is:
   A. Thygeson's superficial punctate keratopathy.
   B. Moren's ulcer.
   C. Superior limbic keratoconjunctivitis (SLK) of Theodore.
   D. Terrien's marginal degeneration.
   E. Neurotrophic keratitis.

49. Mooren's ulcer is characterized by all the following, *except*:
A. Circumferential and central spread of the ulcer.
B. Peripheral ulcer with undetermined central edge of the ulcer (overhanging edge).
C. Chronicity.
D. Pain.
E. Association with collagen vascular disease.

50. The differential diagnosis of nonsyphilitic interstitial keratitis (Cogan's dystrophy) includes all the following, *except*:
A. Lyme disease.
B. Avellino dystrophy.
C. Congenital syphilis.
D. Sarcoidosis.
E. Viral keratitis.

51. As a description of the characteristics of neurotrophic keratitis, which of the following statements is not true?
A. A quiet white eye is usually seen.
B. The condition results from lesions of the fifth cranial nerve.
C. Varicella-zoster and herpes simplex keratitis are the most common causes.
D. Punctate keratitis is seen.
E. Loss of corneal sensation is noted.

52. The therapy for mild neurotrophic keratitis is:
A. Punctal occlusion.
B. Soft contact lens wear.
C. Lateral tarsorrhaphy.
D. Ocular lubrication.
E. Penetrating keratoplasty.

53. Rheumatoid-associated ocular involvement includes all the following characteristics, *except*:
A. Central ulcerative keratitis.
B. Peripheral limbal gutter.
C. Acute corneal stromal keratitis.
D. Keratolysis.
E. Sclerosing keratitis.

54. The pathologic characteristics of paracentral rheumatoid melt include all the following, *except*:
A. Infiltration by monocytes, macrophages, and T-lymphocytes.
B. Strong HLA-DR expression by stromal keratocytes and epithelium.
C. Presence of CD 11 (macrophages) in epithelium and subepithelium at the ulcer edge.
D. Immunoglobulin deposition in corneal epithelium.
E. Stromal infiltration exclusively by neutrophils and eosinophils.

Cornea and External Disease

55. **Bacterial keratitis:**
    A. Is not an important cause of monocular blindness in the developing world.
    B. Is caused by *Streptococcus pneumoniae* and *Serratia marcescens* in the majority of cases.
    C. Occurs in 0.0001–0.0003% of contact lens wearers (10–30 in 100,000).
    D. In patients who have debilitated diseases is caused mainly by *Staphylococcus epidermidis*.
    E. In the eastern and northeastern United States is most commonly caused by pseudomonal infection.

56. **The corneal surface normally is protected by all the following, *except*:**
    A. An intact corneal epithelium.
    B. Stromal antimicrobial substances.
    C. Eyelid blinking which regularly sweeps away debris trapped in the mucin layer.
    D. Tears which contain lysozyme, lactoferrin, 13-lysin, tear-specific albumin, and immunoglobulin.
    E. Immune mediators present in the conjunctiva.

57. **The cardinal sign(s) of bacterial keratitis is (are):**
    A. "dry" satellite stromal lesions.
    B. Satellite lesions plus hypopyon.
    C. Peripheral corneal infiltration and conjunctival injection.
    D. Localized or diffuse central infiltration of the corneal epithelium or stroma.
    E. Ciliary injection and chemosis.

58. **A corneal ulcer is cultured. The organism ferments mannitol. The most probable bacterium present is:**
    A. *Staphylococcus epidermidis*.
    B. *Pseudomonas aeruginosa*.
    C. *Staphylococcus aureus*.
    D. *Neisseria gonorrhoeae*.
    E. *Streptococcus pneumoniae*.

59. **All the following organisms have been associated with infectious crystalline keratopathy. Which is the most common cause?**
    A. *Streptococcus viridans*.
    B. *Streptococcus pneumoniae*.
    C. *Pseudomonas aeruginosa*.
    D. *Haemophilus aphrophilus*.
    E. *Peptostreptococcus*.

60. **Of the following culture media, which is the best for *Neisseria* organisms?**
    A. Blood agar.
    B. Brain heart infusion.
    C. Chocolate agar.

D. Sabouraud dextrose agar.
E. Enriched thioglycollate broth.

61. **Of the following culture media, which is the best for anaerobic bacteria?**
    A. Brain heart infusion.
    B. Blood agar.
    C. Chocolate agar.
    D. Sabouraud dextrose agar.
    E. Enriched thioglycollate broth.

62. **Which of the following is best for the identification of bacteria?**
    A. Giemsa stain.
    B. Grocott–Gomori's methenamine silver stain.
    C. Periodic acid-Schiff stain.
    D. Calcofluor white stain.
    E. Gram-stain.

63. **Definitive diagnosis of bacterial keratitis can be made by:**
    A. Clinical history.
    B. Clinical history and physical examination.
    C. Gram staining of scrapings.
    D. Culture of scrapings.
    E. Giemsa staining of scrapings.

64. **All the following are active in the treatment of gram-negative bacteria and some gram-positive bacteria, *except*:**
    A. Amikacin.
    B. Vancomycin.
    C. Gentamicin.
    D. Tobramycin.
    E. Ofloxacin.

65. **Viruses have all the following attributes, *except*:**
    A. Presence of an intracellular parasite.
    B. Acute sensitivity to treatment with fluoroquinolones.
    C. Only one type of nucleic acid within the infectious unit.
    D. Inability to replicate by binary fission.
    E. Resistance to commonly used topical antibiotics.

66. **All the following belong to the Herpesviridae family, *except*:**
    A. Adenovirus.
    B. Herpes simplex virus.
    C. Varicella-zoster virus.
    D. Epstein–Barr virus.
    E. Cytomegalovirus.

67. **All of the following about Herpesviridae organisms are true, *except*:**
    A. Are deoxyribonucleic acid (DNA) viruses.
    B. Contain a central core surrounded by a protein capsid.

C. Are enclosed within an envelope of glycoprotein, lipid, and carbohydrate.
D. Are one of the leading causes of central corneal blindness in developing countries.
E. Are spread mainly through respiratory droplets.

68. Herpes simplex corneal dendrites tend to have all the following characteristics, *except*:
    A. A fine, lacy appearance.
    B. A linear epithelial defect.
    C. Staining of the base of the defect with fluorescein.
    D. No terminal bulbs.
    E. Staining of diseased border epithelial cells with Rose Bengal.

69. Varicella-zoster virus is all the following, *except*:
    A. Secondary cause of herpes zoster ophthalmicus.
    B. Primary cause of chickenpox.
    C. Primary cause of shingles.
    D. Secondary cause of keratitis.
    E. Secondary cause of iridocyclitis.

70. Ocular findings with Epstein–Barr virus include all of the following, *except*:
    A. Parinaud's oculoglandular syndrome.
    B. Scleromalacia perforans.
    C. Follicular conjunctivitis.
    D. Conjunctival mass.
    E. Subepithelial infiltrates.

71. Which of the following statements does not pertain to cytomegalovirus keratitis?
    A. It has a well-designed protocol for optimal treatment.
    B. It is extremely rare.
    C. It may be associated with human immunodeficiency virus (HIV) infection.
    D. It resembles varicella-zoster keratitis.
    E. Scrapings show multinucleated syncytial giant cells and intranuclear inclusion bodies.

72. All the following are classified as filamentous fungi (septate and nonseptate), *except*:
    A. *Fusarium.*
    B. *Cephalosporium.*
    C. *Aspergillus.*
    D. *Cryptococcus.*
    E. *Alternaria.*

73. All of the following are true about dimorphic fungi, *except*:
    A. Include histoplasma.
    B. Include coccidioides.

C. Include blastomyces.
D. Demonstrate both yeast (in tissues) and mycelial (on saprophytic and culture media surfaces) phases.
E. Include *Candida*.

74. All of the following are true about yeasts, *except*:
    A. Include *Candida*.
    B. Include *Cryptococcus*.
    C. Are unicellular fungi that reproduce by budding.
    D. In tissue may develop elongated buds (pseudohyphae) or real hyphae.
    E. Include *Histoplasma*.

75. Which of the following does not apply to free-living holozoic amebae?
    A. Include *Acanthamoeba*.
    B. Co-contamination with bacteria is a risk factor for adherence to hydrogel lenses.
    C. Include *Vahlkampfia*.
    D. Cannot survive in hot tubs.
    E. Include *Hartmannella*.

76. In the early stages of *Acanthamoeba* keratitis, which of the following is least common?
    A. Epithelial irregularities and infiltration.
    B. Pseudodendrites.
    C. Corneal neovascularization.
    D. Infiltrates around corneal nerves.
    E. Nonspecific stromal or characteristic ring infiltrates.

77. Which of the following statements about microsporidia is incorrect?
    A. Microsporidia are very difficult to culture.
    B. Scrapings from the cornea show gram-positive ovoid intracytoplasmic inclusions.
    C. Weber stain demonstrates dense concentrations of individual intracellular structures.
    D. Polymerase chain reaction (PCR) is useful in differentiation of species.
    E. Microsporidia are only seen in immunocompromised patients.

78. Which of the following statements does not apply to onchocerciasis?
    A. The ocular manifestations are caused by the presence of large worms.
    B. It is the major cause of blindness worldwide.
    C. Because it is transmitted by the *Simulium* black fly which breeds in fast-flowing rivers, it is also called river blindness.
    D. The parasite *Onchocerca volvulus* is a filarial nematode.
    E. Keratitis and secondary angle-closure glaucoma are major causes of blindness.

79. Which one of the following statements does not apply to penetrating keratoplasty (PK)?

- A. It is the most common transplantation procedure.
- B. It is the most successful transplantation procedure.
- C. Because of advances in technology, tissue selection and preservation, and management of postoperative astigmatism, optical results have improved.
- D. PK is performed to restore globe integrity and to restore vision.
- E. It is an old procedure, dating back to the 1920s.

80. **All of the following statements are true about anterior lamellar keratoplasty, *except*:**
    - A. Deep anterior lamellar keratoplasty is effective in patients with keratoconus.
    - B. It is used as a tectonic graft for structural support.
    - C. It carries a higher risk of endothelial rejection than traditional penetrating keratoplasty.
    - D. Complications are less serious than penetrating keratoplasty.
    - E. It is technically more challenging than penetrating keratoplasty.

81. **If globe perforation occurs during a lamellar keratoplasty:**
    - A. Proceed without changing technique.
    - B. Convert to penetrating keratoplasty.
    - C. Suture the perforation site.
    - D. Glue the perforation site.
    - E. Proceed as planned, but begin administering high doses of topical and systemic antibiotics to the patient.

82. **Which of the following complications of lamellar keratoplasty is least common?**
    - A. Perforation of recipient graft.
    - B. Interface scarring.
    - C. Persistent epithelial defect.
    - D. Astigmatism.
    - E. Allograft rejection.

83. **Descemet's stripping automated endothelial keratoplasty is indicated in all the following *except*:**
    - A. Keratoconus.
    - B. Pseudophakic bullous keratopathy.
    - C. Aphakic bullous keratopathy.
    - D. Iridocorneal endothelial syndrome.
    - E. Fuchs' endothelial dystrophy.

84. **In which of the following is penetrating keratoplasty least often indicated?**
    - A. Central cloudy dystrophy.
    - B. Macular corneal dystrophy.
    - C. Corneal scars.
    - D. Chemical burns.
    - E. Herpetic keratitis.

85. Which one of the following is most important in preoperative evaluation for penetrating keratoplasty?
    A. Presence of rosacea.
    B. Corneal scarring with a history of herpes simplex keratitis.
    C. Presence of successfully treated (by laser iridectomy) anatomically narrow angles.
    D. Active uveitis.
    E. Chronic blepharitis.

86. Contraindications to the use of donor tissue for penetrating keratoplasty include all the following, *except*:
    A. Death of unknown cause.
    B. Central nervous system disease (e.g. Creutzfeldt–Jakob disease).
    C. Infections (e.g. HIV).
    D. Corneal disease (e.g. Fuchs' endothelial degeneration).
    E. Epithelial disease (e.g. corneal abrasion).

87. All the following can be considered complications of penetrating keratoplasty, *except*:
    A. Endophthalmitis.
    B. Astigmatism of 2.5 diopters ± 1 diopter.
    C. Graft rejection.
    D. Persistent epithelial defect (longer than 1 week postoperatively).
    E. Flat anterior chamber with increased intraocular pressure.

88. Phototherapeutic keratectomy is indicated in all the following, *except*:
    A. Middle to deep stromal postinflammation scarring.
    B. Granular corneal dystrophy.
    C. Reis–Bückler's dystrophy.
    D. Salzmann's nodules.
    E. Map-fingerprint-dot corneal dystrophy.

89. Absolute contraindications to phototherapeutic keratectomy are all of the following, *except*:
    A. Severe keratoconjunctivitis sicca.
    B. Active uveitis.
    C. Diabetes.
    D. Severe blepharitis.
    E. Systemic immunosuppression.

90. The sclera is composed of all the following, *except*:
    A. Types I, III, IV, VI, and VIII collagen.
    B. Elastin.
    C. Proteoglycans.
    D. Glycoproteins.
    E. Types II and VII collagen.

91. Episcleritis:
    A. Should be treated with topical corticosteroids or nonsteroidal anti-inflammatory agents.

B. Usually (>50%) is associated with a systemic disease that should be treated.
C. Often needs systemic corticosteroids or nonsteroidals.
D. Is almost always a self-limited condition that, if untreated, runs its course in a few days.
E. Causes true ocular pain.

92. Which of the following statements about scleritis is not true?
    A. It is a rare condition.
    B. It may be caused by bacteria or fungi.
    C. Histopathologic studies may show a granulomatous reaction.
    D. Histopathologic studies usually show an acute inflammatory reaction.
    E. Histopathologic studies may show a nongranulomatous reaction.

93. All the following are ocular manifestations of scleritis, *except*:
    A. Unilateral presentation.
    B. Bilateral presentation.
    C. Red eye.
    D. Tenderness to palpation.
    E. Continuous accompaniment by a boring pain.

94. Which one of the following statements about anterior scleritis is not true?
    A. It may appear as a necrotizing scleritis.
    B. It may appear as a nonnecrotizing scleritis.
    C. Necrotizing scleritis usually is minimally to moderately painful.
    D. It may appear as a diffuse process.
    E. It may appear as a nodular process.

95. Which of the following is not usually associated with posterior scleritis?
    A. Pain.
    B. Redness and chemosis.
    C. Blurred vision.
    D. Photophobia.
    E. Chorioretinal changes.

96. Scleromalacia perforans:
    A. Is a type of painless necrotizing scleritis.
    B. Causes an actual perforation in 46% of cases.
    C. Tends to occur in men.
    D. Is not associated with rheumatoid arthritis.
    E. In its early stage causes an acute nonsuppurative inflammation.

97. Which one of the following statements about nanophthalmos is not true?
    A. It is characterized by a smaller than normal crystalline lens.
    B. The condition is bilateral.
    C. It involves short axial length.

D. It is characterized by thick sclera.
E. It is usually autosomal recessive.

98. Concerning the normal tear function, the:
   A. Average tear flow is more than 2.3 µm/min.
   B. Innermost layer of the tear film is the aqueous layer produced by the lacrimal and accessory glands.
   C. Glands of Wolfring and Krause produce the lipid layer.
   D. Tear film is a constantly renewed three part film.
   E. Normal tear film remains intact for less than 5 seconds.

99. Non-Sjögren's tear deficiency is caused by all of the following, *except*:
   A. Graft-versus-host disease.
   B. Sarcoidosis.
   C. Amyloidosis.
   D. Lymphoma.
   E. All of the above.

100. Secondary Sjögren's tear deficiency can be caused by all the following, *except*:
   A. Rheumatoid arthritis.
   B. Primary biliary cirrhosis.
   C. Wegener's granulomatosis.
   D. Dermatomyositis.
   E. Age-related atrophy of the lacrimal glands.

101. All the following are characteristic of trisomy 13, *except*:
   A. Retinal dysplasia.
   B. Cleft lip and palate.
   C. Low-set ears.
   D. Limbal dermoid.
   E. Peters' anomaly.

102. Wilson's disease:
   A. Is X-linked recessive.
   B. Shows excessive secretion of copper from hepatic lysosomes.
   C. Has a gene locus at l3q l4.3-q21.1.
   D. Has a characteristic paracentral Fleischer ring.
   E. Shows typical subcapsular cortical lenticular opacities.

ANSWERS

1. C. A choristoma is a congenital tumor that is composed of dermal and epidermal elements that are not commonly found in the area of involvement. A hamartoma is an abnormal proliferation of tissue that is found in the normal location.
2. E. Goldenhar's syndrome (oculoauriculovertebral dysplasia) is a developmental malformation of the first and second branchial arches resulting in multiple anomalies of the ocular, auditory,

skeletal, cardiac, renal, and/or central nervous system. It is mainly characterized by bilateral limbal dermoids or dermolipomas, preauricular skin tags, blind-ended preauricular fistulas, maxillary and mandibular hypoplasia and other vertebral anomalies. Polydactylism is not associated with this condition.

3. D. Secondary conjunctival localized amyloidosis presents as a yellow-white, waxy, painless nodule. It can occur anywhere on the bulbar conjunctiva but is mostly seen in the inferior fornix. It may occur in association with corneal stromal dystrophies, trachoma, trichiasis, chronic keratitis and keratoconus.

4. A. The most common causes of acute bacterial conjunctivitis are *Staphylococcus aureus, Streptococcus pneumoniae,* and *Haemophilus influenzae. Staphylococcus aureus* is the most common pathogen worldwide.

5. B. Conjunctivitis that persists for longer than 3 weeks is considered chronic. The most common pathogens associated with chronic bacterial conjunctivitis include *Staphylococcus aureus, Moraxella lacunata,* and enteric bacteria such as *Proteus mirabilis, Escherichia coli* and *Klebsiella pneumoniae,* and *Serratia marcescens. Moraxella lacunata* is the most common cause of chronic blepharoconjunctivitis affecting the inner and outer canthal angles.

6. E. Viral conjunctivitis can usually be diagnosed clinically. Viral cultures or subsequent tests are generally not required. It is characterized by a watery discharge and conjunctival hyperemia in one eye followed by the second eye shortly thereafter. Preauricular lymphadenopathy is generally seen on the affected side. Viral conjunctivitis resolves without any treatment within 1-2 weeks.

7. C. Pharyngoconjunctival fever is manifested by pharyngitis, fever and follicular conjunctivitis. It the most common adenoviral infection caused by serotypes 3, 4 and 7. Preauricular lymphadenopathy is seen in about 90% of cases. The condition resolves spontaneously within 2 weeks and requires only supportive treatment with cool compresses and artificial tears as needed for comfort.

8. D. Epidemic keratoconjunctivitis is a highly infectious and more severe form of viral conjunctivitis caused by adenoviruses 8, 19, and 37. It is characterized by copius watery discharge, conjunctival injection, chemosis, and preauricular lymphadenopathy. A mixed follicular and papillary reaction is seen along with subconjunctival hemorrhages. Conjunctival membranes are present in about a third of the cases and may heal with scarring or symblepharon formation. Pseudomembranes can occur as well. Corneal involvement ranges from superficial keratitis in the first week followed by elevated punctate epithelial lesions from day 6-13. Subepithelial opacities are seen from day 14 in 20-50% of cases. These opacities are often visually significant and may persist for months to years. Treatment is symptomatic. Hand hygiene is important for prevention. Topical

steroids can be used with prudence when quick visual recovery is desired. However, it may prolong viral shedding and the resolution of the corneal opacities.

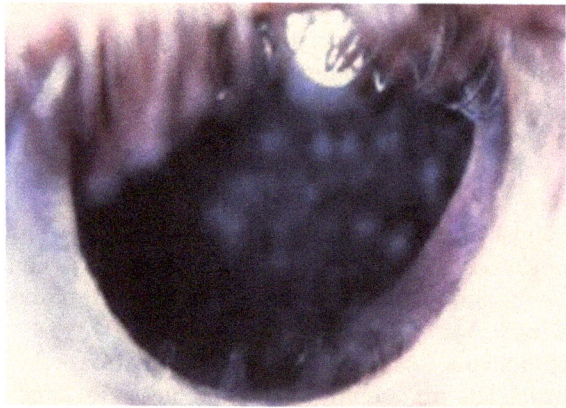

Fig. 4.3: Subepithelial opacities often seen in epidemic keratoconjunctivitis.

9. D. Trachoma, adult inclusion conjunctivitis and neonatal conjunctivitis can all result from infection by *Chlamydia trachomatis*. Serotypes A-C cause trachoma, while serotypes D-K cause adult inclusion conjunctivitis. Both are associated with chronic follicular conjunctivitis. The superficial cornea can be involved in both cases. The deep corneal stroma remains unaffected.

10. C. There are several factors that can result in conjunctivitis of the newborn including organisms harbored in the mother's birth canal, maternal infections, susceptibility of the infant's eye to infection, inadequacy of infant ocular prophylaxis, and ocular trauma during delivery. About 1% buffered silver nitrate solution used for ocular prophylaxis can damage epithelial cells and allow infection by other agents. It is ineffective against *Chlamydia* infections, therefore, prophylaxis by erythromycin ointment is preferred.

11. A. Allergic conjunctivitis is a type I hypersensitivity response mediated by IgE. It is characterized by bilateral, itchy, burning and hyperemic eyes. It may be a localized response or part of a generalized systemic response. Mainstay of treatment includes antihistamines, mast cell stabilizers and combinations of the two. Short-term therapy includes topical corticosteroids and nonsteroidal anti-inflammatory agents.

12. E. Vernal conjunctivitis is a self-limiting, bilateral condition that primarily affects children between 5 years and 20 years (peaks between 11 years and 13 years). It is most commonly seen in the spring and summer months followed by remission during the winter months. There is a male preponderance and a family history of atopy is common. It can occur in palpebral, limbal, and mixed forms. The palpebral form is characterized by cobblestoning of the superior tarsal conjunctiva. The limbal form is characterized by a thickened,

gelatinous, opacification of the superior limbus. Horner-Trantas dots are often seen. They are white dots on the cornea that consist of eosinophils and epithelial debris.
13. B. Giant papillary conjunctivitis (GPC) is due to inflammation of the superior conjunctiva secondary to contact lens wear, ocular prosthesis, or protruding ocular sutures. GPC is seen 10 times more frequently in soft contact lens wearers compared with hard contact lens wearers. Symptoms include itching, mucoid discharge and foreign body sensation. Treatment of this condition involves discontinuing until offending agent till symptoms improve. Mast cell stabilizers and a short course of topical corticosteroids are useful in severe cases.
14. B. Cicatricial pemphigoid is a rare systemic disorder characterized by the formation of blisters on the skin and mucous membranes. It is most commonly seen in older women. Chronic conjunctival inflammation caused subepithelial fibrosis, symblepharon, and blunting of the fornices. In the end stages, there is total loss of fornices, ankyloblepharon, and keratinization of the ocular surface.
15. A. Erythema multiforme is an acute, self-limited inflammatory disorder affecting skin and mucous membranes. Erythema multiforme minor involves only the skin and resolves in 2–3 weeks. Erythema multiforme major (Stevens–Johnson) affects both skin and mucous membranes. Symptoms associated with systemic toxicity include fever, malaise, headache, and fluid imbalance. It can be precipitated by bacteria (typically *Mycoplasma pneumoniae*), viruses (typically *Herpes simplex*), fungi, and drugs (sulfonamides among others). It is rare in children younger than 5 years and adults over 50 years of age.
16. C. Primary acquired melanosis (PAM) appears as a unilateral, flat, patchy brown pigmentation of the bulbar conjunctiva typically adjacent to the limbus. It is secondary to the abnormal production of melanin within epithelial melanocytes, hyperplasia of epithelial melanocytes or both. PAM without atypia is very common and generally benign under the age of 20 years. Malignant transformation of clinically significant PAM is common in older persons. An important prognostic factor for malignant transformation is the presence of atypical melanocytes.

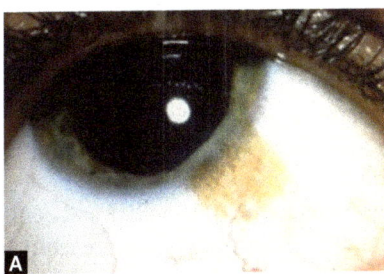 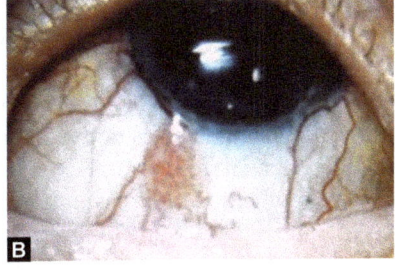

Figs. 4.4A and B: (A) Primary acquired melanosis; (B) Versus carcinoma in situ.

17. E. Conjunctival intraepithelial neoplasia (carcinoma in situ) is a premalignant lesion that is localized to the epithelium. It can involve part of all of the epithelium. It consists of dysplastic malignant epithelial cells that replace normal conjunctival stratified squamous epithelium.
18. D. The corneal epithelium is composed of non-keratinized, non-secretory, squamous epithelium. The most superficial layer of the epithelium consists of 2-3 layers of flat polygonal cells. These cells have extensive microvilli that increase contact with the tear film, as well as tight junctions that decrease permeability of tears into the epithelial cells. Wing cells typically 2-3 cells deep are located directly beneath the superficial layer. They are more round than superficial cells and also possess tight junctions. Basal epithelial cells, a single layer of columnar epithelial cells is found deep to the wing cells and rests on the epithelial basement membrane. The corneal epithelium does not contain any melanotic cells. Langerhans' cells are dendritic leukocytes that may be found in the epithelium.
19. D. After a corneal abrasion, cells at the edge of the epithelial injury begin to cover the defect by a combination of cell migration and cell spreading. This occurs within minutes after a small corneal abrasion and up to 4-5 hours after larger defects. Cell membrane extensions such as lamellipodia, filopodia, and ruffles develop at the leading edge of the wound, while anchoring hemidesmosomes disappear from the basal cells. Cell proliferation only happens 24-30 hours after corneal epithelial injury.
20. E. Recurrent corneal erosion can occur with all these conditions. It is most often seen with map-dot-fingerprint dystrophy, and post-traumatic corneal abrasions but can be associated with all the other conditions.
21. B. Patients with recurrent corneal erosions complain of pain, blurred vision, and occasionally monocular diplopia or ghost imaging. These symptoms most often occur upon awakening in the morning.
22. A. Treatment of recurrent erosion can vary depending on the degree of complaints. Mild pain can be treated with ocular surface lubricants or topical hypertonic solutions. More severe pain can require the use of extended-wear bandage, soft contact lenses. Anterior stromal micropuncture is used for recalcitrant cases. This procedure is generally used in the peripheral cornea due to increased risk of scarring and possible loss of best-corrected visual acuity. Large, loose sheets of devitalized cells are best treated with a cotton swab or blunt instrument so as not to disturb the Bowman's layer.
23. D. Derived from neural crest tissue, the corneal endothelium is a non-replicating monolayer of hexagonal cells. Surface villi are absent on the aqueous side of the endothelium. Adjacent cells share extensive lateral interdigitations, and possess gap and tight junctions along their lateral borders. A high density of Na^+, K^+-ATPase pump sites present

Cornea and External Disease

in the lateral membranes, as well as intracellular carbonic anhydrase pathway, help to control the amount of stromal hydration. Endothelial cells continuously secrete Descemet's membrane throughout life. Specular microscopy is a great tool to image endothelial cells. There are well-defined dark borders with light centers.

24. C. As a result of the characteristics described the water content in the corneal stroma is maintained at around 78%.

25. A. Fuchs' dystrophy is bilateral, noninflammatory, progressive loss of endothelium. It is the most common corneal dystrophy requiring penetrating keratoplasty. It has an autosomal dominant inheritance pattern, but is most commonly symptomatic in females. The key features are central guttae, Descemet's folds, stromal, and microcystic epithelial edema. Endothelial dysfunction results in corneal edema. Other features include prominent corneal nerves, stromal opacification, recurrent corneal erosions, and open-angle glaucoma.

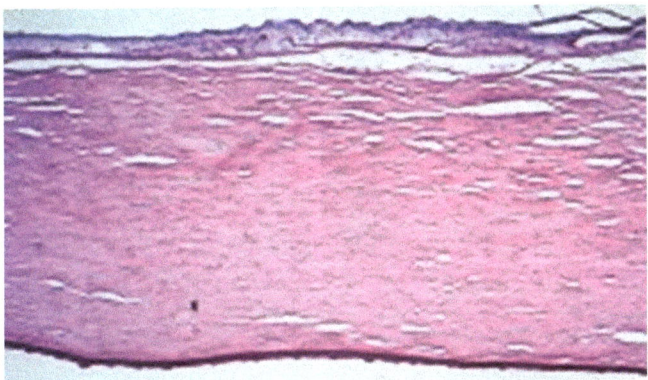

Fig. 4.5: Fuchs' dystrophy. Wart-like excrescences in Descemet's membrane.

26. E. Progressive endothelial dysfunction leads to worsening stromal edema. Symptoms include decreased vision, glare, and halos around lights. Further deterioration of endothelial function causes epithelial edema and disruption of basal adhesion complexes. This results in recurrent erosions, pain, photophobia, and tearing.

27. B. Congenital hereditary endothelial dystrophy (CHED) is characterized by bilateral, symmetric corneal clouding in full-term infants. Dysfunctional endothelium results in the accumulation of abnormal and structurally exaggerated posterior nonbanded Descemet's membrane. The corneal thickness is typically 2 or 3 times normal, but the corneal diameter and intraocular pressure are normal. There are both autosomal dominant and recessive forms. Autosomal recessive inheritance is associated with congenital bilateral corneal edema and nystagmus but without photophobia. Autosomal dominant inheritance is associated with progressive corneal edema after birth (usually by 2 years) and photophobia. Nystagmus is not seen.

28. E. Posterior polymorphous dystrophy (PPMD) is a bilateral, autosomal dominant disorder characterized by transformation of a monolayer of endothelial cells into multilayered epithelial-like cells. Vesicular, curvilinear, and placoid abnormalities are seen on specular microscopy. Iridocorneal adhesions and peripheral anterior synechiae can cause glaucoma which may be difficult to treat.
29. C. Megalocornea is characterized by bilateral enlargement of the corneas with horizontal diameter of more than or equal to 12 mm at birth and more than or equal to 13 mm after 2 years of age. It has both autosomal dominant and X-linked recessive forms. The X-linked recessive form is more common and is associated with ectopia lentis and glaucoma. Endothelium cell density is not affected.
30. B. This condition results from the retention of neural crest cells on the iris and chamber angle.

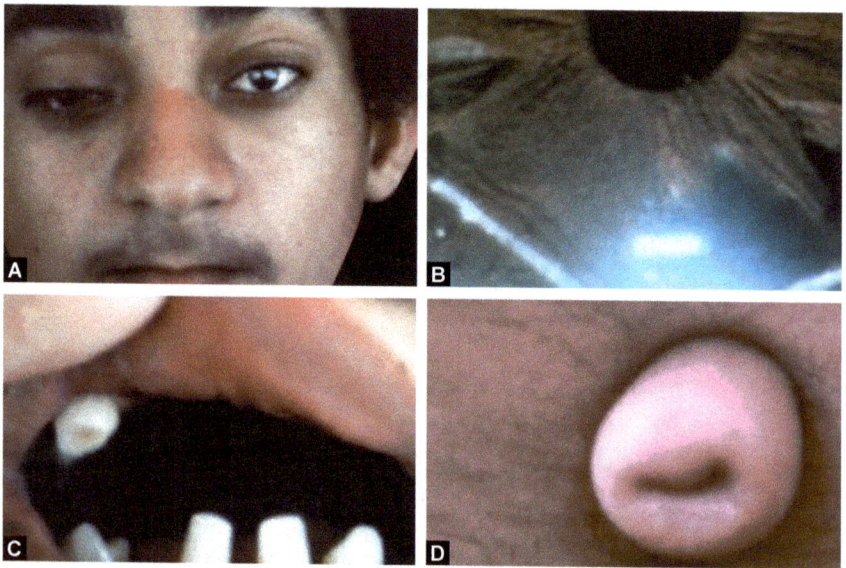

Figs. 4.6A to D: Ocular and systemic manifestations of Axenfeld-Reiger syndrome.

31. D. Peter's anomaly is a form of anterior segment dysgenesis that involves a central or paracentral corneal opacity with adhesions to the iris or lens. Initially, there is a defect of the corneal endothelium and Descemet's membrane below the corneal opacity. Mutations with the *PAX 6 gene* are seen. Peter's anomaly has been reported with fetal alcohol syndrome.
32. E. Reis-Bücklers' dystrophy is a corneal dystrophy characterized by recurrent painful epithelial erosions that begin in the first few years of life. It is caused by a defect in the keratoepithelin gene on chromosome 5q along with lattice type I, Reis-Bücklers', and Avellino dystrophies. It has an autosomal dominant inheritance pattern. Treatment is symptomatic for recurrent erosions.

33. E. Patients with macular dystrophy complain of decreased vision secondary to deposition of anterior stromal opacities from limbus to limbus. The cornea develops a ground-glass appearance over time.
34. B. Lattice type I (Biber-Haab-Dimmer) dystrophy is the most common type of lattice dystrophy. It presents in the first or second decade of life with rod-like glassy deposits that take on linear, often branching appearance. The deposits are most prominent in the anterior stroma. They stain with Congo red, periodic acid-Schiff, and Masson's trichrome. They exhibit dichroism, and birefringence with polarized light. Type II or Merotoja syndrome is associated with familial amyloidosis.
35. A. Granular stromal dystrophy is characterized by crumb-like discrete opacities in the corneal stroma with clear intervening spaces. The deposits consist of hyaline granules that stain red with Masson's trichrome.
36. D. Avellino dystrophy has characteristics of both granular and lattice dystrophies. The discrete anterior stromal deposits stain with Masson's trichrome and the posterior linear, branching, opacities stain with Congo red.
37. C. Granular, Reis-Bücklers', lattice type I, and Avellino dystrophies all map to the *BIGH3*, keratoepithelin gene on chromosome 5q.
38. E. Macular dystrophy results from an abnormality of keratin sulfate. This is due to mutations in the carbohydrate sulfotransferase 6 gene (*CHST6*) on chromosome 16q. Pathology shows deposition of glycosaminoglycans that stain with alcian blue, colloidal iron, and periodic acid-Schiff stains. Penetrating keratoplasty has a good prognosis in these patients.
39. B. A rupture in Descemet's membrane causes acute hydrops in patient with keratoconus.

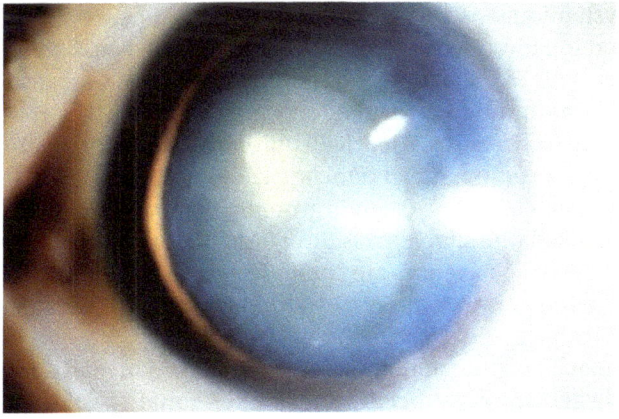

Fig. 4.7: Fleisher ring is seen at the base of the cone in keratoconus.

40. D. Pinguecula are thickening of the bulbar conjunctiva and do not involve the cornea.

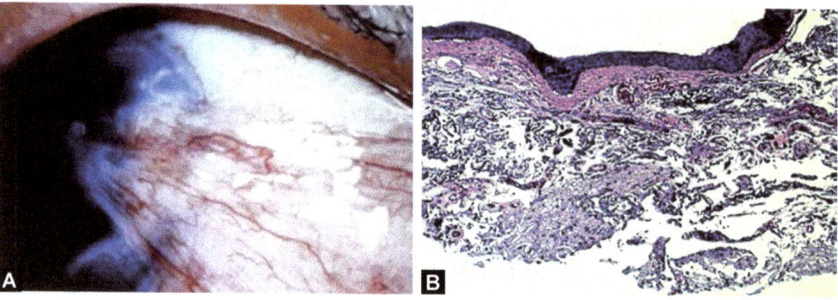

Figs. 4.8A and B: Pterygium. Elastotic degeneration seen in both pterygium and pinguecula.

41. D. Arcus senilis is the most frequent corneal degeneration. The incidence increases with age. There is an association of increased cholesterol levels in patient with arcus who are less than 50 years of age. In asymmetric arcus senilis, the side with less arcus is associated with ipsilateral carotid disease.
42. C. Terrien's marginal degeneration is characterized by bilateral peripheral corneal thinning with neovascularization, and lipid deposition along the leading edge. It starts superiorly and spreads circumferentially over time. This disorder presents in the third to fifth decade of life and slowly progresses over time. There is a male predilection. In younger patients, this condition tends to be more inflammatory. It is unrelated to pellucid marginal degeneration, a disorder that presents with inferior corneal thinning and protrusion.
43. A. Preservatives in pilocarpine have been associated with band keratopathy. This disorder results from deposition of calcium at the level of Bowman's membrane. It is seen most often in eyes with chronic disease such as uveitis, glaucoma, keratitis, and trauma. Systemic diseases with elevated serum calcium can also result in band keratopathy. Treatment is with disodium ethylenediaminetetraacetic acid (EDTA) chelation or laser phototherapeutic keratectomy.
44. A. Salzmann nodular degeneration is seen in patients with a prior history of keratitis, especially phlyctenular keratitis, vernal keratitis, Thygeson's superficial punctate keratitis, and interstitial keratitis. It is more commonly seen in women. Symptomatic nodules may be removed with simple excision or laser phototherapeutic keratectomy, however, recurrences are common.
45. C. Hyaline granules are deposited in the corneal stroma in granular dystrophy.
46. B. Broad spectrum antibiotics are mainly used in infectious keratitis.
47. E. Thygeson's superficial punctate keratopathy is bilateral corneal disease marked by inflammation, with long duration of exacerbations and remissions. It is seen mostly in the second and third decade of life. There is a slight female predilection. Small, round or oval, granular, white-gray, intraepithelial dot-like opacities are typically

seen in a white and quiet eye. Subepithelial opacities are common. Topical corticosteroids are the mainstay of treatment. Topical 2% cyclosporine and phototherapeutic keratectomy have also been used.

48. C. Superior limbic keratoconjunctivitis (SLK) of Theodore is a bilateral, recurrent inflammation of the superior limbus, tarsal and bulbar conjunctiva. It is seen more commonly in women 30–55 years of age. SLK is associated with thyroid and collagen vascular diseases. Silver nitrate (0.5%) solution has been used in the past. Resection or recession of the abnormal conjunctiva is very successful. Cryotherapy and thermotherapy have also been used. Bandage contact lenses, and pressure patching may be helpful in temporarily relieving symptoms.

49. E. Mooren's ulcer is an autoimmune reaction to the corneal stroma that is characterized by a painful peripheral ulcer with an overhanging edge. There are two types. One is seen in older patients tends to be unilateral and is more responsive to therapy. The other seen in younger patients mainly of African origin tends to be bilateral and resistant to systemic immunosuppression. It may be associated with hepatitis C.

50. B. Interstitial keratitis is not present in Avellino dystrophy. Hyaline and amyloid deposits are seen in Avellino dystrophy.

51. A. Lesions of the fifth cranial nerve cause loss of corneal sensation resulting in corneal inflammation ranging from punctate keratitis to frank epithelial defect, and eventually to stromal loss and even perforation. An oval ulcer with rolled edges is seen in the lower half of the cornea in a red eye. Varicella-zoster and herpes simplex keratitis are the most common causes.

52. D. Mild neurotrophic keratitis can be treated with ocular lubrication. Other treatments including punctual occlusion, bandage contact lens, and lateral tarsorrhaphy are useful in more severe cases. Penetrating keratoplasty may be needed in severe stromal loss leading to corneal perforation.

53. A. Rheumatoid arthritis is associated with peripheral ulcerative keratitis. Paracentral defects may be seen in association with dry eyes.

54. E. Rheumatoid-associated corneal melt is an inflammatory disorder mediated by monocytes, macrophages, and T-lymphocytes. Neutrophils and eosinophils are generally not seen.

55. C. Bacterial infection is the leading cause of unilateral blindness in the developing world. In the United States, the incidence of contact lens-associated bacterial keratitis is 10–30 persons per 100,000. Pseudomonal and staphylococcal infections are implicated in the majority of cases followed by *Serratia marcescens*. The incidence of bacterial keratitis varies by region with staphylococcal species most commonly seen in the eastern and northeastern United States.

Pseudomonas infection is more common in the southern United States. Infections associated with *Moraxella* are seen in patients who have debilitating diseases such as malnutrition, alcohol abuse and diabetes.

56. B. Stromal antimicrobial substances are not part of the normal protective mechanisms in the cornea.
57. D. The cardinal sign of bacterial keratitis is a localized or diffuse central infiltration of the corneal epithelium or stroma generally with an overlying epithelial defect. Depending on the cause of infection, there may also be a stromal abscess with an intact epithelium. There is conjunctival injection and chemosis. Satellite lesions are a hallmark of fungal infections.
58. C. *Staphylococcus aureus* is a gram-positive, coagulase positive cocci that can ferment mannitol.
59. A. Needle-like opacities at all levels of the corneal stroma are seen in the setting of infectious crystalline keratopathy. *Streptococcus viridans* is the most common cause. It is typically seen in corneal grafts.
60. C. *Neisseria* is gram-negative, intracellular diplococci that grows well on chocolate agar. *Haemophilus* and *Moraxella* also have grown well on chocolate agar.
61. B. Blood agar is best for aerobic bacteria (37°C) and saprophytic fungi (room temperature). Brain heart infusion can be useful in bacterial and fungal infections. Sabouraud dextrose agar is best for fungi. Small inocula of aerobic and anaerobic bacteria can be isolated from enriched thioglycollate broth.
62. E. Gram-stain is useful to identify bacteria and yeasts. Giemsa stain is used to visualize cytology and to identify bacteria, fungi, and chlamydial inclusions. They all stain blue. Periodic acid-Schiff, Grocott-Gomori methenamine silver- and calcofluor white stains are all useful to identify fungi.
63. D. A culture of corneal scrapings is the best way to establish the definitive diagnosis.
64. B. Vancomycin inhibits cell-wall synthesis in gram-positive organisms including methicillin-resistant staphylococci.
65. B. There is no role for antibiotics in the treatment of viral keratitis.
66. A. Adenovirus does not belong to the Herpesviridae family.
67. E. Herpesviridae is generally spread through close contact either through fluid exchange (sexual, saliva, blood) or respiratory droplets depending on the specific virus.
68. D. Herpes simplex dendrites are fine, linear, branching epithelial lesions with terminal bulbs at the end of each branch. The central epithelial defect stains with fluorescein. The borders of herpetic dendrites are raised due to the presence of swollen epithelial cell and stain with Rose Bengal or lissamine green.

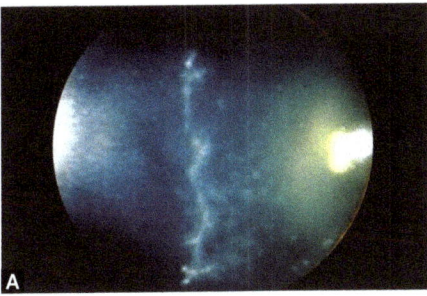 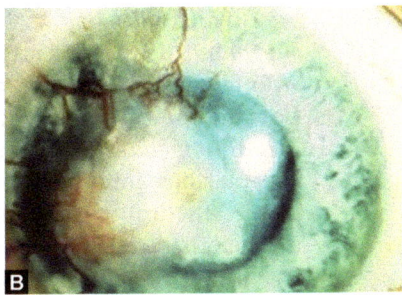

Figs. 4.9A and B: (A) Herpes simplex dendrites; (B) Stromal keratitis.

69. C. Primary infection with Varicella-zoster virus is seen as chickenpox typically before the age of 10 years. The virus then becomes dormant in the sensory ganglia. During times of decreased virus-specific cell mediated immunity, the virus can reactivate and present as shingles or herpes zoster ophthalmicus (HZO). HZO can affect all ocular and adnexal tissues including keratitis, and iridocyclitis. It may occur at the time of the cutaneous eruptions or years later.

70. B. Epstein–Barr virus is a double-stranded deoxyribonucleic acid (DNA) virus that is transmitted through exchange of bodily fluids. It can cause a variety of ocular problems including follicular conjunctivitis, iritis, mucosa-associated lymphoid tissue (MALT)-related lymphomas, conjunctival Burkitt's lymphoma, and Parinaud's oculoglandular syndrome. Discreet subepithelial infiltrates similar to those caused by adenoviral infections are also seen in Epstein-Barr virus (EBV) infections.

71. A. Rarely, cytomegalovirus can produce a linear, branching epitheliopathy that is similar to Varicella-zoster keratitis. Scrapings showing multinucleated syncytial giant cells and intranuclear inclusion bodies confirm the diagnosis. Treatment remains a diagnostic and therapeutic challenge as immune recovery syndrome is more common with the introduction of highly active antiretroviral therapy (HAART).

72. D. *See answer 74.*
73. E. *See answer 74.*
74. E. Fungi can be divided into filamentous, yeast, and diphasic forms. Filamentous fungi are further subdivided into septate and nonseptate organisms. *Fusarium, Cephalosporium, Aspergillus, Curvularia,* and *Alternaria* species are septate, while *Mucor* and *Rhizopus* are nonseptate. Yeasts such as *Candida* and *Cryptococcus* are unicellular fungi that reproduce by budding. They may present with hyphae or develop elongated buds known as pseudohyphae. *Histoplasma, Coccidioides,* and *Blastomyces* are dimorphic fungi. They present as yeast in tissue, and as mycelia on saprophytic and culture media.

75. D. Free-living amoebae such as *Acanthamoeba, Vahlkampfia*, and *Hartmannella* thrive in soil and water environments such as ponds, swimming pools, hot tubs, and contact lens saline solutions.
76. D. Corneal neovascularization is uncommon. Early stages of *Acanthamoeba* keratitis may be confined to the epithelium with irregularities, infiltration or pseudodendrites. Perineural invasion results in prominent corneal nerves. Nonspecific stromal or characteristic ring infiltrates are seen as the diseases progresses.

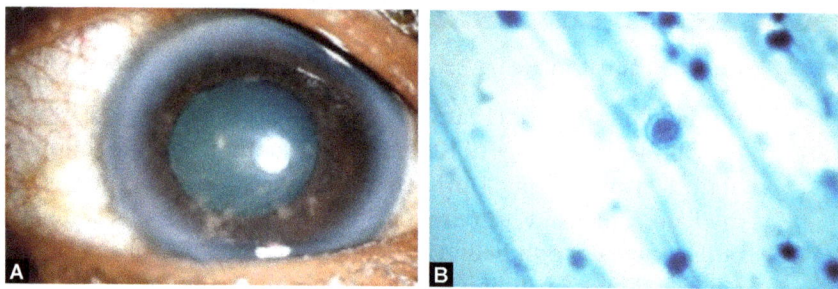

Figs. 4.10A and B: Early stage of *Acanthamoeba* keratitis: (A) and double-wall cyst; (B) Confirms the diagnosis.

77. E. Microsporidia are seen in both immunocompromised and immunocompetent patients. Stromal keratitis is seen in immunocompetent individuals, whereas conjunctivitis and epithelial keratitis are typical in immunocompromised patients.
78. A. Inflammatory response to the nematodes results in eye disease. Various ocular structures can be affected including conjunctival epithelium, corneal stroma, iris, ciliary body, sclera, extraocular muscles, and optic nerve sheath. Oral ivermectin 150 µg/kg given as a single dose and repeated yearly is the treatment of choice.
79. E. Corneal grafting techniques date back to the latter part of the 19th century and early part of the 20th century.
80. C. Since the host endothelium is intact, there is much less risk of allograft rejection in anterior lamellar keratoplasty.
81. B. Anterior lamellar keratoplasty can be technically challenging. Traditionally, a trephine was used to create a partial thickness trephination to the desired location and a microkeratome or blade was used to extend the dissection plane. In deep anterior lamellar keratectomy, aqueous is first replaced with air for better endothelial visualization. Viscoelastic material is used to dissect out a deep stromal pocket followed by trephination of the anterior stromal tissue. If inadvertent globe perforation occurs, the procedure is converted to penetrating keratoplasty.
82. E. Since the host endothelium is intact, there is much less risk of allograft rejection in anterior lamellar keratoplasty.
83. A. Descemet's stripping automated endothelial keratoplasty (DSAEK) has been successfully used to treat a variety of corneal endothelial

disorders such as pseudophakic and aphakic bullous keratopathy, Fuchs' dystrophy, iridocorneal endothelial syndrome (ICE), and posterior polymorphous dystrophy (PPMD). DSAEK has a higher complication rate in patients with ICE and PPMD.

84. A. Central cloudy dystrophy of Francois is a dominantly inherited corneal dystrophy that is characterized by central stroma haze in a mosaic pattern. Patients are asymptomatic and do not require any surgical intervention.

85. C. Presence of successfully treated anatomically narrow angles does not affect the outcome of penetrating keratoplasty. The rest of the conditions are associated with a higher rate of graft failure.

86. E. Epithelial defect in the donor tissue usually heals within a week and is not a contraindication to use of the donor tissue.

87. B. Postoperative astigmatism is expected after penetrating keratoplasty and is not considered a complication. It is an important factor in determining visual acuity. Serial corneal topography and suture management can be performed starting 6-8 weeks after surgery. Single interrupted sutures can be selectively removed, and continuous sutures adjusted to minimize astigmatism.

88. A. Phototherapeutic keratectomy is useful in the treatment of various pathologies confined to the epithelium, Bowman's membrane or anterior stroma including granular and Reis-Bückler's dystrophies, Salzmann's nodules, or map-dot-fingerprint dystrophy. It is not indicated for deep stromal pathology since at least 350 µm of residual stroma is required for corneal stability after the procedure.

89. C. Absolute contraindications to phototherapeutic keratectomy (PTK) include severe keratoconjunctivitis sicca, active uveitis, severe blepharitis, lagophthalmos, and systemic immunosuppression. Relative contraindications include neurotrophic corneas, collagen vascular disease, and diabetes because of poor wound healing.

90. E. The sclera is composed of types I, III, IV, V, VI, and VIII collagen, elastin, proteoglycans, and glycoproteins.

91. D. Episcleritis is the inflammation of the connective tissue between the conjunctiva and sclera. It can present with either nodular or diffuse inflammation. This self-limited condition typically resolves in a few days. Nodular episcleritis presents with more discomfort and takes longer to resolve. No systemic cause is found in two-third of the cases.

92. D. *See answer* 93.

93. E. Scleritis is a rare condition that can be unilateral, bilateral or alternate from one eye to the other. It is characterized by inflammation of the sclera and episclera and presents with a violaceous hue. Topical phenylephrine (2.5 or 10%) does not blanch tissue. It can be either diffuse or sectoral. The eye is tender to palpation. Patients report deep, boring pain that wakes them up from sleep. Systemic autoimmune disease is present in 50% of cases. Associated conditions include rheumatoid arthritis, Wegener's granulomatosis, polyarteritis

nodosa, systemic lupus erythematosus, and relapsing polychondritis. Psoriatic arthritis, ankylosing spondylitis, and inflammatory bowel disease may also be seen. Infectious causes include *Pseudomonas, Aspergillus,* and tuberculosis.

94. C. Anterior scleritis can be present as necrotizing or non-necrotizing scleritis. Necrotizing scleritis is a very painful condition that presents with sclera thinning, staphyloma formation and exposure of bare uvea.

95. B. Posterior scleritis is the inflammation of the eye posterior to the equator. Anterior segment findings such as redness and chemosis are typically seen when accompanied by anterior scleritis.

96. A. Scleromalacia perforans is a type of painless necrotizing scleritis. It is seen mostly in women with a history of rheumatoid arthritis. Yellow sclera nodules develop in the absence of any symptoms.

97. A. Nanophthalmos is a rare, bilateral condition that is characterized by short axial length, thickened sclera and high lens/eye ratio. Both autosomal recessive and autosomal dominant forms have been reported.

98. D. The tear film is a three-part layer of mucin, aqueous, and lipid. Produced by the conjunctival goblet cells, the mucin layer adheres to the hydrophobic corneal epithelium and renders it hydrophilic. The aqueous layer secreted by the main lacrimal gland, accessory glands of Krause and Wolfring, rests on the mucin layer. The outermost layer is the lipid layer produced by the meibomian glands. It stabilizes the tear film by increasing surface tension and decreasing evaporation. The average tear flow is 1.2 µm/min. Normal tear film remains intact for more than 10 seconds.

99. E. Non-Sjögren's tear deficiency is dry eye without a systemic autoimmune cause. It typically results from infiltration and damage to the lacrimal gland and can be seen in lymphoma, sarcoidosis, hemochromatosis, amyloidosis, human immunodeficiency virus infection, and graft-versus-host disease.

100. E. Dry eye associated with a systemic autoimmune condition is termed Sjögren's tear deficiency. Secondary causes include rheumatoid arthritis, systemic lupus erythematosus, polyarteritis, Wegener's, scleroderma, polymyositis, dermatomyositis, and primary biliary cirrhosis.

101. D. Ocular manifestations of Trisomy 13 (Patau syndrome) include microphthalmos, corneal opacity, Peters' anomaly, cataract and retinal dysplasia. Systemic findings include microcephaly, low-set ears, cleft lip and palate. Limbal dermoids are seen in Goldenhar's syndrome.

102. C. Wilson's disease is an autosomal recessive disease resulting from defective excretion of copper from hepatic lysosomes. It has a gene locus at 13q14.3–q21.1. Kayser–Fleischer ring is seen in the periphery of Descemet's membrane. Copper deposits within the lens capsule give the characteristic appearance of this sunflower cataract.

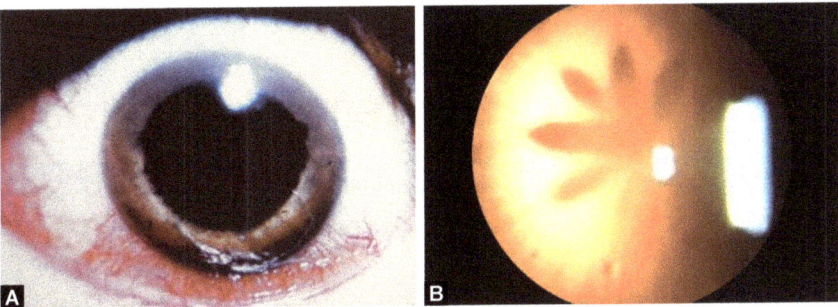

Figs. 4.11A and B: (A) Kayser–Fleischer ring; (B) Sunflower cataract in Wilson's disease.

CHAPTER 5

Refractive Surgery

An Vo

QUESTIONS

Identify the correct answer for all questions (unless instructed otherwise)

1. About two-third of refraction of the eye occurs at:
   A. The anterior epithelial surface.
   B. Bowman's membrane.
   C. The air-tear interface.
   D. The level of Descemet's membrane.
   E. The nodal point of the eye.

2. Photorefractive keratectomy:
   A. Uses the 248 nm ultraviolet laser.
   B. Gives excellent results from myopia of 3-9 diopters.
   C. Acts by steepening differentially the corneal meridians.
   D. Uses a treatment zone of 4.5 mm.
   E. Has results comparable to those of radial keratotomy or LASIK in low myopia.

3. With laser-assisted in situ kratom-ileus is (LASIK):
   A. An Nd:YAG laser is applied to midstroma under a corneal flap.
   B. A 193 nm ultraviolet laser is applied to midstroma under a corneal flap.
   C. A 248 nm ultraviolet laser is applied to midstroma under a corneal flap.
   D. At least 4 sutures are needed to reapply the corneal flap.
   E. More postoperative pain results than with photorefractive keratectomy.

4. The main advantage of photorefractive keratectomy over LASIK is that it:
   A. Causes less postoperative pain.
   B. Has better results with high myopia.
   C. Involves quicker visual rehabilitation.
   D. Is technically quicker and easier to perform.
   E. Is better for hyperopia.

5. **In astigmatic keratotomy:**
   A. The desired effect is produced by an uncoupling effect 180° away from the transverse incision.
   B. An arcuate or straight incision is made parallel to the steep meridian of the astigmatism.
   C. The incisions are made perpendicular to the steep meridian of the astigmatism.
   D. The incisions are made parallel to the flat meridian of the astigmatism.
   E. The incisions are made perpendicular to the flat meridian of the astigmatism.

6. **In thermokeratoplasty:**
   A. Solid-state lasers [e.g. holmium:yttrium-aluminum-garnet (Ho:YAG)] appear to be the lasers of choice.
   B. A 193 nm laser is used to shrink posterior corneal stroma.
   C. Excellent results can be achieved in correcting hyperopia up to 9 diopters.
   D. Excellent results can be achieved for low degrees of with-the-rule myopic astigmatism.
   E. Presbyopia cannot be corrected.

7. **Relative contraindications to photorefractive surgery include all the following, *except*:**
   A. Immunologic disease.
   B. Pregnancy or nursing.
   C. Diabetes mellitus.
   D. Age >66 years.
   E. History of abnormal wound healing.

8. **Relative ophthalmic contraindications to photorefractive surgery include all the following, *except*:**
   A. Severe dry eyes.
   B. Herpes zoster ophthalmicus/herpetic keratitis during the prior 6 months.
   C. Keratoconus.
   D. Neurotrophic keratitis.
   E. Choroidal nevus >2 disk diameters in size.

9. **Mandatory preoperative examination consists of all the following, *except*:**
   A. Manifest and cycloplegic refraction.
   B. Schirmer's test.
   C. Slit-lamp examination.
   D. Fundoscopy.
   E. Topography.

10. **Which of the following is correct regarding radial keratotomy?**
    A. The age of the patient is not a factor.
    B. Incisions directed toward the central cornea (centripetal) cause the most predictable deep incisions.

C. Pachymetry is not necessary.
D. Incisions directed toward the peripheral cornea (centrifugal) cause the most predictable deep incisions.
E. A 2.5 optical zone is optimal for myopia <4 diopters.

11. Wound healing after radial keratotomy is divided into 4 stages. Which of the following is incorrect?
    A. Stromal phase.
    B. Cross-linking and initial stabilization phase.
    C. Endothelial Descemet's phase.
    D. Epithelial phase.
    E. Remodeling and strengthening phase.

12. In the early (12–48 hours) epithelial phase following radial keratotomy:
    A. Sliding and replication result in complete coverage of the stromal incisional edges.
    B. The epithelium slides over, not into the stromal incision to cover the wound.
    C. A new basement membrane does not form (formation does not occur for at least 3 months).
    D. Cross-linked collagen is produced within the first 12 hours.
    E. Epithelial heparin is produced to reduce plug formation.

13. Which statement about radial keratotomy technique is incorrect?
    A. For safety reasons, the thickest part of the cornea should be incised first.
    B. It is important to extend the incision to or just beyond the limbus.
    C. Incisional depth usually is between 90% and 95% of corneal depth.
    D. The diamond knife needs to be calibrated at the start of the procedure.
    E. The incision must stop just peripheral to the central clear zone.

14. Astigmatic keratotomy:
    A. Aims to eliminate the entire astigmatic error with a single procedure.
    B. Usually is performed within the 5 mm optical zone.
    C. Causes a flattening in the meridian of the incision.
    D. Has increased effectiveness up to 110° of arc.
    E. Is not affected by wound healing or age.

15. Which is the least likely potential complication of refractive surgery?
    A. Decreased day vision.
    B. Halo effect.
    C. Diurnal visual fluctuation.
    D. Starburst effect.
    E. Early regression.

16. Which of the following is least likely to have an adverse effect on the visual result of refractive keratotomy?
    A. Using the corneal light reflex for the physiologic visual axis.
    B. An incision that invades the optical zone.

C. Corneal perforation.
D. Optic nerve damage caused by retrobulbar anesthesia.
E. Diamond blade chip.

17. All the following are known postoperative complications of refractive keratotomy. Which is the most serious?
    A. Corneal endothelial cell loss.
    B. Diminished corneal strength.
    C. Epithelial basement membrane disorders.
    D. Induced regular astigmatism.
    E. Infectious keratitis.

18. Excimer laser photorefractive keratectomy:
    A. Is excellent for hyperopia up to 5 diopters.
    B. Is best for myopia between 2 and 6 diopters.
    C. Uses a 248 nm excimer laser.
    D. Should be used to correct astigmatism up to 4.5 diopters.
    E. Does not cause stromal haze when used in myopia between 2 and 4 diopters.

19. The excimer (which stands for excited dimer) laser, as commonly used for photorefractive keratotomy:
    A. Uses the XeF laser.
    B. Uses the ArCl laser.
    C. Uses the XeCl laser.
    D. Uses the ArFl laser.
    E. Has a moderate mitogenic effect.

20. The advantages of the excimer laser include all the following, *except* which one?
    A. It involves intense, pure wavelength.
    B. It allows amplification to occur at three wavelengths.
    C. It uses a highly directional beam.
    D. It uses a coherent, monochromatic beam.
    E. It can be considered to have wave-like or particle-like properties.

21. In general, the amount of corneal tissue removed by each pulse of the excimer laser is:
    A. 0.25 μm.
    B. 0.5 mm.
    C. 0.52 μm.
    D. 0.25 mm.
    E. 0.75 μm.

22. The amount of corneal tissue that must be removed by photorefractive keratotomy to achieve a certain refractive result depends mainly on the:
    A. Thickness of the corneal epithelium.
    B. Anterior curve of the cornea.
    C. Optical zone size.

D. State of the corneal endothelium.
E. Total thickness of the cornea.

23. Which one of the following statements is incorrect?
A. Corneal epithelium ablates at a faster rate than corneal stroma.
B. Bowman's layer ablates at a slower rate than corneal stroma.
C. Fluorescein has no effect on the ablation rate.
D. The transition zone between treated and untreated areas of the cornea needs to be as smooth as possible.
E. The depth of ablation is directly proportional to the optical zone.

24. With-the-rule astigmatism is:
A. A negative cylinder at 180°.
B. A positive cylinder at 180°.
C. A negative cylinder at 90°.
D. Less common than against the rule astigmatism.
E. Easier to correct by photorefractive keratotomy than is myopia.

25. In performing photorefractive keratotomy or LASIK:
A. The corneal epithelium should never be removed with the excimer laser only.
B. Ablation is delayed for 4 minutes after epithelial removal to obtain the proper corneal hydration.
C. The state of corneal hydration plays an important role during the procedure.
D. The visible beam of the ultraviolet laser is used for centration.
E. Excess corneal surface fluid is important for proper focusing.

26. After photorefractive keratotomy or LASIK, which one of the following complications is least serious?
A. Infectious keratitis.
B. Recurrent erosion syndrome.
C. Significant overcorrection at 1 month.
D. Loss of the "flap" during LASIK.
E. Endothelial cell loss in a previously normal cornea.

27. The benefits of LASIK over photorefractive keratectomy include all the following, *except*:
A. Less healing response.
B. Shorter visual rehabilitation.
C. Relative painlessness.
D. Ease of performance.
E. Greater range of treatable refractive errors.

28. Which one of the following is *least* correct for LASIK?
A. It can be used to correct up to 4 diopters of astigmatism.
B. It should be used in patients 18 years of age and older.
C. It can be used to correct irregular astigmatism.
D. It can be used to correct 0.5–6 diopters of hyperopia.
E. It can be used to correct 0.5–15 diopters of myopia.

29. Absolute contraindications to LASIK include all the following, *except*:
    A. Keratoconus.
    B. Posterior corneal crocodile shagreen.
    C. Active corneal ulcer.
    D. Pregnancy.
    E. Lactation.

30. A relative contraindication to LASIK is:
    A. A history of recurrent erosion.
    B. Being older than 65 years.
    C. 12.5 diopters of myopia.
    D. Wearing of soft contact lenses more than 6 days before surgery.
    E. Active Wegener's granulomatosis in the preoperative eye.

31. Which one of the following complications is least important to the visual outcome of LASIK?
    A. Contaminants at the time of LASIK (e.g. talc, blood, stainless steel fragments).
    B. Epithelial cyst or ingrowth.
    C. Decentered ablation.
    D. Malpositioned flap.
    E. Postoperative infection.

32. In general, the day after LASIK:
    A. A "boring" pain is present that should disappear within 2 days.
    B. A mild midstromal haze is seen.
    C. Moderate stromal edema is noted.
    D. The epithelium is 75% regenerated.
    E. The uncorrected visual acuity is 20/40 (6/12) or better.

33. Holmium:yttrium-aluminum-garnet conductive keratoplasty to correct hyperopia and hyperopic astigmatism:
    A. Uses a wavelength of 1.93 µm.
    B. Penetrates the cornea to a depth of 360–380 µm.
    C. Produces an "hourglass" temperature profile range.
    D. Uses a wavelength of 2.06–2.12 µm.
    E. Is used in the continuous rather than in the pulsed mode.

34. Intrastromal corneal ring implants have all the following advantages *except* which one?
    A. They protect against induced irregular astigmatism.
    B. The correction is reversible.
    C. The correction is titratable.
    D. Postoperative time for visual rehabilitation is minimal.
    E. Normal corneal asphericity is maintained.

35. Intrastromal corneal ring implantation:
    A. Most commonly involves a sutureless technique.
    B. Uses an incision 3–4 mm from the center of the cornea.

C. Can be performed with use of topical anesthesia.
D. Needs a retrobulbar anesthesia.
E. Protects against postoperative infection.

36. **Phakic intraocular lenses to correct refractive errors:**
    A. Are best in terms of risk/benefit for low degrees of myopia and hyperopia.
    B. Use a large optical diameter (>6 mm).
    C. Avoid the postoperative problem of glare.
    D. Are reversible through lens removal and lens exchange.
    E. Require the surgeon to learn an entirely new technique.

37. **All the following phakic intraocular lenses have been used, *except*:**
    A. In-the-bag lens.
    B. Nonmultiplex anterior chamber lens.
    C. Posterior chamber lens.
    D. Iris fixation lens.
    E. Multiplex anterior chamber lens.

38. **The most commonly performed refractive surgery is:**
    A. Radial keratotomy.
    B. LASIK.
    C. Cataract surgery.
    D. Photorefractive keratectomy.
    E. Thermal keratoplasty.

39. **Which one of the following *does not* occur in cataract surgery?**
    A. The cornea steepens adjacent to and 180° away from tight limbal sutures, and it flattens 90° away.
    B. The cornea steepens over any incision.
    C. The cornea flattens directly over any sutured incision.
    D. Radial corneal incisions flatten the adjacent cornea and the cornea 90° away.
    E. The cornea flattens adjacent to and 180° away from loose limbal sutures, and it steepens 90° away.

ANSWERS

1. C. Two-third of the refraction of the eye occurs at the air–tear interface.
2. E. Photorefractive keratectomy (PRK) uses the 193 nm ultraviolet argon fluoride excimer laser. This laser penetrates tissue very poorly and is ideally suited to work on the surface of the cornea. Myopia is corrected by ablating tissue in the center of the visual axis, while hyperopia is corrected by removing tissue in a ring around the visual axis. Patients with low myopia do equally well with PRK or LASIK. Higher levels

of myopia are complicated by corneal haze in PRK. Treatment zone can vary depending on several considerations including degree of correction needed and pupil size. Smaller ablation zones are complicated by glare and halos.

3. B. As in PRK, LASIK uses the 193 nm ultraviolet argon fluoride excimer laser. However, in LASIK, midstromal tissue is ablated under a corneal flap. No sutures are necessary to keep the flap in place. Since the epithelium remains intact, LASIK patients experience very little postoperative pain, if any.

4. D. In PRK, corneal epithelium is removed and surface corneal tissue is ablated by excimer laser. In LASIK, a corneal flap has to be created first either with a microkeratome or a femtosecond laser before application of the laser. Complications can arise during flap creation. LASIK is generally preferred by patients due to less postoperative pain and faster visual recovery. Studies have also shown better results with LASIK in patients with high myopia.

5. C. The incisions are made perpendicular to the steep meridian of the astigmatism.

6. A. Solid-state infrared lasers, e.g. Ho:YAG laser are used in thermokeratoplasty to treat hyperopia of ≤2.50 diopters.

7. D. Age is not a contraindication for PRK. However, some older patients may have decreased best corrected visual acuity due to the presence of cataract. These patients may benefit from cataract surgery to correct their refractive error.

8. E. Any condition that affects normal wound healing is a relative contraindication to PRK. Choroidal nevus is not a contraindication to PRK.

9. B. Manifest and cycloplegic refraction, slit-lamp examination, fundoscopy, and corneal topography are essential components of preoperative evaluation for refractive surgery. Schirmer's test may be beneficial in evaluating patients who have dry eyes. It does not need to be performed routinely.

10. B. Incisions directed toward the central cornea cause the most predictable deep incisions. The goal is to create incisions that are roughly 90–95% corneal depth. Generally, a clear optical zone of 3–4 mm is maintained. An optical zone over 6 mm does not have much effect in reducing the refractive error. Pachymetry is needed to ensure that the surgeon does not inadvertently enter the eye.

11. C. Wound healing after radial keratotomy is divided into 4 stages: (1) epithelial phase, (2) stromal phase, (3) cross-linking and initial stabilization phase, and (4) remodeling and strengthening phase.

12. A. The epithelial phase begins about 12-48 hours after radial keratotomy. A new basement membrane is deposited and epithelial cells fill the stromal incisional edges by sliding and replication. The stromal phase occurs 1-6 weeks postoperatively. During this phase, activated keratocytes migrate into the wound, bridge the gap between the wound edges and pull the wound closed. 2 to 6 months later, cross-linked collagen provides stability and strength to the wound. The remodeling and strengthening phase occurs many months after radial keratotomy. Collagen synthesis, breakdown and cross-linking continue during this last phase.

13. D. The diamond knife does not need to be calibrated at the start of each procedure. Blade chipping and thickness can affect the incisions. Thinner blades are preferred because there is less resistance and better penetration of tissue. However, thinner blades are more prone to chipping.

14. C. Arcuate or tangential incisions made in astigmatic keratotomy cause maximal flattening in the meridian of the incision when they are placed within 5-7 mm of the optical zone. These incisions can be lengthened up to 90° of arc to produce greater degrees of astigmatic corrections. The effect of astigmatic incisions is influenced by wound healing and patient age. Older patients experience greater effects from the same incision length than younger patients. In astigmatic keratotomy, the goal is to correct about two-third of the astigmatic error. Therefore, more than one procedure may be needed to eliminate the entire astigmatism.

15. A. Decreased day vision is not common.

16. A. The corneal light reflex is used to approximate the physiologic visual axis.

17. E. Infectious keratitis can cause loss of vision due to corneal scarring and stromal melt.

18. B. Photorefractive keratectomy is best for low levels of myopia <6 diopters. With higher levels of myopia, the incidence of stromal haze is greater.

19. D. Excimer laser is an argon fluoride (ArFl) laser.

20. B. By definition, laser allows amplification at only one wavelength.

21. A. Approximately 0.25 µm of corneal tissue is ablated with each laser pulse.

22. C. The optical zone determines the amount of corneal tissue that must be removed by PRK.

23. C. Fluorescein decreases the ablation rate by about 40%.

24. A. In with-the-rule astigmatism, the vertical meridian has more power than the horizontal meridian. A negative cylinder will correct the

cylinder when placed at 180°. A positive cylinder placed at 90° will also correct the astigmatism.

25. C. The state of corneal hydration can affect the rate of ablation in laser surgery. For a given laser pulse, the greater the hydration, the less the ablation. The surgeon should wipe the corneal surface with either a slightly moist or dry Weck-Cel sponge. Corneal epithelium in PRK can be removed either mechanically or with a laser (epi-LASEK). The ablation is performed immediately after epithelial removal. Iris registration or limbal registration systems are used by newer lasers for centration. Decentration reduces the effectiveness of higher-order aberration treatment.

26. E. About a 5% endothelial cell loss is seen after PRK or LASIK and usually does not affect the stability of the cornea.

27. D. LASIK is technically more challenging than PRK due to the creation of a corneal stromal flap.

28. C. LASIK is not indicated for the treatment of irregular astigmatism.

29. B. Posterior corneal crocodile shagreen is a benign condition that does not affect vision. It is not an absolute contraindication to LASIK.

30. A. A history of recurrent erosion is a relative contraindication for LASIK. Active uveitis as in the Wegener's granulomatosis is an absolute contraindication.

31. A. Epithelial cysts or ingrowth, postoperative infection, decentered ablations and malpositioned flaps can all lead to poor visual outcomes. Malpositioned flaps can cause poor flap adhesion and increase the likelihood of epithelial cyst formation and epithelial ingrowth. Decentered ablation affects the visual outcome by reducing the treatment of higher order aberrations. Postoperative infections can cause corneal scarring and reduce best corrected visual acuity. Contaminants at the time of LASIK rarely cause problems with vision.

32. E. Since the epithelium is intact, patients experience very little pain after LASIK. The uncorrected visual acuity is generally excellent at least 20/40 or better.

33. D. Conductive keratoplasty (CK) is a corneal steepening procedure used in the correction of hyperopia and presbyopia. A Ho:YAG solid-state laser is used. It emits light in the wavelength of approximately 2.1 µm and penetrates corneal stroma to a depth of around 450 µm. A cylindrical thermal footprint is seen in CK.

34. A. Currently, Intacs is mainly used to reduce myopia associated with keratoconus and corneal ectasia. Two curved clear plastic segments are implanted in the periphery of the cornea to reduce myopia. It does not protect against irregular astigmatism.

35. C. Intacs can be performed under topical anesthesia. A channel is created for the two arcuate segments in the periphery of the cornea leaving a large, clear central optical zone. After placement of the segments, the incisions are closed with 10-0 nylon sutures. This procedure can be complicated by postoperative infections.
36. D. Phakic intraocular lenses (IOLs) are artificial lenses implanted in the anterior or posterior chamber of the eye to correct refractive errors. They may be indicated in patients who are poor candidates for excimer laser surgery. Accommodation is preserved since the natural crystalline lens is retained. One of the other advantages of phakic IOLs is its reversibility.
37. A. Phakic IOLs can be anterior chamber angle-supported, anterior chamber iris-fixated, or posterior chamber IOLs. They cannot be placed in the bag since the natural lens is retained.
38. C. Cataract surgery is the most commonly performed refractive surgery.
39. B. There is a flattening effect over incisions. This effect is exploited to reduce astigmatism in limbal relaxing incisions and astigmatic keratotomy.

CHAPTER 6

Lens

Myron Yanoff, Nicole Pumariega

QUESTIONS

Identify the correct answer for all questions (unless instructed otherwise).

1. **Adult lens:**
   A. Shows a greater curvature of the anterior surface than the posterior surface.
   B. Shows an average thickness (anterior to posterior) of 4.0 mm.
   C. Is held in place by zonular fibers arising from the posterior iris.
   D. Has an equatorial diameter of about 10.5 mm.
   E. Is a biconvex disk.

2. **Capsule of the normal adult lens:**
   A. Is the thickest basement membrane in the body.
   B. Is produced continuously for only approximately the first 35 years of life.
   C. Is thickest at the posterior pole of the lens.
   D. Includes these major structural proteins—type IV collagen, laminin, heparan sulfate proteoglycan, osteoid, and entactin.
   E. May reach a thickness of about three red blood cells.

3. **Epithelium of the normal adult lens:**
   A. Ends just short of the posterior pole.
   B. Is multilayered 3.0 mm lateral to the anterior pole need a period after pole.
   C. Proliferates under pathologic conditions.
   D. May form a tumor called a phakoma.
   E. Secretes a yellow pigment into the interior lens with aging.

4. **During aging of the lens:**
   A. The lens shrinks in all dimensions because of increased density.
   B. The oldest lens fibers are externalized.
   C. Absorption of ultraviolet wavelengths increases.
   D. A yellow pigment is deposited in the posterior cortex.

E. Posterior migration of lens epithelium causes nuclear sclerotic changes.

5. **Which one of these anomalies of lens growth *does not* occur at birth?**
   A. Duplication of the lens.
   B. Microspherophakia.
   C. Lenticonus.
   D. Phakoma.
   E. Ectopia lentis.

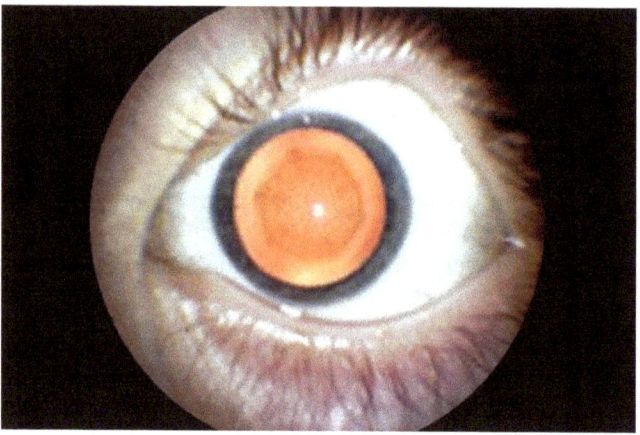

Fig. 6.1: Congenital nuclear cataract.

6. **Lens epithelial changes can cause cataracts by:**
   A. Metaplastic changes resulting in anterior subcapsular cataract.
   B. Migration posteriorly resulting in equatorial subcapsular cataract.
   C. Production of toxins causing nuclear sclerosis.
   D. Anterior migration causing posterior cortical cataract.
   E. Degeneration resulting in Phacoanaphylactic endophthalmitis.

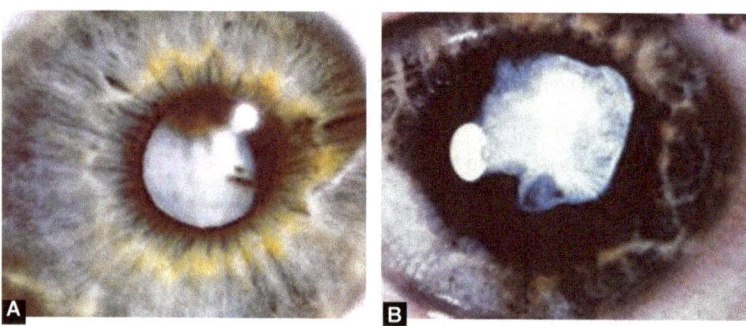

Figs. 6.2A and B: Anterior subcapsular cataract: (A) Undilated; (B) Dilated.

7. **Which of the following is not associated with cataract formation?**
   A. Radiation.
   B. Trauma.
   C. Waardenburg syndrome.

D. Lowe's syndrome.
E. Retinitis pigmentosa.

8. A child is noted to have cataracts at 3 weeks of age. A deficiency of galactose-1-phosphate uridylytransferase is found. Which of the following answers is *true*?
   A. The cataract is predominantly nuclear in its early stage.
   B. Without treatment, the cataract usually progresses for only a few weeks.
   C. A less severe adult form does not exist.
   D. Change of diet does not affect the progression.
   E. It is inherited in an autosomal recessive pattern.

9. A patient has been on systemic corticosteroids for years. He notes blurred vision. Which of the following findings are most likely related to the drug?
   A. Anterior subcapsular cataract.
   B. Posterior subcapsular cataract.
   C. Corneal edema.
   D. Iris neovascularization.
   E. Nuclear cataract.

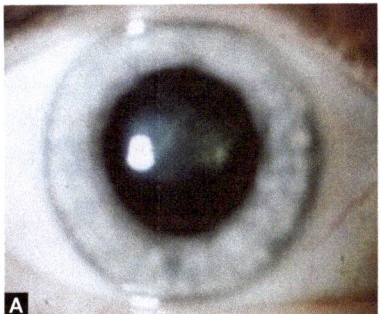 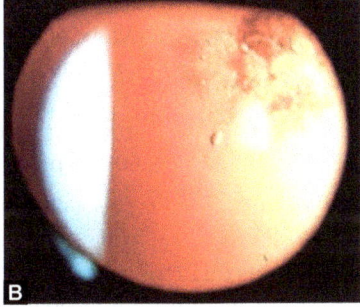

Figs. 6.3A and B: (A) Opacity in lens; (B) Red reflex appearance of early opacity just anterior to the posterior capsule.

10. Probable risk factors for cataract include all the following, *except*:
    A. Sunlight.
    B. Aspirin.
    C. Smoking.
    D. Age.
    E. Diabetes.

11. A boy is born with bilateral cataracts. He then develops glaucoma and kidney problems at age of 2. He probably will show:
    A. An autosomal dominant inheritance pattern.
    B. Decreased contrast sensitivity.
    C. Snowflake vitreal opacities.
    D. A single defect in the *OCRL1* gene.
    E. Systemic alkalosis.

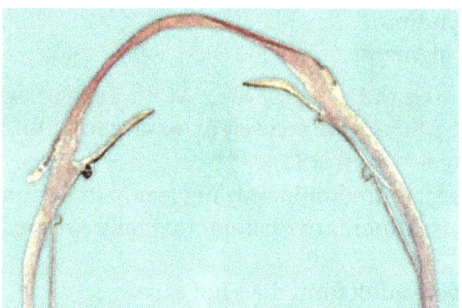

Fig. 6.4: Patient had congenital glaucoma and a small discoid lens.

12. **Lowe's syndrome is suspected as a cause of bilateral cataracts in a child. Which of the following tests would be *most* helpful?**
    A. Urine assay for reducing substances after milk feeding.
    B. Random blood sugar.
    C. Plasma calcium and phosphorus.
    D. Red blood cell transferase and galactokinase serum levels.
    E. Screening for aminoaciduria.

13. **After cataract extraction, a woman develops a posterior capsular opacification. This probably:**
    A. Is related to the woman's age.
    B. Develops from pre-existing lens fibers.
    C. Is caused by growth factors (e.g. acidic and basic fibroblastic).
    D. Is caused by a proliferation of remaining lens epithelium.
    E. Occurs in over 60% of patients.

14. **A Scandinavian patient develops glaucoma. Examination is likely to find all *but* one of the following:**
    A. Pupils dilate poorly.
    B. Central anterior lens opacity.
    C. Peripheral anterior lens deposit of a coarse, granular, white material.
    D. Dandruff-like deposit on the pupillary iris.
    E. No pigment in the anterior chamber angle.

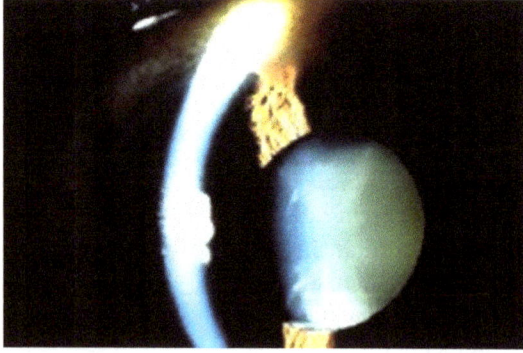

Fig. 6.5: Opacity on anterior surface of the lens.

15. **Pseudoexfoliation syndrome is diagnosed in a patient. All *but* one of the following is true:**
    A. The condition is found worldwide.
    B. The peak age is 45.
    C. It is rare in blacks.
    D. It is bilateral in over 50% of patients.
    E. Glaucoma will develop in about 15% of patients in 10 years.

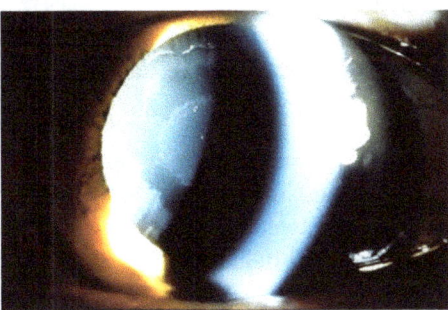

Fig. 6.6: Opacity on anterior surface of lens both centrally and peripherally.

16. **A 55-year-old ex-boxer complains of decreased vision, gradually worsening over the last few years. Examination is most likely to find as a cause of the decreased vision:**
    A. An anterior subcapsular cataract.
    B. Retinal detachment.
    C. Glaucoma.
    D. Corneal edema.
    E. Vitreous syneresis.

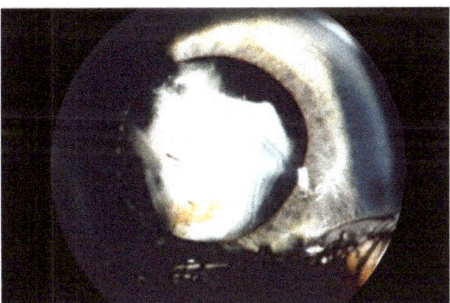

Fig. 6.7: Anterior surface of lens shows wrinkles and opacity.

17. **A patient complains of decreased vision. Findings are a posterior subcapsular cataract. Which of the following is *least* likely to be found?**
    A. Bone–corpuscular retinal pigmentation.
    B. Pale, waxy disc.
    C. Retinal neovascularization.
    D. Attenuation of retinal blood vessels.
    E. Night blindness.

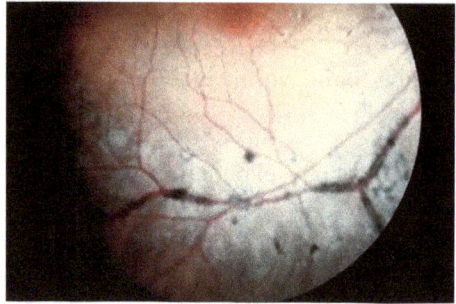

Fig. 6.8: Pigmentation around retinal vessels and "moth-eaten" appearance to retina.

18. **Soemmering's ring and Elschnig's pearl formation have in common:**
    A. No relationship to ocular trauma.
    B. The need for a seal between the anterior and posterior capsule.
    C. Proliferation of lens epithelial cells.
    D. No effect on visual acuity.
    E. The fact that both are within the visual axis.

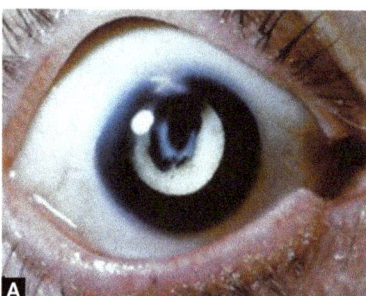
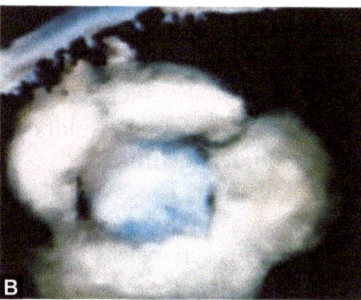

Figs. 6.9A and B: Residual cataract in peripheral lens: (A) Clinical; (B) Gross.

19. **The difference in magnification between an intraocular lens and the original crystalline lens is approximately:**
    A. 3.5%.
    B. 7%.
    C. 1.5%.
    D. 0.5%.
    E. 4%.

20. **A patient has an anterior chamber intraocular lens placed into the eye after a complicated phacoemulsification procedure. 3 months later, the uveitis–glaucoma–hyphema (UGH) syndrome results.**
    All the following *except* one may be found as part of the syndrome:
    A. Anterior uveitis.
    B. Hyphema.
    C. Glaucoma.
    D. Corneal edema.
    E. Retinal detachment.

21. Two days after cataract surgery, a patient develops pain, ciliary injection, chemosis, hypopyon, and blurred vision. A vitreous culture is performed. All of the following may be found, *except*:
    A. *Staphylococcus aureus*.
    B. *Pseudomonas aeruginosa*.
    C. *Propionibacterium acnes*.
    D. *Neisseria gonorrhoeae*.
    E. *Streptococcus pneumoniae*.

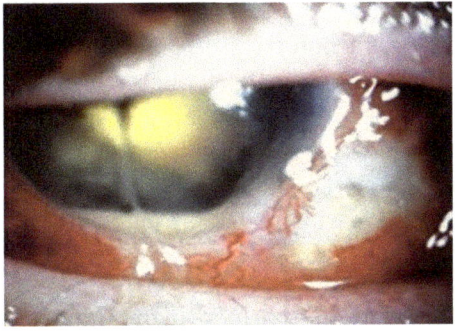

Fig. 6.10: Chemosis, hypopyon, ciliary injection, and pain developed 1 day after cataract surgery.

22. Successful cataract surgery was performed with postoperative vision of 20/20. 7 weeks later, the patient presents with blurred vision. Examination may show all of the following findings, *except*:
    A. Vitreous culture showing the presence of *Staphylococcus aureus*.
    B. Plaque-like material on the posterior capsule.
    C. Generalized opacification of the posterior capsule.
    D. Vitreous culture showing the presence of a fungus.
    E. Vitreous culture showing the presence of *Propionibacterium acnes*.

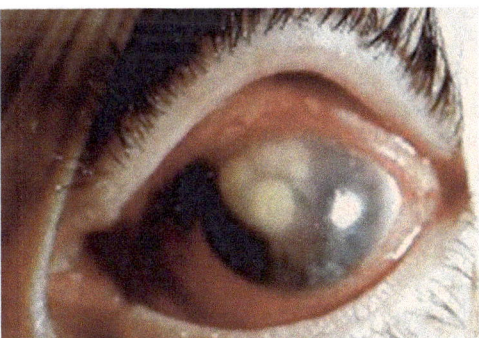

Fig. 6.11: About a month after cataract surgery pain, chemosis, hypopyon, and ciliary injection developed.

23. With posterior chamber implantation of intraocular lenses in patients with Fuchs' corneal dystrophy, which of the following is *least* common?

A. Corneal decompensation.
B. Bullous keratopathy.
C. Glaucoma.
D. Retinal neovascularization.
E. Microhyphema.

24. To calculate the proper power of the intraocular lens, which measurement is most essential?
    A. Horizontal "white-to-white" corneal measurement.
    B. Axial length.
    C. Preoperative refraction.
    D. Streak retinoscopy.
    E. Corneal thickness.

25. Traditional formulas for calculating intraocular lens power are most accurate in:
    A. A normal-size eye with moderate astigmatism.
    B. High hyperopia.
    C. High myopia.
    D. Astigmatism with-the-rule more than 6 diopters.
    E. Astigmatism against the rule more than 6 diopters.

26. The main disadvantage of iris-supported intraocular lenses is:
    A. Increased incidence of anterior uveitis.
    B. Inability to place the optic in front of the pupil.
    C. Increased incidence of ocular pain in response to touch.
    D. Increased incidence of corneal edema.
    E. Increased incidence of posterior lens capsular opacification.

27. Subsequent to in-the-bag intraocular lens (IOL) placement after cataract extraction, a planned −0.5 diopter result becomes a +5 overcorrection. The phakic other eye has no significant cataract. Both patient and surgeon would like to see a postoperative refraction of −0.5 diopter. The best way to correct this is:
    A. Photorefractive keratectomy.
    B. Removal and exchange of the posterior chamber in-the-bag IOL.
    C. A sulcus-placed "piggyback" IOL.
    D. Radial keratotomy.
    E. A corneal lenticular implant.

28. Which of the following *least* accurately estimates corneal topography?
    A. Keratometry.
    B. Photokeratoscopy.
    C. Videokeratoscopy.
    D. IOLMaster.
    E. Comparison with convex mirrors of known curvature.

29. Corneal topography before cataract surgery:
    A. Measures the needed power of the intraocular lens.
    B. Provides a measurement of the corneal curvature.
    C. Does not demonstrate an irregular astigmatism.

D. Is not as valid as keratometry in patients who have had previous corneal refractive surgery.
E. Is mandatory in all cases.

30. Corneal topography before cataract surgery:
A. Is helpful in planning correction of pre-existing astigmatism.
B. Can be used to correct irregular astigmatism.
C. Is contraindicated in corneas that have undergone radial keratotomy.
D. Should be restricted to patients who have had prior laser-assisted in situ keratomileusis (LASIK).
E. Helps to demonstrate endothelial viability.

31. Corneal topography after cataract surgery helps identify all the following, *except*:
A. Tight sutures.
B. Evaluative evidence when best visual acuity is less than expected without obvious cause.
C. Presence of an irregular astigmatism.
D. Decentration of the intraocular lens.
E. Presence of persistent refractive error.

32. Indications for lens surgery may include all the following, *except*:
A. Vision-decreasing cataract.
B. Phacolytic glaucoma.
C. Dense nuclear opacity in a sightless eye.
D. Phacoanaphylactic endophthalmitis.
E. Poorly visualized diabetic retinopathy.

33. A subluxated lens:
A. If visually significant, may be an indication for surgery.
B. Will always progress and should be removed.
C. Is located outside the posterior chamber in the anterior chamber or vitreous compartment.
D. If removed, will protect against the development of angle-recession glaucoma.
E. Should always be approached through a superior clear corneal incision.

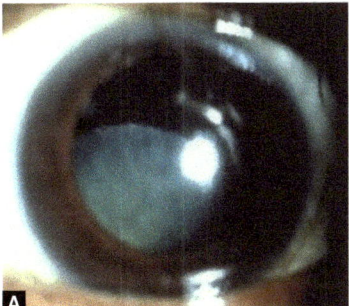 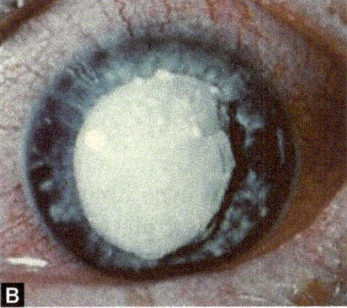

Figs. 6.12A and B: (A) Cataractous lens in posterior chamber but not in normal position (subluxated); (B) Cataractous lens out of posterior chamber into anterior chamber (dislocated).

34. A 40-year-old man has a significantly subluxated cataractous lens. If you were limited to one of the following approaches, which one would you use?
   A. Capsulorhexis and nuclear expression.
   B. Capsulorhexis and phacoemulsification.
   C. Capsulorhexis and nuclear expression.
   D. Pars plana lensectomy.
   E. Can-opener capsulectomy and phacoemulsification.

35. Which one of the following is *not* an important routine preoperative test for cataract surgery?
   A. Corrected and uncorrected visual acuity.
   B. Color vision.
   C. Ultrasound measurement of axial length.
   D. Biomicroscopy through a dilated pupil.
   E. Evaluation for the presence or absence of glaucoma.

36. Before surgery, the patient should be informed of all the following issues *except* which one?
   A. Purpose of the surgery.
   B. Potential serious complications.
   C. Guaranteed good visual outcome.
   D. Refractive requirements after surgery (e.g. spectacles).
   E. Benefits of successful surgery.

37. Before cataract surgery, the patient should be informed of all the following, *except*:
   A. Description of the surgical procedure.
   B. Anesthetic requirements.
   C. Potential temporary postoperative visual problems.
   D. Alternative ways to manage the cataract (e.g. observation).
   E. Visual acuity of 20/20 to 20/30 on the 1st postoperative day.

38. All the following are important physical advances in achieving modern cataract surgery, *except*:
   A. Intraoperative keratometry.
   B. Operating microscopes with coaxial illumination.
   C. Ultrasharp metal and diamond knife development.
   D. Viscoelastic agents.
   E. Intraocular lenses of superb optical and physical qualities.

39. Ophthalmic viscosurgical agents:
   A. In general are interchangeable.
   B. Most have in common that they consist of long-chain biopolymers.
   C. Are all supercohesive (high zero-shear viscosity).
   D. Include supercohesive viscoelastics which are best for selective isolation of areas.
   E. Consist of hyaluronic acid or hydroxyacetyl propyl cellulose.

40. Postoperative medications administered after cataract surgery most often consist of:
  A. Systemic and topical antibiotics only.
  B. Corticosteroids and nonsteroidal anti-inflammatory drugs only.
  C. Topical corticosteroids or nonsteroidal anti-inflammatory drugs along with topical antibiotics only.
  D. Topical and systemic corticosteroids only.
  E. Topical and systemic corticosteroids and topical antiglaucoma medication only.

41. In determining the type of anesthesia for cataract surgery:
  A. History is not important.
  B. With widespread use of topical anesthesia, concomitant disease conditions are irrelevant.
  C. It should be noted that all patients can have topical anesthesia only.
  D. General anesthesia continues to have a role.
  E. Age is no consideration.

42. As a rule, general anesthesia is least indicated in all the following, *except*:
  A. Uncooperative patients (e.g. those with mental impairment).
  B. Uncontrolled coughing or sneezing.
  C. Inability to speak the same language as the operating room team.
  D. Severe claustrophobia.
  E. Refusal of local anesthesia.

43. Which of the following is both an advantage and a disadvantage of topical anesthesia during cataract surgery?
  A. The patient is fully alert.
  B. It eliminates the risk of retrobulbar hemorrhage.
  C. No postoperative diplopia is referable to akinesia.
  D. Along with clear corneal incision, it minimizes the risk of periocular hemorrhage.
  E. Functional vision is maintained in monocular patients.

44. A Phaco handpiece:
  A. Contains an ultrasonic transducer that passes through mechanical energy.
  B. Has a tip design that does not play an important role in the effectiveness of acoustic and cavitational forces.
  C. Newer models have been designed to eliminate piezoelectric (electrostrictive) or magnetostrictive transducers.
  D. Converts electrical energy into mechanical vibratory energy.
  E. Uses a frequency that is standard for all handpieces regardless of the design and materials used.

45. When applied to the physical aspects of phacoemulsification, which statement is *incorrect*?

A. Flow means evacuation of fluid from the eye.
B. Vacuum refers to the present preset maximum vacuum level indicated on the console.
C. Power is expressed as a proportion of the maximum power available.
D. Inflow means flow into the eye.
E. Occlusion means stoppage of the venturi pumping system.

46. The advantages of temporal clear corneal incisions for cataract surgery include all the following, *except*:
    A. Since the incisions are in the farthest area from the visual axis, there is less transmission of astigmatic forces.
    B. They eliminate the need to work over the brow.
    C. They facilitate removal of temporal cortex.
    D. They eliminate the need for "bridle suture".
    E. The lateral canthal angle facilitates drainage of fluids from the operative site.

47. At the end of temporal clear corneal small incision cataract surgery, the surgeon notices wound leakage. Which of the following is *true*?
    A. The wound should always be sutured.
    B. Stromal hydration by injecting balanced salt solution often solves the problem.
    C. It can be ignored because it always stops.
    D. It may herald an expulsive hemorrhage.
    E. Viscoelastic material should be injected into the anterior chamber to seal the wound.

48. Which of the following is *true* regarding hydrodissection during cataract surgery?
    A. Balanced salt solution (BSS) is injected into the most anterior nucleus.
    B. BSS is injected until the nucleus emerges anteriorly out of the capsular bag.
    C. It should not be injected forcefully enough to result in a fluid "wave".
    D. Hydrodissection mobilizes the nucleus within the capsular bag enhancing nuclear rotation.
    E. Hydrodissection causes an intracortical plane away from the capsule.

49. Which of the following is *true* regarding hydrodelineation during cataract surgery?
    A. Balanced salt solution is injected into the substance of the nucleus.
    B. It is injected into the cortex until the nucleus emerges anteriorly out of the capsular bag.
    C. It should be injected into the posterior cortex.
    D. Hydrodelineation causes an intracortical plane away from the capsule.
    E. Hydrodelineation mobilizes the cortex within the capsular bag enhancing nuclear rotation.

Lens

50. A surgeon is deciding between irrigation and aspiration (I and A) alone or phacoemulsification plus I and A in removing a cataract. Which of the following will *not* help in making the decision?
    A. The patient is 25-year-old.
    B. The patient is 35-year-old.
    C. The patient is 15-year-old.
    D. The patient is 5-year-old.
    E. The patient is 55-year-old.

51. During capsulorhexis, the capsule abruptly changes direction and goes out toward the pupil:
    A. More viscoelastic should be added to further dilate the pupil. The capsule should be redirected 90° from the prior direction.
    B. The procedure should be converted to a nuclear expression.
    C. A new capsulorhexis should be started in a different area.
    D. The capsulorhexis immediately should be converted to a "can-opener" incision.
    E. The wound should be closed and the case canceled.

52. A 67-year-old man has been treated for years with pilocarpine for control of glaucoma and has a small pupil that does not dilate well before cataract surgery. Which of the following is *true*?
    A. A superior iridectomy is the procedure of choice before phacoemulsification.
    B. The pupil usually can be mechanically dilated (pupil expansion) at the time of surgery to allow for adequate visualization during phacoemulsification.
    C. Pilocarpine should not be stopped before surgery because of the risk of high pressure.
    D. Extracapsular cataract extraction/nuclear expression is indicated.
    E. A combination of ketorolac 0.5%, phenylephrine 2.5%, tropicamide 1%, and cyclopentolate 1% will probably provide adequate dilation of the pupil.

53. A man has been on tamsulosin (Flomax) to improve urination for over a year. He needs cataract surgery. Which of the following should be done?
    A. Stop the tamsulosin for at least 3 weeks and proceed with the surgery.
    B. Preoperatively just before surgery double the dose of dilators.
    C. Stop the tamsulosin for at least 3 months and proceed with the surgery.
    D. Use your standard procedure but with pupil expanding device to stabilize the iris.
    E. Use your standard procedure but with a more viscous viscoelastic agent.

54. Extracapsular cataract extraction/nuclear expression:
    A. Always requires a large incision.
    B. Is the procedure of choice in the United States.

C. Should be performed with the patient under general anesthesia.
D. Always requires at least 5 sutures.
E. Is one of the most commonly used procedures used worldwide.

55. **The main advantage of large incision extracapsular cataract extraction/nuclear expression is:**
    A. Decreased with-the-rule astigmatism.
    B. Less chance of wound leakage.
    C. Lower incidence of bullous keratopathy.
    D. Low cost and need for only minimal instrumentation.
    E. Minimization of complications in pseudoexfoliation cataract.

56. **All the following may be indications for cataract surgery combined with other procedures, *except*:**
    A. Glaucoma.
    B. Corneal opacity.
    C. Effects of penetrating trauma.
    D. Galactosemia.
    E. Vitreoretinal disorders.

57. **Which of the following is not true following combined small incision keratoplasty and cataract extraction?**
    A. Variability of refractive outcome is noted as compared with cataract surgery alone.
    B. There is delayed rehabilitation compared with cataract surgery alone.
    C. Additional risk of cystoid macular edema is noted as compared with cataract surgery alone.
    D. There is an increased risk of intraoperative complications compared with cataract surgery alone.
    E. Increased risk of graft failure is noted as compared with two separate procedures.

58. **A 28-year-old woman has chronic idiopathic iridocyclitis, cataract, and a small bound down pupil. Cataract phacoemulsification surgery is scheduled. Which of the following is *true*?**
    A. Active inflammation has no influence in the timing of surgery.
    B. Oral corticosteroids are always contraindicated.
    C. Posterior synechiolysis is contraindicated.
    D. If possible, an anterior chamber intraocular lens (IOL) should be avoided in favor of an in-the-bag IOL.
    E. A superior iridectomy should be performed routinely for better visualization.

59. **An 89-year-old aphakic patient is scheduled for a secondary lens implant. All the following options are viable, *except*:**
    A. Sulcus placement.
    B. Anterior chamber placement.
    C. Transscleral sutured posterior chamber placement.
    D. Iris-sutured posterior chamber placement.
    E. Canceling surgery and trying a continuous wear contact lens.

60. In the immediate postoperative period after small incision, sutureless cataract surgery, which of the following is *usually* done?
    A. A mandatory eye pad is worn for 30 hours.
    B. Topical mydriatics are given twice a day.
    C. Topical antibiotics and corticosteroids (or nonsteroidal anti-inflammatory drugs) are administered 3 or 4 times a day.
    D. Topical antiglaucoma medicine is started on day 1.
    E. Oral acetazolamide is given immediately after surgery, the first night after surgery, and the next morning.

61. The pars plana approach for removal of cataracts in children is best for:
    A. Poor pupil dilation.
    B. Neonates and infants younger than 2 years.
    C. All children.
    D. Children older than 7 years.
    E. No children; it is contraindicated in those younger than 16 years.

62. The limbal approach for the removal of cataracts in children over 2 years of age:
    A. Should not be combined with posterior capsulectomy and anterior vitrectomy in any child.
    B. Has a postoperative course that is generally less complicated than that of the pars plana approach.
    C. Is the most versatile technique for pediatric surgery.
    D. Is always combined with a posterior capsulectomy.
    E. Is contraindicated for those younger than 16 years.

63. Phacoemulsification that is sutureless and involves a small self-sealing, tunnel-like, temporal, clear cornea cataract incision has the disadvantage of:
    A. Significant postoperative against-the-rule astigmatism.
    B. Delayed visual rehabilitation.
    C. Achieving 20/40 or better visual acuity in less than 85% of patients.
    D. All of the above.
    E. None of the above.

64. To prevent a radial tear during capsulorhexis, or if a tear occurs and starts to extend beneath the iris, all the following may be useful, *except*:
    A. Injecting more viscoelastic agent.
    B. Switching to a Westcott scissors and cutting the capsular flap.
    C. Redirecting the tear in a more central direction.
    D. Restarting the capsulorhexis from its origin in an opposite direction.
    E. Retracting the iris to note the extent of the radial tear.

65. If significant iris prolapse is noted early in cataract surgery, which one of the following approaches would *not* be useful?
    A. Suturing the incision and moving to a new location.
    B. Considering the possibility of preoperative tamsulosin use as the cause.

C. Injecting a viscoelastic agent posterior to the iris in the region of the prolapse.
D. Performing a peripheral iridectomy at the site of prolapse.
E. Proceeding with the surgery, if easy introduction of instruments into the eye is not impeded.

66. All the following factors predispose to postcataract surgery corneal edema, *except*:
    A. Prior corneal endothelial disease.
    B. Intraoperative mechanical endothelial trauma.
    C. Excessive postoperative inflammation.
    D. Prolonged postoperative elevation of intraocular pressure.
    E. Incomplete removal of the viscoelastic agent at the end of surgery.

67. Which of the following statements about postcataract extraction cystoid macular edema (CME) is *not true*?
    A. Prostaglandin analogs are the drugs of choice to control postoperative elevation of intraocular pressure elevation.
    B. Fluorescein angiographic evidence of CME is present less than 40% of the time.
    C. Clinical CME is present in less than 10% of patients.
    D. It does have a higher incidence in diabetic patients.
    E. Typically CME has its onset within 6-10 weeks after cataract surgery.

68. Objective measures of cataract surgery outcomes include all the following, *except*:
    A. High contrast visual acuity.
    B. Contrast sensitivity and threshold.
    C. Dark adaptation.
    D. Glare disability.
    E. Color vision.

69. Subjective measures of cataract surgery outcomes:
    A. Are evaluated best through interviews and questionnaires.
    B. Are always unreliable.
    C. Have the poorest reliability in terms of patient satisfaction.
    D. Are best measured through the biomicroscopic examination of the eye.
    E. Are initiated by the surgeon.

70. Cataract surgery, a form of refractive surgery causes induced refractive changes by all the following mechanisms, *except*:
    A. Intraocular lens placement.
    B. Intraoperative incisional corneal changes.
    C. Postoperative wound healing.
    D. Cataract removal.
    E. The type of viscoelastic agent used in the anterior chamber during surgery.

71. During cataract surgery, a piece of the cataract falls posteriorly through a posterior capsular tear. Postoperatively, the lens remnant is noted in the inferior vitreous compartment in a "quiet" eye. The best immediate course of action is:
    A. Vitrectomy and lensectomy.
    B. Continuation of routine corticosteroid eyedrop therapy and close observation.
    C. Intravitreal injection of a corticosteroid.
    D. High-dose systemic corticosteroid therapy.
    E. Laser break-up of the lens remnants.

72. The intraocular pressure on the 1st postoperative day is 38 mm Hg. The best course of action is:
    A. Take the patient back to the operating room and explore the wound.
    B. Give intravenous acetazolamide.
    C. Do nothing and see the patient in follow-up the next day.
    D. "Burp" the wound so that a small amount of aqueous is removed.
    E. Put in one drop of 1% pilocarpine and see the patient the next day.

73. A 46-year-old patient presents with acute, unilateral ocular pain, cloudy cornea, mature cataract, milky substance in the anterior chamber, and intraocular pressure of 48 mm Hg. He gives a vague history of ocular trauma to the eye. Which of the following is *true*?
    A. He is at a high-risk for cataract surgery.
    B. He should be treated conservatively until the intraocular pressure normalizes perhaps in a week.
    C. One suspects a traumatic ruptured lens capsule.
    D. He should be treated with oral acetazolamide and antiglaucoma drops and be seen the next day.
    E. He should have cataract surgery on an urgent basis.

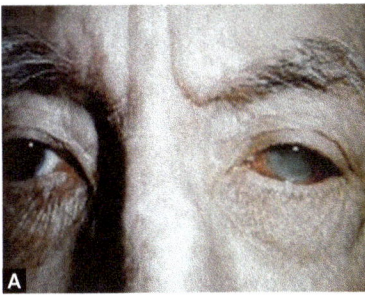
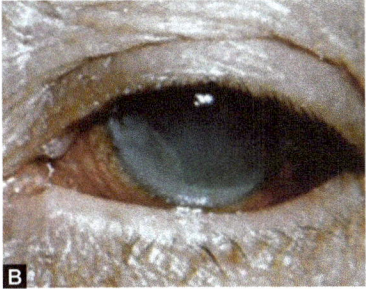

Figs. 6.13A and B: Red left eye with opalescent corneal and milky material in anterior chamber without keratic precipitates.

74. A penetrating injury of the eye through the central cornea and into the lens is repaired by suturing of the cornea followed by atropine drops local and systemic antibiotics. About 3 weeks later, a severe anterior

uveitis develops. The intraocular pressure is slightly elevated. Which of the following should be done?
   A. Atropine should be restarted.
   B. A vitreous tap should be performed and cultured.
   C. Phacoantigenic endophthalmitis must be considered.
   D. Amphotericin B should be started.
   E. Sympathetic uveitis is probable.

75. **A 68-year-old patient comes in with decreased vision of the right eye, correctable to 20/30 with refraction (−1.75 sphere). 2 years ago, the refraction was −0.50 sphere. 1 year ago, the refraction was −1.25 sphere. The most likely diagnosis is:**
   A. Nuclear cataract.
   B. Anterior cortical cataract.
   C. Posteriorly subluxated lens.
   D. Fuch's corneal dystrophy.
   E. Amyloidosis of the vitreous.

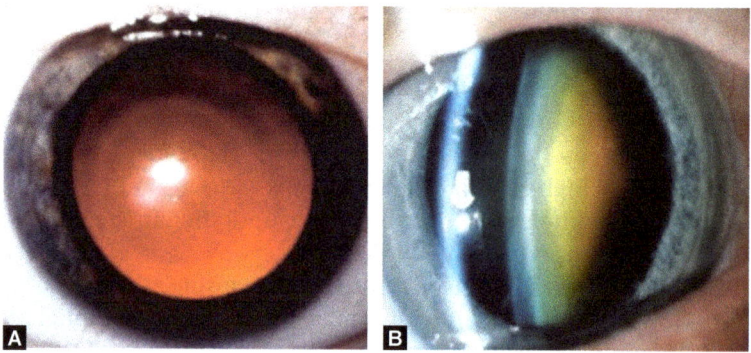

Figs. 6.14A and B: (A) "Oil-droplet" lens reflex; (B) Yellow pigment in central lens.

ANSWERS

1. A. The adult lens is a transparent, biconvex structure reaching 4.75–5 mm in thickness and 9–10 mm in diameter. The zonules arise from the region of the ciliary epithelium.
2. A. Descemet's membrane is the second thickest basement membrane in the body. The lens capsule is composed of type IV collagen and other matrix proteins. Thickest in the anterior and posterior pre-equatorial regions and thinnest posteriorly (2–4 mm). The anterior lens capsule continues to thicken throughout life.
3. C. The unilayered, lens epithelium posterior to the anterior lens capsule ends at the equator and turns inward toward the equator differentiating into fibers. Although, neoplasms of the lens epithelium do not occur, proliferations are common (posterior and anterior

subcapsular cataracts). With aging yellow-pigmented proteins accumulate in the nucleus.
4. C. As the lens epithelia turn inwards at the equator, elongate, and constantly differentiating into new lens fibers, they internalize the older lens fibers. Posterior migration of lens epithelium causes posterior subcapsular cataracts. Yellow pigment is deposited in the nucleus and can absorb ultraviolet light.
5. D. Proliferations of the lens epithelium are common (e.g. posterior and anterior subcapsular cataracts), but neoplasms such as phakomas do not occur at birth.
6. A. Anterior trauma, blunt injury, or anterior uveitis can cause metaplastic changes resulting in anterior subcapsular cataract. Anterior migration of lens epithelium results in anterior subcapsular cataract, while posterior migration of lens epithelium results in posterior subcapsular cataract. Nuclear cataracts are produced by compaction of lens fibers and deposition of yellow pigment not from toxins.

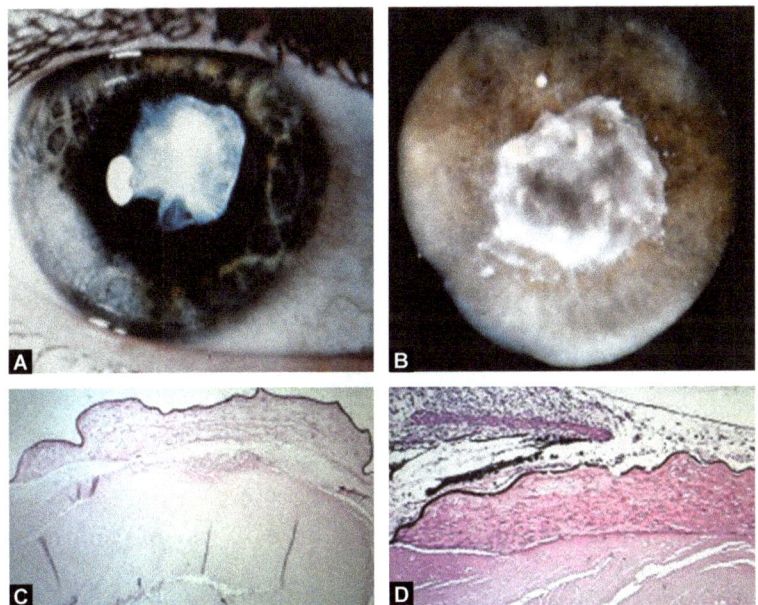

Figs. 6.15A to D: (A and B) Clinical and gross appearance of anterior subcapsular cataract; (C) Large, fibrous plaque lies between anterior lens capsule and cortex; (D) Plaque results from fibrous metaplasia of anterior capsular lens epithelium.

7. C. Radiation, trauma, Lowe's syndrome, and retinitis pigmentosa are often associated with cataract. Waardenburg syndrome is not.
8. E. The cataract formation in galactosemia (autosomal recessive) usually is an anterior and posterior subcapsular opacity. The cataract can

become nuclear before it matures. A forme fruste type of galactosemia can occur in young adults (35–55 years of age) caused by a partial deficiency of galactose-1-phosphate uridylytransferase, resulting in a posterior subcapsular opacity at an early age. Prompt treatment involving dietary restrictions of milk products can reverse early cataract formation.

9. B. Long-term use of systemic corticosteroids often causes posterior subcapsular cataracts and may cause glaucoma.
10. B. Sunlight, smoking, age, and diabetes all have been implicated as risk factors for cataract development.
11. D. Lowe's (oculocerebrorenal) syndrome is a severe X-linked recessive disorder caused by mutations in the *OCRL1* gene. Because of this defective gene, an essential enzyme called PIP2-5-phosphatase found in the trans-Golgi network is not produced. The syndrome results in bilateral congenital cataracts, brain abnormalities associated with intellectual disabilities, hypotonia, renal tubular acidosis (renal Fanconi syndrome), aminoacidosis, and hypophosphatemic rickets.

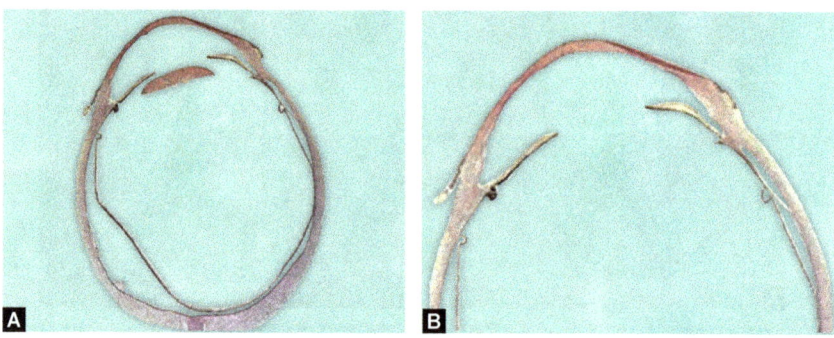

Figs. 16A and B: Lowe's syndrome. Note the small disk-like cataract and the "pulling" on the zonules—(A) Section of whole eye; (B) Section of anterior half of eye.

12. E. Screening for aminoaciduria is an easy way of confirming the diagnosis.
13. D. Although most of the cataract is removed during cataract surgery, some lens epithelial cells may be left behind. These lens epithelial cells can proliferate and cause an opacification of the posterior lens capsule.
14. E. Pseudoexfoliation (PEX) syndrome is a systemic abnormality involving deposition of abnormal basement membrane and elastic fibers in several bodily organs as well as the eyes. The glaucoma is an open-angle glaucoma and the trabecular meshwork is heavily pigmented resembling the pigment dispersion syndrome. The prevalence of PEX syndrome increases markedly with age.

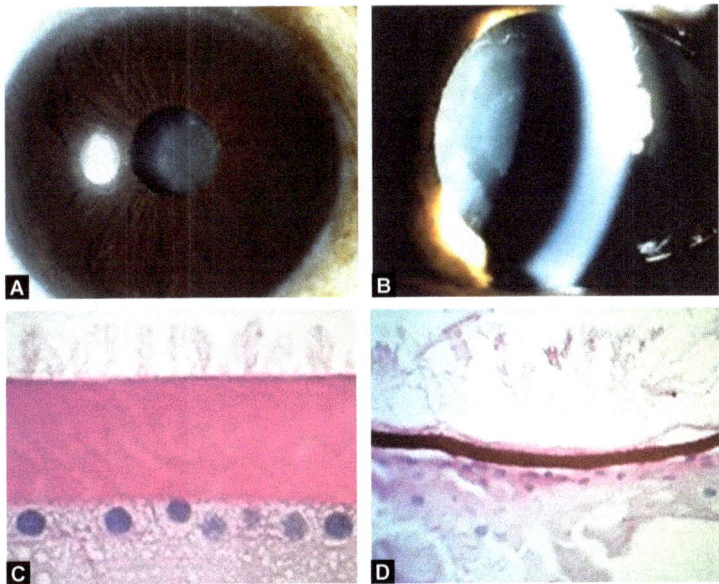

Figs. 6.17A to D: Pseudoexfoliation syndrome. (A) Early clue to diagnosis of PEX is "dandruff" material on pupillary iris; (B) A central disk and peripheral deposition both on the anterior lens surface are characteristic of PEX; (C) Central disk shows "lining up" of deposition; (D) Peripheral deposition random and widespread.

15. B. It is unusual for PEX to be diagnosed before the age of 50 years.

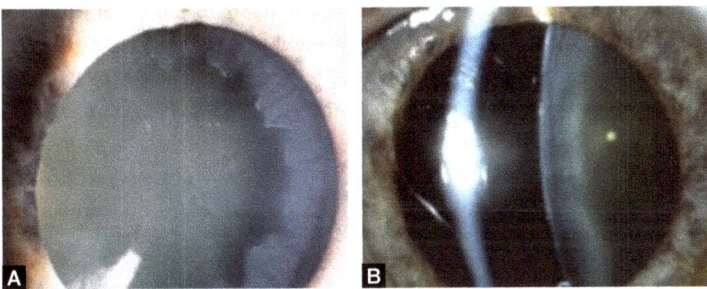

Figs. 18A and B: (A) Large deposition in periphery; (B) Slit-lamp shows central and peripheral deposition.

16. A. Any injury to the anterior lens (traumatic or noxious, e.g. iritis or keratitis) can result even years later in an anterior subcapsular cataract.
17. C. Retinitis pigmentosa is a bilateral, symmetric, and progressive disease that starts in early adult life. The inheritance pattern may be autosomal dominant or recessive, X-linked, digenic, mitochondrial, or sporadic. Night blindness, bone-corpuscular retinal pigmentation, pale, waxy disc, attenuation of retinal blood vessels, and a posterior subcapsular cataract are characteristic. Cystoid macular edema also may be present.

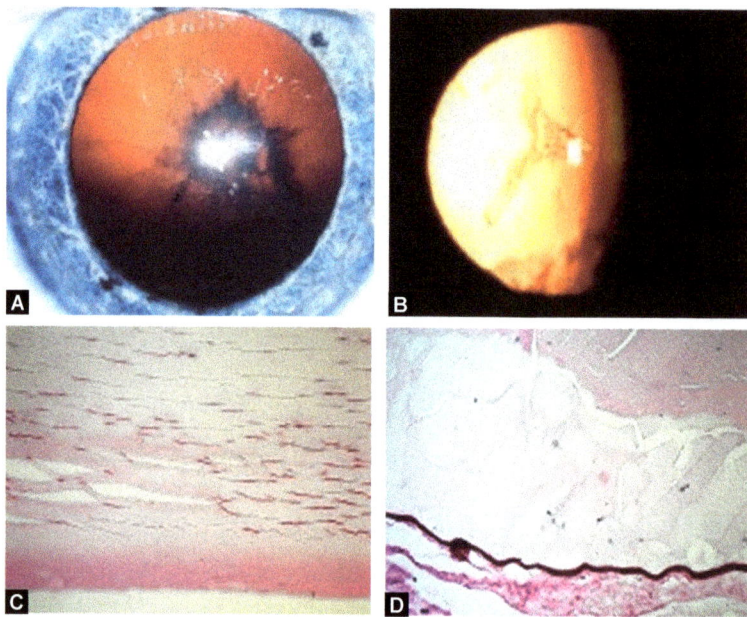

Figs. 19A to D: (A and B) Clinical and red reflex view of posterior subcapsular cataract (PSC); (C) Any capsular lens nuclei seen on the posterior surface of the lens is abnormal and an early sign of PSC; (D) The lens nuclei posteriorly tend to enlarge (bladder or Wedl cells) and move anteriorly.

18. C. Lens epithelium cells can proliferate in several patterns after removal of nucleus and cortex. Elschnig's pearl formation results from aberrant attempts by remaining lens epithelial cells to form new lens fibers. Soemmering's ring cataract results with loss of nucleus and anterior and posterior cortex (nonsurgical or surgical trauma), but retention of equatorial cortex. Also, the remaining lens epithelial cells tend to form new lens fibers in the region.

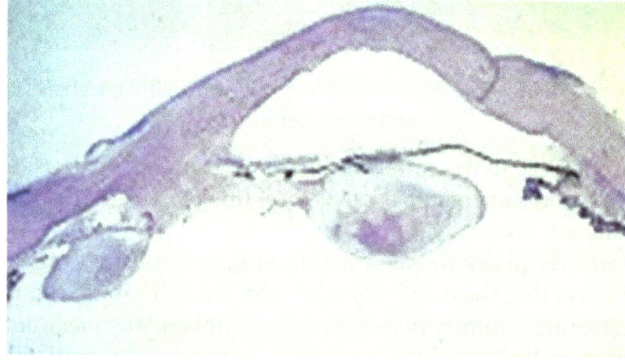

Fig. 6.20: Peripheral perforating corneal scar is present. The nucleus and anterior cortex extruded from the eye at the time of trauma. Cortical material was trapped in the peripheral lens bag, resulting in a Sommering's (2 "m" and 2 "r") ring cataract.

19. C. A posterior IOL in-the-bag has an average power of 12.5 diopters. The average magnification of an IOL in this position is 1.5% compared to the original crystalline lens.
20. E. The uveitis, glaucoma, and hyphema (UGH) syndrome is caused by mechanical excoriation of the angle or iris, or both by the haptics or optic of an IOL and consists of UGH. The inflammation is restricted to the anterior segment of the eye yet cystoid macular edema may develop.
21. C. Inflammation in the eye in the immediate postoperative period (within the first few postoperative days) must be considered as an acute bacterial endophthalmitis until proven otherwise. Endophthalmitis caused by fungi or *Propionibacterium acnes* usually occurs in the delayed postoperative period typically after the 1st postoperative month.
22. A. The onset of blurred vision 7 weeks after cataract surgery in a "quiet" eye is suggestive of a posterior lens capsule opacification. *Propionibacterium acnes* endophthalmitis may occur in a quiet eye put typically it occurs in a symptomatic eye as does fungal endophthalmitis.
23. D. Corneal decompensation, even bullous keratopathy, glaucoma, and microhyphema all can occur in postoperative cataract surgery in patients who have Fuchs corneal dystrophy. Retinal neovascularization is unrelated to Fuchs corneal dystrophy.
24. B. The 6 important variables in calculating IOL power are: (1) Net corneal power; (2) Axial length; (3) IOL power; (4) Effective lens position; (5) Desired refraction; and (6) Vertex distance.
25. A. The anterior and posterior segments of the eye often are not proportional in size which can cause significant error in the prediction of the IOL power in high hyperopia and high myopia, as well as in significant astigmatic errors. Current IOL formulas take this into consideration. The most accurate calculations occur a normal-size eye with moderate astigmatism.
26. D. Corneal edema is the most common complication of iris-supported intraocular lenses. Chronic corneal edema in this situation can lead to corneal decompensation, bullous keratopathy, and even cystoid macular edema.
27. C. Trying to place the second IOL in-the-bag several weeks after the primary surgery is difficult. Placing the second IOL in the sulcus is easier, and there is a less chance of posterior displacement of the first IOL.
28. E. Keratometry, photokeratoscopy, videokeratoscopy, and IOL master are all useful methods.
29. B. The curvature of the corneal surface determines the refractive power it provides. Corneal topography assesses the corneal curvature. Corneal topography can be helpful in patients who had previous refractive surgery especially with the more recent development

involving measurement of both anterior and posterior corneal curvature preventing refractive surprises following IOL placement. Keratometry determines the refracting power of the cornea.

30. A. Corneal topography provides a representative measure of the corneal curvature or power necessary to calculate the IOL power.
31. D. Topography will not give information of the lens position. Intraocular lens tilt and decentration postoperatively has been investigated using Purkinje meter systems.
32. C. The age-old adage, "the only surgery that should be performed on a sightless eye is enucleation", still applies.
33. A. A subluxated lens is still in the posterior chamber but not in its normal position. A dislocated lens is out of the posterior chamber and into the vitreous compartment or anterior chamber. Dislocation into the anterior chamber could result in pupillary block and angle-closure glaucoma.

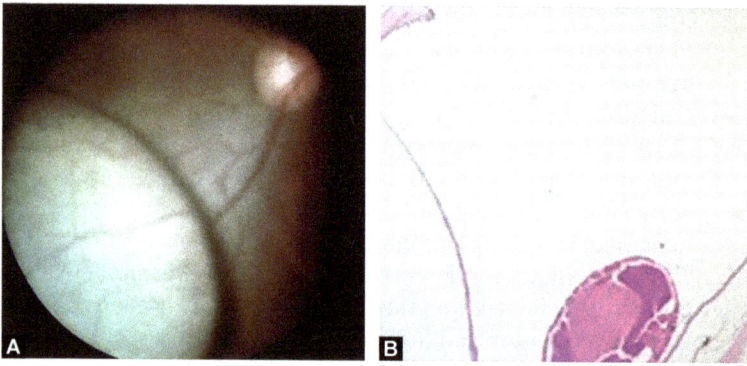

Fig. 6.21: (A and B) show clinical and histological appearance of a dislocated lens. The lens is no longer in the posterior chamber but has been dislocated into the vitreous compartment. If the lens remains in the posterior chamber but out of its normal position, it is termed subluxated.

34. D. Although many different techniques have been described for removal of a subluxated cataractous lens, pars plana lensectomy is the safest with the best results in cases of severe instability. Capsular hooks or capsular tension rings can provide support for safe phacoemulsification with poor capsular support.
35. B. Color vision is not an important indicator of postcataract surgery vision or helpful in determining the power of an IOL.
36. C. No matter how competent the surgeon and how favorable the type of cataract and anatomy of the eye, ultimate visual outcomes can never be predicted with certainty.
37. E. Again, no matter how competent the surgeon and how favorable the type of cataract and anatomy of the eye, short-term or ultimate visual outcomes can never be predicted with certainty.
38. A. It is difficult to believe that before the mid 1980s intracapsular cataract extraction using loop magnification was the norm and viscoelastic

agents, operating microscope, phacoemulsification, and posterior chamber IOLs were used in only a few centers.

39. B. Most viscoelastic agents have in common that they are solutions of long-chain biopolymers consisting of one or more substances, including chondroitin sulfate, sodium hyaluronate, and hydroxypropyl methylcellulose. Different agents, however, have diverse properties, and one agent may be more advantageous in certain situations than another agent. The goal of varying viscoelastic agents is to keep the anterior chamber well formed and protecting the corneal endothelium during surgery.

40. C. Generally, postoperative cataract surgery medications consist of short-term topical antibiotics to prevent infection along with topical corticosteroids and/or nonsteroidal anti-inflammatory agents to reduce and eliminate inflammation.

41. D. Obviously, anesthesia needs to be tailored to the individual patient. Age of patient, a history of existing diseases, the patients' desires, and other factors need to be considered. General anesthesia still has a role in selected patients.

42. C. Inability to speak the same language as the operating room team is not a contraindication. The family and interpreters should be used preoperatively to bring the patient thoroughly up to speed as to what to expect in the operating room.

43. A. A fully alert patient is advantageous because of its safety, the surgeon's ability to offer instructions (e.g. look to the left) during surgery, quick recovering time, and no risk of problems from insertion of a needle into the orbit. Disadvantages are the patient's remembering inadvertent, unwise conversation, more stress for the surgeon, and difficulties in university settings with resident surgery.

44. D. Phacoemulsification uses ultrasound technology with key components including the handpiece, irrigation system, vaccum pump, and foot pedal. The Phaco handpiece houses an ultrasound transducer which is a device that converts electrical energy into mechanical vibratory energy.

45. E. Occlusion results in a high vacuum that causes the pump to work harder. This will continue until the lens particles are evacuated or the vacuum will reach a preset value on the Phaco machine determined by the surgeon.

46. C. The temporal cortex is the most difficult cortex to remove with a temporal incision because this cortex is just under the incision and difficult to engage. Many surgeons may choose an aspiration cannula >45° to better reach the subincisional cortex.

47. B. Generally, a small amount of wound leakage will stop by itself. To be certain, however, stromal hydration by injecting balanced salt solution with a blunt 25–30-G irrigating tip often solves the problem.

It is indeed rare that suturing of the main wound is needed. The surgeon will often use a Weck-Cel sponge to apply a small amount of force to the edge of the incision to assess for a leak. If there is a wound leak uncontrolled by BSS hydration, surgeons can use a 10–0 nylon suture for secure closure. Wound sealants such as glues or adhesives, may be used; however, viscoelastic material should not be injected into the anterior chamber at the conclusion of the case.

48. D. Hydrodissection involves elevation of the anterior capsular leaf and injection of balanced salt solution into the anterior cortex to cause cortical cleavage, thereby mobilizing the nucleus.

49. A. In hydrodelineation, unlike hydrodissection, the fluid is injected into the substance of the nucleus separating softer epinucleus from the harder endonuclear mass (often resulting in a "golden ring").

50. E. As a general rule most, but not all, cataracts in patients who have cataracts and are 30-year-old or younger have "soft" cataracts that can be removed by irrigation and aspiration (I and A) alone. After the age of about 45 years, most nuclei are "hard" and need to be removed by phacoemulsification plus I and A. From the ages of 30–45 years, some nuclei are still soft, but this can only be determined during the surgical procedure.

51. A. It is important to maintain a deep anterior chamber during capsulorhexis to prevent tension on the anterior zonules which can occur if the anterior chamber shallows. Also, with a deep anterior chamber the lens is pushed backwards, facilitating the capsulorhexis and helping to prevent accidental radial capsular tears. If, during capsulorhexis, a radial tear is detected, the anterior chamber should be deepened with a viscoelastic. The leading edge (flap) of the capsulorhexis should be carefully and completely unfolded and then redirected (by cystotome or forceps) 90° from the prior direction. A can-opener capsulotomy creates multiple punctures or small incisions around the anterior capsule with a cystotome or bent needle. Unfortunately, there is a higher chance of posterior extension using the can-opener technique.

52. B. Small pupils use to be a relative contraindication for phacoemulsification. Today, however, with the use of pupil-expanding techniques proper visualization should be available for both capsulorhexis and phacoemulsification.

53. D. Tamsulosin is a selective alpha-blocker and current or prior use is commonly associated with intraoperative floppy iris syndrome (IFIS). No known dosage or duration of therapy exist to prevent IFIS. Without proper aid, iris floppiness and prolapse can cause great difficulties; however, with the use of iris hooks and pupil expansion devices, the iris can be stabilized and both capsulorhexis and phacoemulsification can be carried out with excellent results.

54. E. Although extracapsular cataract extraction/nuclear expression is not used near as much as phacoemulsification in much of the world, it is still used commonly in some parts of the world as well as being used when conditions dictate conversion from standard phacoemulsification procedures.
55. D. Large incision extracapsular (nuclear expression) cataract surgery is still performed in parts of the world where resources are scarce. The procedure has the advantage of low cost and need for only minimal instrumentation.
56. D. The cataracts in galactosemia, in general, are not associated with other ocular abnormalities that would require combined procedure. See answer choice #8.
57. E. Actually, there is an increased risk of graft failure with two procedures rather than one combined procedure.
58. D. The timing of cataract surgery should be such as to perform the surgery when the uveitis has been quiescent without the use of topical corticosteroids for at least 3 months. Oral steroids can be administered the week before surgery and then tapered over the next 2–3 weeks. Topical nonsteroidal anti-inflammatory drugs are recommended at least 3 days preoperatively for patients with chronic uveitis to prevent cystoid macular edema postoperatively. Synechialysis is usually performed. With the use of pupil expanding techniques, the iris can be stabilized and both capsulorhexis and phacoemulsification can be carried out along with in-the-bag placement of the IOL.
59. A. Placing an IOL in the sulcus in an aphakic eye will not work because of the lack of posterior support and the probability that the IOL will end up in the vitreous compartment.
60. C. In most patients, cataract surgery is performed using topical anesthesia, so that the corneal reflex is intact after the procedure. An eye pad therefore is not necessary.
61. B. The pars plana approach is best in neonates and infants under 2 years of age. The limbal approach is preferred for children 2 years of age or older.
62. C. The pars plana approach is best in neonates and infants under 2 years of age. In children, 2 years of age or older, the limbal approach allows for better preservation of the capsular bag for in-the-bag placement of the IOL.
63. E. The standard clear corneal, temporal, sutureless cataract surgery most often results in little or no effect on the preoperative astigmatism, prompt visual rehabilitation, and achieving a visual acuity of 20/40 or better in over 90% of patients.
64. B. It is important to maintain a deep anterior chamber during capsulorhexis to prevent tension on the anterior zonules which can occur if the anterior chamber shallows. Also, with a deep anterior

chamber, the lens is pushed backwards facilitating the capsulorhexis and helping to prevent accidental radial capsular tears. If a radial tear occurs, the deepening of the anterior chamber also usually results in increased iris dilatation, so that the extent of the radial tear can be better visualized.

65. C. Some of the causes of intraoperative iris prolapse include entering the anterior chamber too posteriorly near the iris root, the patient's use of systemic medications such as tamsulosin for urinary problems, or extremely rarely impending choroidal effusion or expulsive hemorrhage. Injecting a viscoelastic agent posterior to the iris compounds the problem.

66. E. Incomplete removal of the viscoelastic agent in some cases can lead to problems with elevated intraocular pressures, but not to corneal endothelial cell loss causing corneal edema.

67. A. Prostaglandin analogs have been associated with cystoid macular edema in some postoperative cataract surgical patients. Prostaglandin analogs, therefore, should not be the first drug of choice. If, however, other antiglaucoma drops do not work, prostaglandin analogs can be used with caution.

68. C. Dark adaptation is not a useful test as a parameter to measure cataract surgery outcomes.

69. A. There are not many ways to subjectively evaluate cataract surgery outcomes. Subjective findings are best evaluated using interviews or questionnaires.

70. E. The type of viscoelastic agent used in the anterior chamber during surgery has no effect on the final refractive change.

71. B. More often than not, lens remnants in the vitreous compartment, even when quite large will reabsorb although it can take many months. As long as there is no sign of inflammation (e.g. impending phacoantigenic endophthalmitis or Phacolytic glaucoma) and the patient can reliably be followed, conservative therapy with topical corticosteroids often works quite well.

72. D. Most patients with a 1st day elevation of pressure will respond nicely to "burping" the wound and draining aqueous fluid. After the procedure, the patient should be seen again in 1–2 hours. If the pressure is normal, the patient should be sent home on antiglaucoma drops and seen again in a few days to a week. If the pressure is not normal, the burping procedure should be repeated one time. This usually solves the problem.

73. E. The signs and symptoms are highly suggestive of phacolytic glaucoma. Keratic precipitates are rare in this condition. Cataract surgery using routine phacoemulsification and in-the-bag IOL on an urgent basis is the best course of therapy.

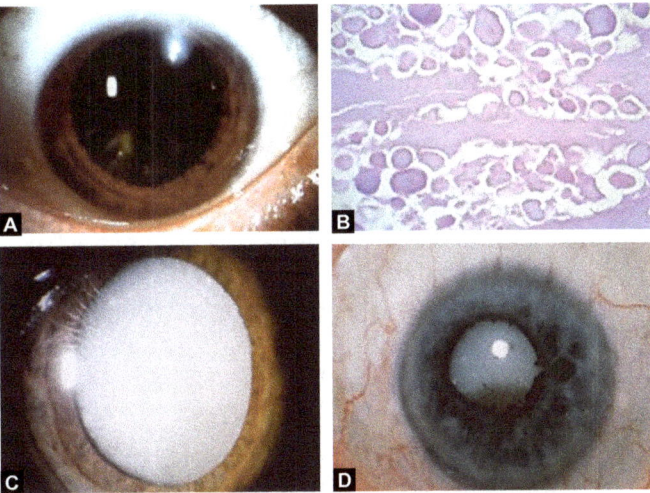

Figs. 22A to D: Evolution of Phacolytic glaucoma. (A) Cortical spokes result from morgagnian (liquefaction) degeneration of the cortex; (B) When the entire cortex undergoes morganian degeneration, the cataract becomes a mature cataract; (C) The lens often swells becoming an intumescent cataract. The nucleus can settle inferiorly; (D) In the liquefied cortex. Lens material which is no longer antigenic can escape through an intact lens capsule resulting in a hypermature cataract.

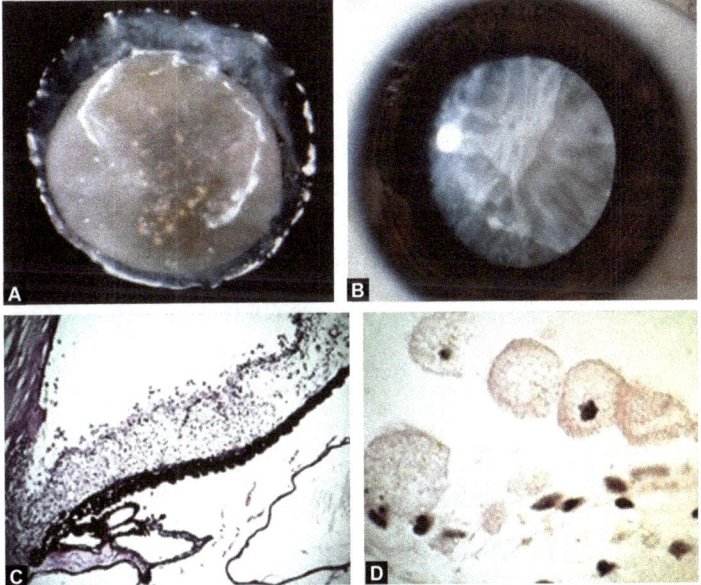

Figs. 23A to D: Evolution of Phacolytic glaucoma. (A) Gross photo of hypermature cataract with the nucleus displaced inferiorly; (B) Clinically, a hypermature cataract shows a wrinkled anterior lens capsule; (C) The nonantigenic liquefied cortex passes through an intact capsule and causes a macrophagic response. The macrophages clog an open-angle and cause secondary open-angle glaucoma; (D) The macrophages are engorged with liquefied cortical material.

122 Ophthalmology Review

74. C. Sympathetic uveitis would indeed be rare in a penetrating wound into the eye through the cornea that does not involve uveal tissue. The timeline is such that it is too late for a bacterial endophthalmitis and too soon for a fungal endophthalmitis. Phacolytic glaucoma does not cause a severe anterior uveitis, but does cause a marked rise in intraocular pressure.
75. A. Nuclear sclerosis of the lens often causes a slowly increasing myopia (myopic shift) in patients. This can give rise to the "second sight" phenomena where the patient is able to read without glasses.

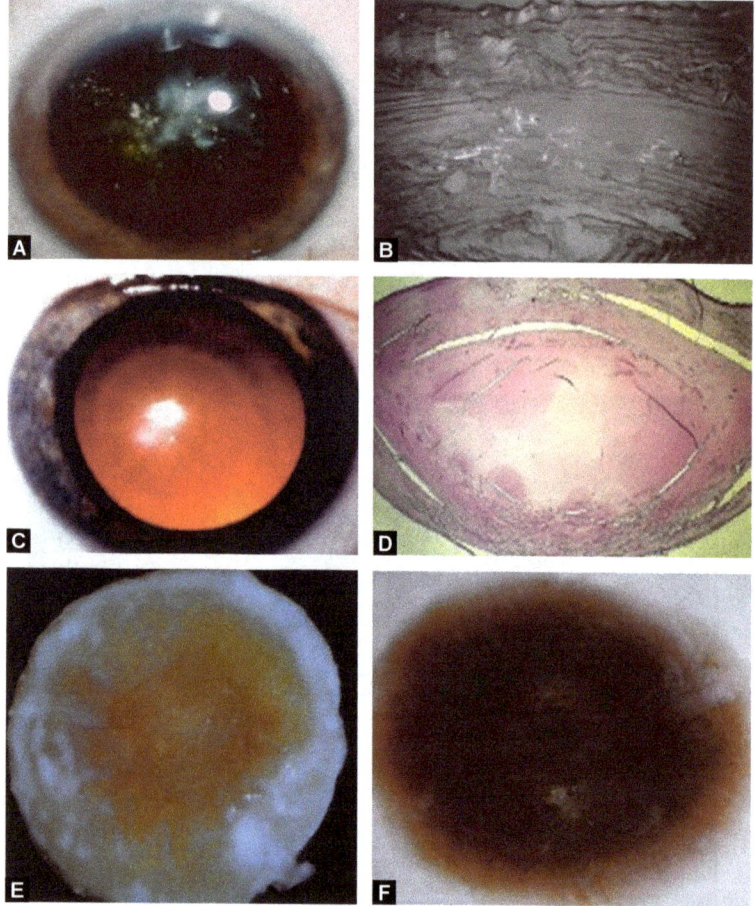

Figs. 24A to F: Nuclear sclerosis. (A) In addition to yellow pigment, other materials can deposit in the nucleus, e.g. cholesterol in "Christmas tree" cataract; (B) Polarized, frozen section of nucleus in (A) shows the birefringent cholesterol; (C) The "oil droplet" reflex is characteristic of nuclear sclerosis, but can also occur in keratoconus and lenticonus; (D) The homogeneity and lack of the usually found "crack artifacts" are characteristic histologically of nuclear sclerosis; (E) Gross photo showing yellow-pigment buildup in a cataracta brunescens; and (F) In a cataract nigra.

CHAPTER 7

Orbit and Oculoplastics

Vincent B Lam, Ryan McGuire, Nida Khan

QUESTIONS

Identify the incorrect answer for all questions.

1. **The orbital septum:**
   A. Inserts on the orbital rim.
   B. Is separated from the levator aponeurosis by orbital fat.
   C. Is firmly attached to Whitnall's ligament.
   D. Fuses with the capsulopalpebral fascia in the lower lid.
   E. Inserts on the levator aponeurosis about 3-5 mm above the tarsal plate.

2. **The tarsal plates:**
   A. Contain the eccrine meibomian glands.
   B. Of the upper lid are about 10 mm in height.
   C. Of the lower lid are about 4 mm in height.
   D. Impart structural integrity to the eyelids.
   E. Do not contain lash follicles.

3. **The orbital floor is:**
   A. Thinnest just medial to the infraorbital canal.
   B. Composed primarily of the maxillary bone.
   C. Composed of the zygomatic and palatine bones.
   D. Separated from the lateral wall by the inferior orbital fissure.
   E. The largest of the orbital walls, running to the orbital apex.

4. **The lateral orbital wall:**
   A. Is the safest wall to remove in an orbital decompression.
   B. Contains the frontozygomatic suture below the lateral orbital tubercle (of Whitnall).
   C. Is the thickest orbital wall.
   D. Is composed of the greater wing of the sphenoid bone and the zygomatic bone.
   E. Is located adjacent to the middle cranial fossa.

5. The ophthalmic artery:
A. Terminates as the supratrochlear artery.
B. Crosses over the optic nerve in 85% of individuals.
C. Enters the orbit through the optic canal.
D. Gives off the lacrimal artery as its first orbital branch.
E. Gives off the central retinal artery which runs under the optic nerve.

6. Thyroid eye disease:
A. Is six times more common in females compared to males.
B. Parallels the serum level of free thyroxine (T4) and triiodothyronine (T3).
C. The order for surgical intervention is first orbital decompression followed by strabismus surgery and finally eyelid surgery.
D. Causing strabismus should be surgically corrected only using muscle recessions.
E. Has muscle enlargement caused by increased glycosaminoglycan (GAG) synthesis by extraocular muscle fibroblasts.

7. Neurogenic causes of eyelid retraction include:
A. Tertiary lues (syphilis).
B. Dorsal midbrain syndrome.
C. Wernicke's encephalopathy.
D. Palatal myoclonus.
E. Impending tentorial herniation.

8. Myogenic causes of eyelid retraction include:
A. Myasthenia gravis.
B. Thyroid eye disease.
C. Familial periodic paralysis.
D. Congenital myasthenia gravis.
E. Down syndrome.

9. Congenital myopathic ptosis:
A. Is less marked in downgaze.
B. Is associated with an indistinct or absent upper eyelid crease.
C. Coexists with hypotropia in about 30% of patients.
D. Causes occlusive amblyopia in about 20% of patients.
E. Is unilateral in about 70% of patients.

10. Blepharophimosis, ptosis and epicanthus inversus syndrome:
A. Is a dysmorphic syndrome of the midface.
B. Also consists of telecanthus and epicanthus inversus.
C. Is commonly associated with mental retardation.
D. Is caused by mutations of the FOXL2 gene.
E. Is seen in 6% of children who have congenital ptosis.

11. Avulsion of the medial canthus:
A. Is caused by large amounts of vertical tension on the eyelid.
B. Is associated with rounding of medial canthal angle.

C. An isolated anterior tendon avulsion should be sutured to ligament remnant.
D. Is associated with acquired telecanthus.
E. Examination should always include evaluation of lacrimal drainage apparatus.

12. **Dehiscence of the levator aponeurosis:**
    A. Is typically associated with poor levator function.
    B. Is associated with an abnormally high or indistinct upper eyelid crease.
    C. Occurs in 6% of patients after cataract surgery.
    D. May be caused by contact lens wear.
    E. Is the most common cause of acquired ptosis.

13. **Entropion:**
    A. Is often caused by attenuation of the capsulopalpebral fascia and orbital septum.
    B. May be caused by age-related horizontal lower lid laxity.
    C. Is commonly caused by enophthalmos.
    D. May be caused by an overactive orbicularis muscle.
    E. May be caused by reduced posterior lid lamellar support.

14. **Which statement is *incorrect* regarding the repair of eyelid defects?**
    A. Small eyelid defects (<30%) can undergo primary closure.
    B. Large (>50%) defect in the upper eyelid can be repaired with a Cutler–Beard procedure.
    C. Split thickness grafts should be used.
    D. A (30–50%) defect in the lower eyelid can be repaired with a rotational flap.
    E. Closure of large defects with local skin flaps usually provides best tissue match.

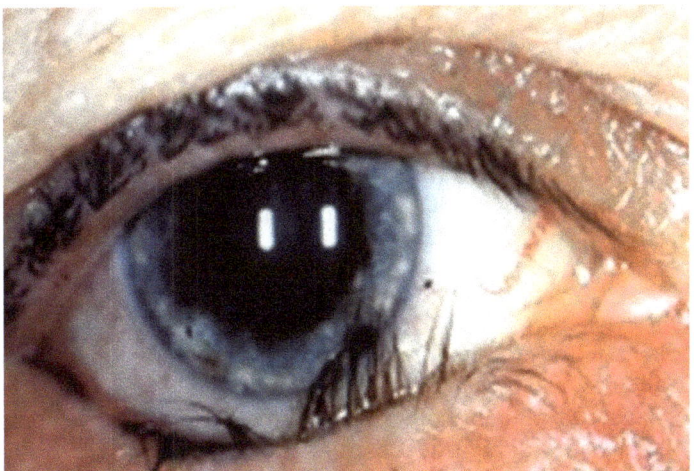

Fig. 7.1: Lower eyelid is turned inward.

15. Techniques for entropion repair include:
A. Lid retractor reattachment.
B. Botulinum toxin injection.
C. Quickert–Rathbun sutures.
D. Transverse tarsorrhaphy.
E. Kuhnt–Szymanowski procedure.

16. Epicanthal folds:
A. Will improve with facial bone growth.
B. Are a common cause of pseudostrabismus.
C. Epicanthus inversus is normal variant of Asian eyelids.
D. Equally involving upper and lower eyelids are called epicanthus palpebralis.
E. Are found in 60% of patients with Down syndrome.

17. Techniques available for correction of ectropion include:
A. Lateral tarsal strip procedure.
B. Full-thickness wedge excision.
C. Y-plasty.
D. Medial canthal tendon resection.
E. Medial canthal tendon plication.

18. Complications of lower eyelid blepharoplasty include:
A. Superior rectus muscle weakness.
B. Epiphora.
C. Lower lid retraction.
D. Injury to inferior oblique muscle.
E. Loss of vision.

19. Laser skin resurfacing:
A. Should not be performed within 6 months of isotretinoin use.
B. Should be avoided in keloid-forming patients.
C. Can eliminate wrinkles and skin imperfections.
D. Gives best results in patients with low Fitzpatrick skin type.
E. May cause reactivation of herpes simplex.

20. Essential blepharospasm:
A. Is more common in women than in men.
B. Usually occurs in patients older than 50 years.
C. May be associated with phenothiazine use.
D. Does not abate during sleep.
E. Is usually bilateral.

21. Granulomatosis with polyangiitis:
A. Is a syndrome of small vessel vasculitis, granulomatous inflammation, and tissue necrosis.
B. Has serum autoantibodies against proteinase 3 and myeloperoxidase.
C. Is treated with high-dose steroids alone.
D. Has orbital involvement in 50% patients throughout disease course.
E. Untreated has a mortality rate of 80%.

22. Methods of treating essential blepharospasm include:
A. Surgical myectomy of affected areas.
B. Chemical injection with doxorubicin.
C. Botulinum toxin chemodenervation.
D. Oral benzodiazepines.
E. Lid crutches.

23. Cutaneous horns:
A. May develop from seborrheic keratosis.
B. May develop from basal cell carcinoma.
C. May develop from keratoacanthoma.
D. It is a projection of packed keratin.
E. Should undergo biopsy.

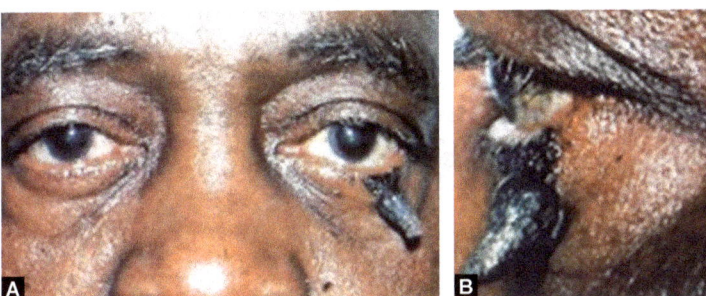

Figs. 7.2A and B: Large cutaneous horn of left lower lid.

24. Keratoacanthoma:
A. Usually develops over a period of weeks.
B. Does not exhibit cellular atypia.
C. May be associated with systemic malignancy.
D. Usually undergoes spontaneous involution.
E. Is usually umbilicated.

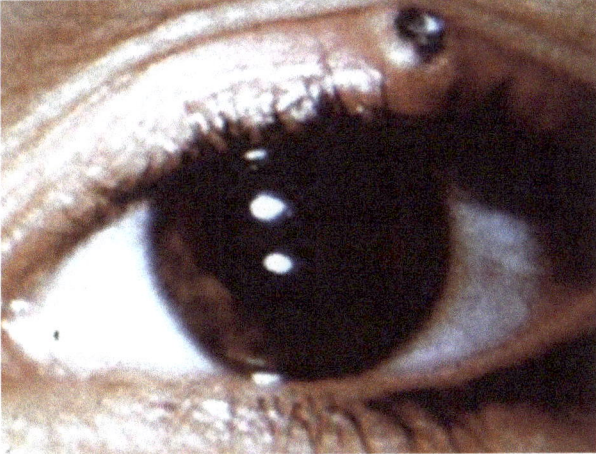

Fig. 7.3: Umbilicated lesion has had rapid growth over the prior 3 months.

25. **Actinic keratosis:**
    A. Requires biopsy or excision for cytopathologic study.
    B. Develops into squamous cell carcinoma in about 20% of lesions.
    C. Exhibits hyperkeratosis, dyskeratosis and parakeratosis.
    D. Commonly affects the eyelids.
    E. Is the most common premalignant skin condition.

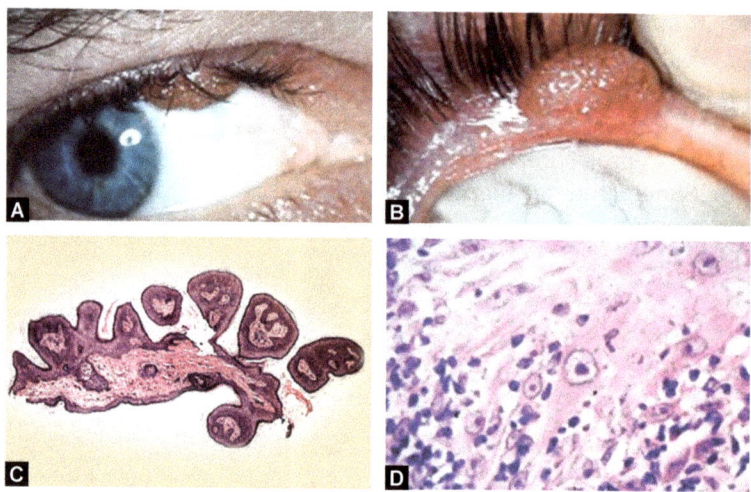

Figs. 4A to D: (A and B) Papillary lesions can be confused with actinic keratosis; (C) Lesion has a papillary configuration; (D) Acanthosis and intranuclear eosinophilic bodies show this to be a verruca vulgaris.

26. **Capillary hemangiomas:**
    A. Are usually present at birth.
    B. Regress by age 7 years in 75% of affected individuals.
    C. May be associated with the Kasabach–Merritt syndrome.
    D. Represent the most common type of orbital tumor in children.
    E. Localized eyelid lesions can be treated with topical beta-blockers.

27. **Erdheim–Chester disease:**
    A. Is characterized by progressive fibrosclerosis of the orbit and internal organs.
    B. Often leads to vision loss.
    C. Is associated with asthma.
    D. Is the most devastating form of adult xanthogranuloma.
    E. Requires aggressive therapies.

28. **Floppy eyelid syndrome:**
    A. Leads to chronic papillary conjunctivitis.
    B. Is associated with obesity, keratoconus, eyelid rubbing and sleep apnea.
    C. Patients may have a history of sleeping supine.
    D. Has a superior tarsal plate that is soft, rubbery and flaccid.
    E. Treatment can include horizontal tightening of the eyelid.

29. The nevus of Ota:
A. Is known as oculodermal melanocytosis if episclera is involved.
B. Is usually unilateral and congenital.
C. Often undergoes malignant degeneration in blacks.
D. Involves the ophthalmic and maxillary trigeminal divisions.
E. Arises from dermal melanocytes.

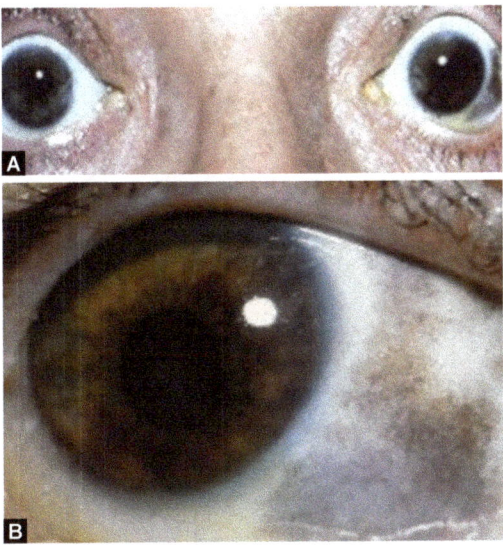

Figs. 7.5A and B: (A) Patient shows heterochromia iridum (left iris darker); (B) Subtle pigmentation of left eyelids (nevus of Ota) both present since childhood.

30. Molluscum contagiosum:
A. Usually results from sexual contact and transmission in adults.
B. May produce a follicular conjunctival reaction.
C. May be confluent in immunocompromised patients.
D. Usually spontaneously resolves in 3–12 months.
E. Is caused by a large RNA poxvirus.

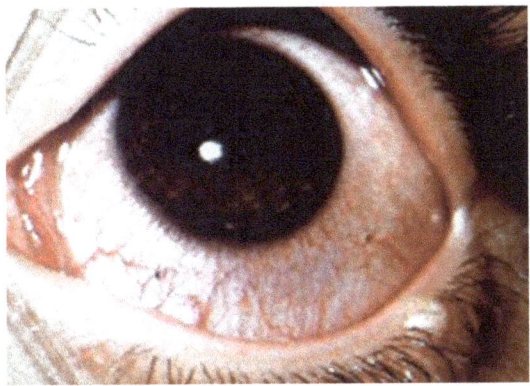

Fig. 7.6: Lesion of left lower lid has caused a reactive conjunctivitis.

31. Basal cell carcinoma:
  A. Commonly metastasizes.
  B. May be pigmented.
  C. Affects the lower lids in two-third of patients.
  D. Is related to ultraviolet light exposure in fair-skinned individuals.
  E. Comprises 90–95% of eyelid malignancies.

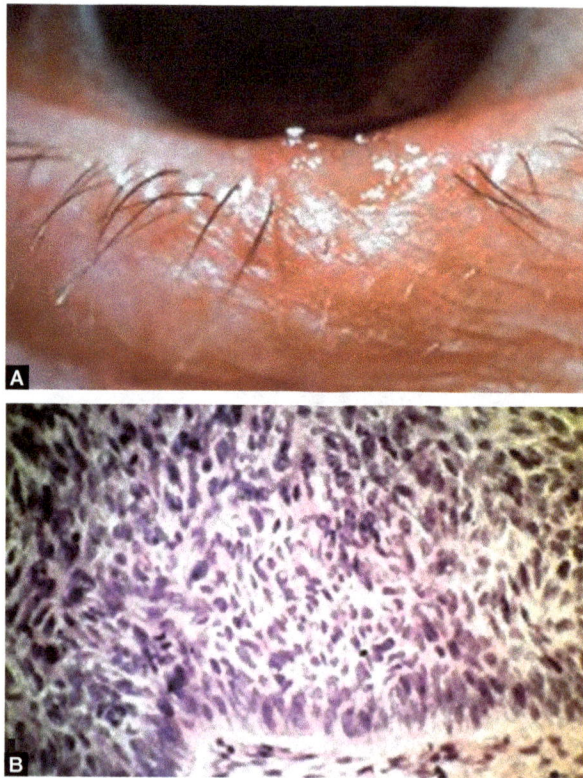

Figs. 7.7A and B: (A) Indurated, painless lesion slowly growing over prior year; (B) Proliferation of basal cells showing characteristic, peripheral palisading

32. Basal-cell nevus syndrome (Gorlin syndrome):
  A. Is inherited as an autosomal dominant trait.
  B. Includes jaw cysts.
  C. Includes mental retardation.
  D. Occurs in roughly 1% of patients who have basal cell carcinoma.
  E. Generally appears before age 10 years.

33. Acceptable treatment techniques for basal cell carcinoma include:
  A. Cryotherapy.
  B. Mohs' micrographic surgery.
  C. Initial radiation therapy.

D. Radiation therapy to advanced or recurrent lesions.
E. Excisional biopsy with frozen section control.

34. Squamous cell carcinoma of the eyelids:
   A. Is more aggressive than basal cell carcinoma.
   B. Is more common in lightly pigmented individuals than in darker pigmented ones.
   C. May be potentiated by immunodeficiency.
   D. Does not arise from actinic lesions.
   E. Often metastasizes along nerves.

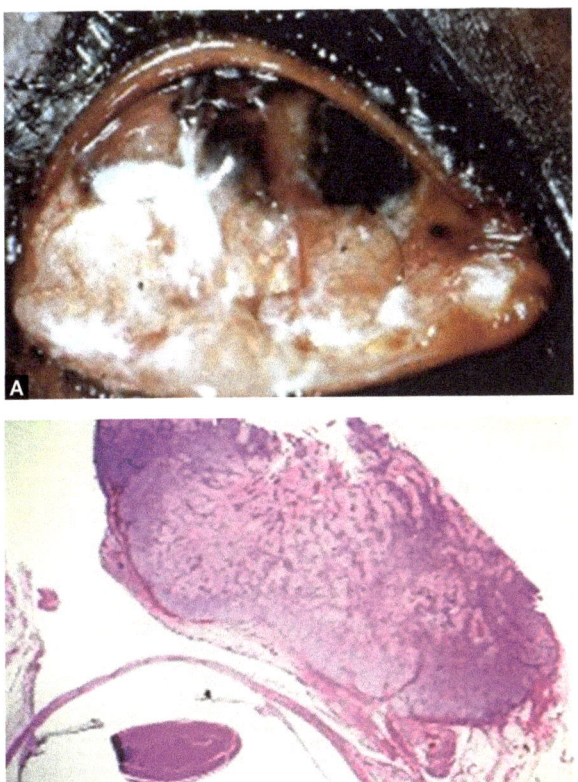

Figs. 8A and B: (A) Advanced lesion that started in the lower lid a few years ago; (B) Proliferating squamous cells have practically replaced the lid.

35. Sebaceous adenocarcinoma of the eye lids:
   A. Is the third most common eyelid malignancy.
   B. Is more common in women than in men.
   C. Is more common on the upper eyelids.
   D. Must be confirmed by full-thickness wedge biopsy.
   E. Arises from the meibomian and Moll's glands.

132 Ophthalmology Review

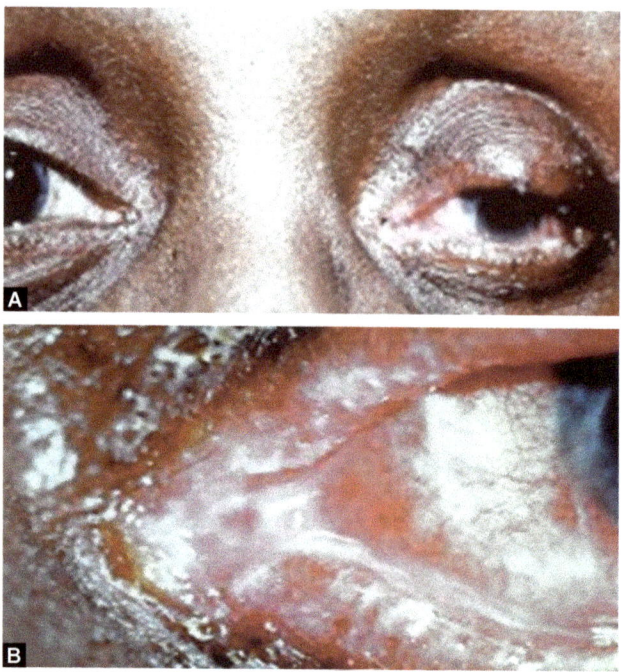

Figs. 7.9A and B: (A) Patient noted an irritated left eye with loss of eyelashes; (B) Two years later, the condition has progressed.

36. Malignant melanoma of eyelid skin:
A. Is usually nodular.
B. May arise from lentigo maligna.
C. Is more common in fair-skinned individuals.
D. May arise from acquired melanosis.
E. May be successfully treated with cryotherapy.

37. Eyelid burns:
A. Require aggressive lubrication.
B. Require frequent evaluation.
C. Lead to cicatricial changes.
D. May need tarsorrhaphies that are less extensive that seems to be immediately necessary.
E. May require early use of full-thickness skin grafting and amniotic membranes.

38. Nonspecific orbital inflammation:
A. Is also known as orbital pseudotumor.
B. Is a diagnosis of exclusion.
C. May have thickening of extraocular muscle tendons of insertion.
D. Improves with systemic steroids.
E. Is painless.

39. Pleomorphic adenoma of the lacrimal gland (benign mixed cell tumor):
A. Occurs mainly in the palpebral lobe.
B. Represents 50% of epithelial lacrimal gland tumors.
C. Most commonly occurs in the fourth to fifth decades of life.
D. Is slowly progressive over 12 months or more.
E. Is circumscribed by a pseudocapsule.

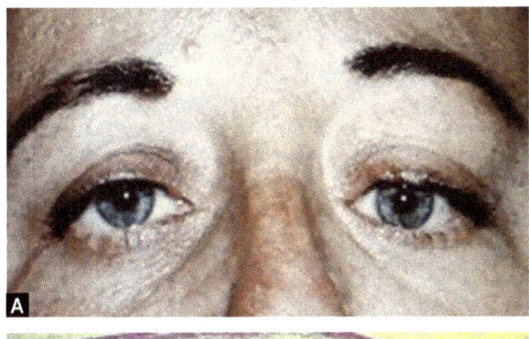
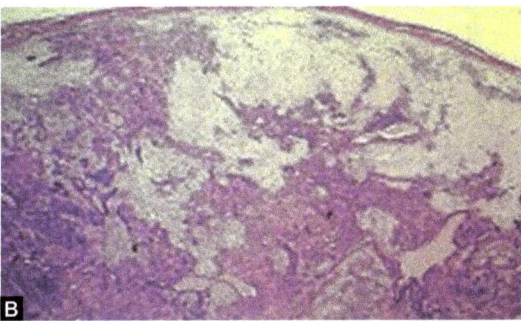

Figs. 7.10A and B: (A) Patient had slowly progressive left exophthalmos; (B) Diphasic pattern, pale background with highly cellular component, characteristic of pleomorphic adenoma (benign mixed tumor)

40. Adenoid cystic carcinoma of the lacrimal gland:
A. Has short duration of symptoms often 6 weeks or less.
B. Is rarely painful.
C. Has a dismal prognosis even with treatment.
D. Usually extends into the posterior orbit.
E. Is the most common epithelial malignancy of the lacrimal gland.

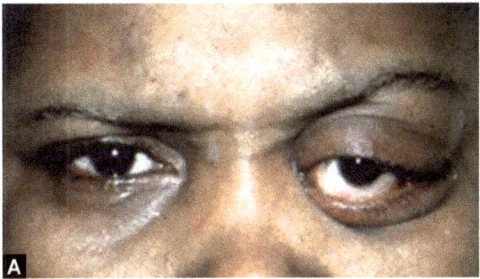

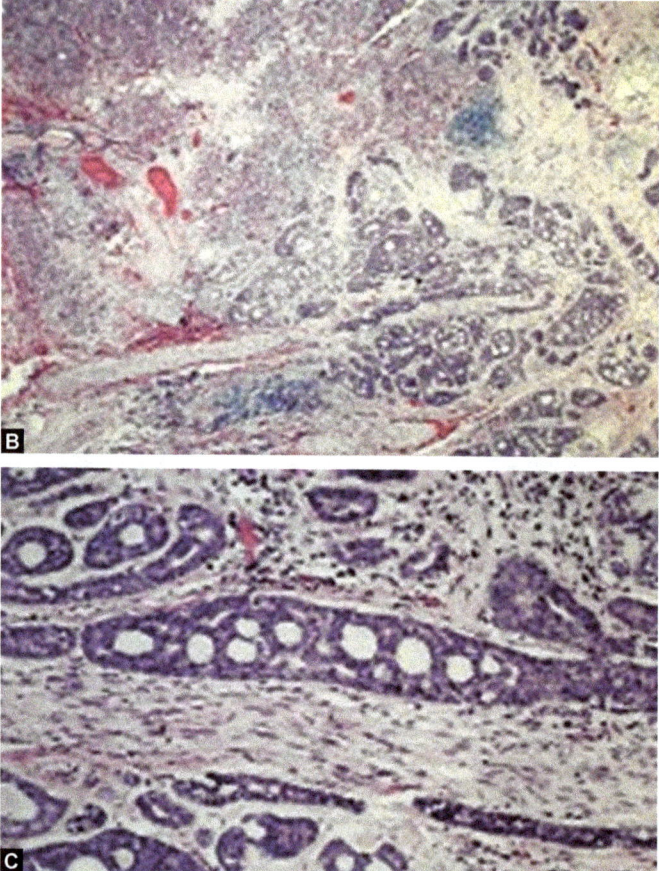

Figs. 7.11A to C: (A) Patient presented with slowly developing proptosis of left eye; (B) Low power view shows lacrimal gland and adenoid cystic carcinoma; (C) Adenoid cystic carcinoma surrounds a ciliary nerve.

41. **Fibrous dysplasia of the orbit:**
    A. May cause vision loss from compression of the optic nerve in the optic canal.
    B. Shows dural enhancement on MRI.
    C. Most commonly involves the frontal bone.
    D. Replaces normal bone with immature bone and osteoid.
    E. Can be monostotic or polyostotic.

42. **Rhabdomyosarcoma:**
    A. Requires immediate biopsy to confirm the diagnosis.
    B. Is most commonly in the embryonal form.
    C. Involves a 5-year survival rate in 45% of affected individuals.
    D. Affects boys more frequently than girls.
    E. Is the most common primary orbital childhood malignancy.

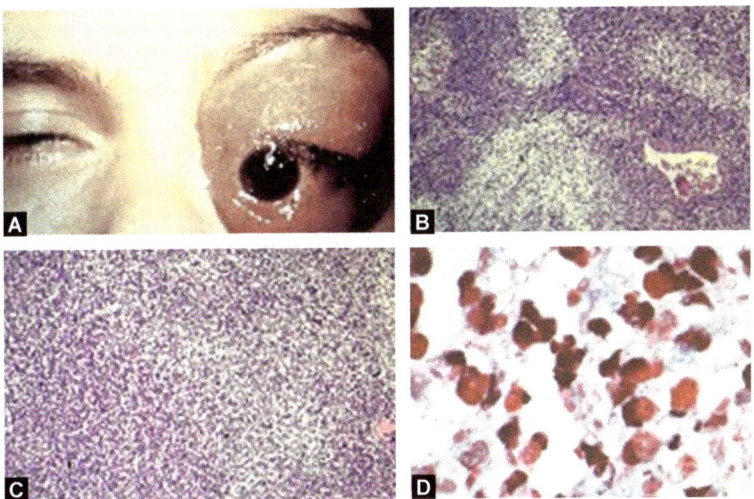

Figs. 12A to D: (A) Rapidly developing left exophthalmos in a young child; (B) Low power view shows an embryonic pattern; (C) Characteristic of embryonal rhabdomyosarcoma; (D) Rhabdomyoblasts are present.

43. **Plexiform neurofibroma:**
    A. Is the most common benign peripheral nerve tumor involving the eyelids and orbit.
    B. Is characteristic of neurofibromatosis type 1.
    C. Is noninfiltrative.
    D. Is not metastatic.
    E. Has a propensity for sensory nerves.

44. **Cavernous hemangioma:**
    A. Is composed of large cavernous spaces containing red blood cells.
    B. May increase in size during pregnancy.
    C. Is the most common benign neoplasm of the orbit in adults.
    D. Commonly involutes spontaneously.
    E. Affects women more than men.

45. **Merkel cell carcinoma:**
    A. Can mimic other malignant lesions.
    B. Has a 5-year survival rate of 50%.
    C. Arises from dermal melanocytes.
    D. Requires early consideration for radiation and/or chemotherapy.
    E. Can have overlying telangiectatic blood vessels.

46. **Orbital dermoid cysts:**
    A. May be subtotally resected with good results.
    B. May lie deep in the orbit.
    C. Are lined with epithelium and filled with keratinized material.
    D. Are choristomas.
    E. Most commonly occur in the area of the lateral brow.

47. Orbital floor fractures:
A. Most frequently occur medial to the infraorbital canal.
B. Associated with significant enophthalmos demand urgent repair, preferably within 2 weeks.
C. Of the medial wall are associated with orbital emphysema.
D. Associated with hypesthesia of the cheek and upper gum suggest infraorbital nerve damage.
E. Associated with a positive forced duction test always have extraocular muscle entrapped in the fracture.

48. Hydroxyapatite orbital implant after enucleation:
A. Can be wrapped in donor sclera.
B. Receives the four rectus muscles.
C. Can add a peg to produce maximal movement of the implant.
D. May be rejected by the body's immune system.
E. Generally undergoes drilling 6–12 months after placement.

49. Evisceration:
A. Is contraindicated in cases of suspected intraocular malignancy.
B. Always requires corneal removal.
C. Does not obviate the risk of sympathetic ophthalmia.
D. May be technically more difficult than enucleation in phthisical eyes.
E. Is contraindicated if precise histopathologic examination of the globe is needed.

50. Complications of exenteration include:
A. Severe blood loss.
B. Cerebrospinal fluid leakage.
C. "Phantom limb" pain from the cut optic nerve.
D. Skin graft infection.
E. Chronic sino-orbital fistulas.

51. Dacryocystography:
A. Can define the site of complete lacrimal system obstruction.
B. Can visualize a filling defect in patients who have a lacrimal sac tumor.
C. May evaluate lacrimal system physiologic function.
D. Can define the site of incomplete lacrimal system obstruction.
E. Can image compression or deflection of the lacrimal sac or duct.

52. Congenital nasolacrimal obstruction:
A. Should usually be treated by about age 1 year with irrigation and probing.
B. Should be treated with silicone intubation after two failed probing attempts.
C. Should be treated with dacryocystorhinostomy if nasal probing cannot be performed.
D. Associated with amnioceles requires probing at an early age.
E. Spontaneously resolves in more than 90% of patients by age 1 year.

53. Dacryocystorhinostomy:
A. Should be performed after active infection is treated.
B. Can have an intranasal or transcutaneous approach.
C. May require incision of the anterior limb of the medial canthal tendon.
D. Anastomoses the lacrimal sac to the nose.
E. Usually requires silicone tube placement.

ANSWERS

1. C. The orbital septum is a thin, fibrous, multilayered membrane that begins anatomically at the arcus marginalis along the orbital rim. It inserts on the levator aponeurosis about 3–5 mm above the tarsal plate. In the lower eyelid, the septum fuses with the capsulopalpebral fascia. The septum is not firmly attached to Whitnall's ligament.
2. A. Within each tarsus, there are the meibomian glands, numbering about 25 in the upper lid and 20 in the lower lid. These are holocrine-secreting sebaceous glands that are not associated with lash follicles.

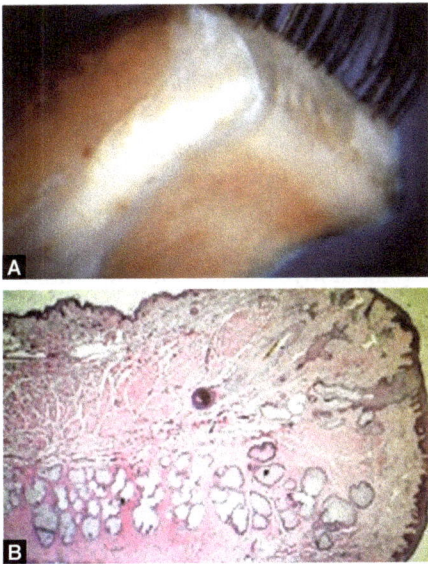

Figs. 7.13A and B: (A) Gross appearance of cut-section of lid viewed from below. The tarsal plate is clearly seen containing white meibomian glands; (B) Histology of cross-section of lid. The large meibomian glands occupy the lower third of the lid. A hair follicle is seen centrally above the tarsal plate.

3. E. The orbital floor is the shortest of all the orbital walls. It extends back only 35–40 mm from the inferior rim. The orbital floor is composed primarily of the maxillary bone. The zygomatic bone forms the anterolateral portion and the palatine bone lies at the posterior extent of the floor. The orbital floor is thinnest just medial to the infraorbital canal which is the most common site for blow-out fractures.

4. B. The lateral orbital wall is composed of the zygomatic bone and the greater wing of the sphenoid. The frontozygomatic suture is located approximately 1 cm above the lateral orbital tubercle of Whitnall. It is the strongest wall of the orbit and is adjacent to both the temporal fossa as well as the middle cranial fossa. In orbital decompression, the lateral orbital wall is the safest wall to access and remove. This is followed by the medial and inferior orbital walls, respectively.

5. D. Shortly after the ophthalmic artery enters the orbit, it gives off a number of branches. The central retinal artery is usually the first branch.

6. B. The severity and clinical course of thyroid eye disease (TED) is not correlated with plasma free T4 and T3 levels. Symptomatic double vision or head posturing postorbital decompression should be corrected in patients after 6 months of stable misalignment. Eyelid malpositions are often altered with surgical manipulation of the vertical extraocular muscles. Thus, any eyelid correction is reserved until after any strabismus surgery. Due to the neural crest origin of the orbital fibroblasts, these cells can undergo adipocyte differentiation resulting in the synthesis of glycosaminoglycan in the extraocular muscles.

7. C. Wernicke's encephalopathy begins abruptly usually with eye movement disorders such as nystagmus, gaze palsies, and ophthalmoplegia or eye paralysis (especially of the lateral rectus muscles) and other symptoms such as gait ataxia, confusion, confabulation, and short-term memory loss. It is not a neurogenic cause of eyelid retraction. Tertiary syphilis, dorsal midbrain syndrome, palatal myoclonus, and impending tentorial herniation are all neurogenic causes of eyelid retraction.

8. E. Down syndrome is classified under miscellaneous causes of eyelid retraction. This miscellaneous category has been developed for cases in which eyelid retraction is reported but no clear explanation of cause and effect can be determined. Optic nerve hypoplasia, microphthalmos, essential hypertension, hepatic cirrhosis, meningitis, sphenoid wing meningioma, and lymphoma in the superior cul-de-sac are diseases also listed under the miscellaneous causes of eyelid retraction.

9. D. Simple congenital ptosis is unilateral in 69% of cases. Bilateral involvement may be symmetrical or asymmetrical in appearance. Coexisting strabismus is present in approximately 30% of children. Hypotropia is common and may be a possible manifestation of developmental failure affecting both the superior rectus and levator muscles. Anisometropia is present in 12% of patients with simple congenital ptosis. Strabismus and anisometropia may lead to amblyopia which is found in 20% of patients who have simple congenital ptosis. Occlusion amblyopia is less common and should be considered a diagnosis of exclusion. In downgaze, the ptosis is

reduced or absent because the fibrotic levator muscle cannot stretch. Early surgery is indicated in cases with obstruction of the visual axis. Treatment is otherwise delayed until the late preschool years.

10. C. Blepharophimosis–ptosis–epicanthus inversus syndrome (BPES) is not commonly associated with mental retardation. It is an autosomal dominant disease with 50% of new cases arising from sporadic mutations. The genetic defect is in the FOXL2 gene on chromosome 3 which encodes for a DNA-binding transcription factor.

11. A. Avulsion of the medial canthus is usually the result of increased horizontal tension on the eyelid; the prototypical example is of a finger or blunt object pulling on the lower eyelid. Clinical signs include rounding of the medial canthal angle and acquired telecanthus. Isolated avulsion of the anterior portion can be reattached to the tendon stump while an isolated avulsion of the posterior tendon requires wire refixation to the posterior lacrimal crest. Avulsion associated with nasal bone fracture may require plating with wire fixation.

12. A. In ptosis caused by dehiscence of the levator aponeurosis, the levator function is not reduced. Loss of the aponeurotic attachment results in an abnormally high or indistinct upper eyelid crease.

13. C. Enophthalmos alone may be insufficient to cause entropion.

14. D. Small (<30%) upper and lower eyelid defects usually can be repaired with direct closure. Moderate defects (30–50%) are repaired with advancement of the lateral segments with rotational or semicircular flaps. Large upper eyelid defects (>50%) are repaired with full thickness lower eyelid advancement graft (Cutler–Beard procedure). Large lower eyelid defects (>50%) are repaired with tarsoconjunctival flap from the upper eyelid with skin graft (modified Hughes procedure).

15. E. The Kuhnt–Szymanowski procedure is used as a technique primarily for involutional ectropion repair. It is useful when there is an excess of lower lid skin in addition to generalized horizontal lid laxity.

16. C. Epicanthal folds are formed due to poorly developed facial bone structure and soft tissue. There are four classifications based on clinical appearance of most prominent region of the fold. Epicanthus tarsalis has more prominent upper eyelid fold, and is a normal variant in Asian populations. Epicanthus inversus has greater involvement of the lower eyelid fold and usually requires surgical repair. Epicanthus palpebralis has equal involvement of the upper and lower eyelids and epicanthus supraciliaris originates above the eyebrow.

17. C. Some of the techniques available for correction of ectropion include the lateral tarsal strip procedure, full-thickness wedge excision, medial canthal tendon resection, medial canthal tendon plication, and the Z-plasty. A Z-plasty is a flap rearrangement procedure used to correct skin shortening due to a focal linear scar. The Z-plasty may have to be combined with other procedures to correct ectropion effectively. The Y-V plasty is a surgical technique used in the correction of epicanthal folds.

18. A. In lower eyelid blepharoplasty, injury to the extraocular muscles can occur where the inferior oblique and inferior rectus are prone to damage with exploration of the medial fat pad. In these instances, a follow-up of at least 6 months is necessary prior to considering surgical interventions, as spontaneous resolution is fortunately the rule. Loss of vision secondary to postoperative retrobulbar hemorrhage is the most feared complication associated with lower eyelid blepharoplasty. Excessive excision of skin in the lower lids can lead to lower lid retraction.

19. C. With laser skin resurfacing, wrinkles and skin imperfections can be reduced but not eliminated. The best candidates for laser skin resurfacing are patients with a lower Fitzpatrick scale. The lower scale correlates with skin pigmentation. The more pigmented the skin, the greater is the risk of development of hyperpigmentation after resurfacing. Patients who have a history of keloid formation are at greater risk for scarring. Patients with a history of herpes simplex virus infections are at risk for recurrent infection with scarring. Recent use of isotretinoin, laser resurfacing, chemical peeling or radiation therapy within the past 6 months should be considered contraindications for this procedure.

20. D. One of the distinguishing features of essential blepharospasms is that they abate during sleep. Spasms may spread to involve the midface over a variable period of time. This progression of essential blepharospasm to include adjacent focal oromandibular dystonia is referred to as Meige's syndrome. Other adjacent dystonias such as dystonic activity of the neck muscles (craniocervical dystonia) and dystonic activity of the vocal cords (spastic dystonia) can be seen in association with essential blepharospasm.

21. C. Granulomatosis with polyangiitis (GPA) is a systemic disorder with high degree of ocular involvement. This disease associated with necrotizing granulonephritis and necrotizing granulomas of the sinus cavities and lung. On presentation, 15% of patients can be noted to have ocular involvement and this proportion increases up to 50% throughout the disease course. There is a high untreated mortality rate and treatment requires aggressive immunosuppression classically with cyclophosphamide and steroids. Serum autoantibodies to proteinase 3 [cytoplasmic-antineutrophil cytoplasmic antibody (c-ANCA)] and myeloperoxidase (MPO)-ANCA have high specificity for the diagnosis.

22. E. Lid crutches are not used in the treatment of essential blepharospasm. Botulinum toxin is currently the initial treatment of choice for benign essential blepharospasm (BEB). Oral pharmacological agents often are helpful for milder cases of BEB or as adjunctive therapy. Myectomy usually is reserved for those individuals who respond poorly to more conservative therapy or for those patients who have anatomical problems such as ptosis which need correction. Chemomyectomy

is another type of myectomy in which local injections of doxorubicin produce permanent orbicularis oculi weakness.

23. C. Cutaneous horn is not a distinct pathological entity but may develop from a variety of underlying lesions including seborrheic keratosis, actinic keratosis, inverted follicular keratosis, verruca vulgaris, basal cell carcinoma, squamous cell carcinoma, and other epidermal tumors. Because definitive therapy is dependent on the underlying cause, biopsy of the cutaneous horn (including the underlying epidermis) is required to obtain a histological diagnosis.

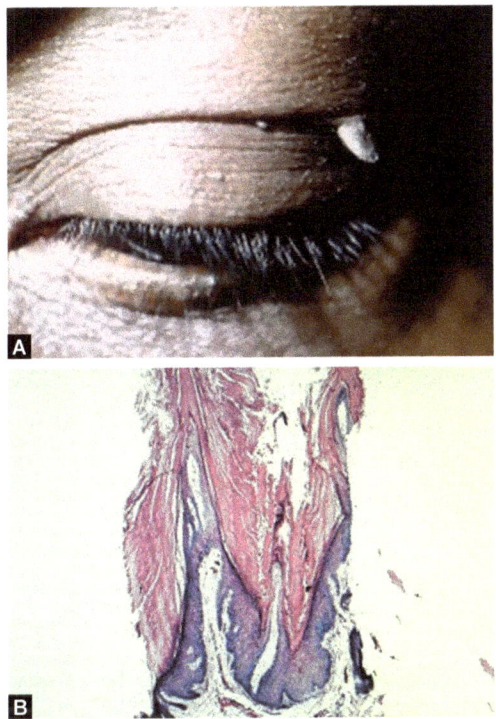

Figs. 7.14A and B: (A) Cutaneous horn seen clinically; (B) Acanthosis and hyperkeratosis are characteristic.

24. B. Keratoacanthoma most commonly appears as a solitary, rapidly growing nodule on sun-exposed areas of middle-aged and older individuals. The nodule is usually umbilicated with a distinctive central crater filled with a keratin plug. Microscopically, the base is usually noninfiltrating and often demarcated from the underlying dermis by an inflammatory reaction. Cellular atypia may be present making differentiation from squamous cell carcinoma (SCC) difficult. Many pathologists consider keratoacanthoma as a type of low-grade SCC. Patients with Muir–Torre syndrome may develop in association with internal malignancy, multiple keratoacanthomas and sebaceous neoplasms.

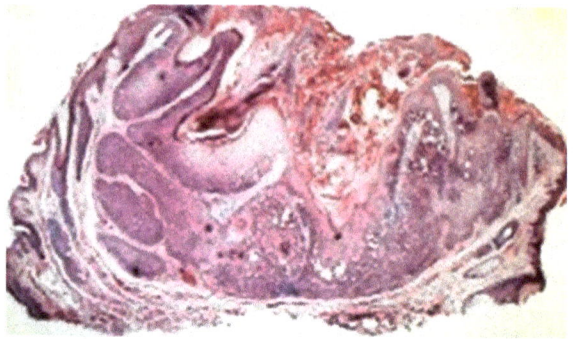

Fig. 7.15: Keratoacanthoma shows umbilicated configuration. The base is blunt and noninvasive.

25. D. Actinic keratosis is not truly a benign condition, being the most common premalignant skin lesion. The lesions develop on sun-exposed areas and commonly affect the face, hands, and scalp and less commonly, eyelid.

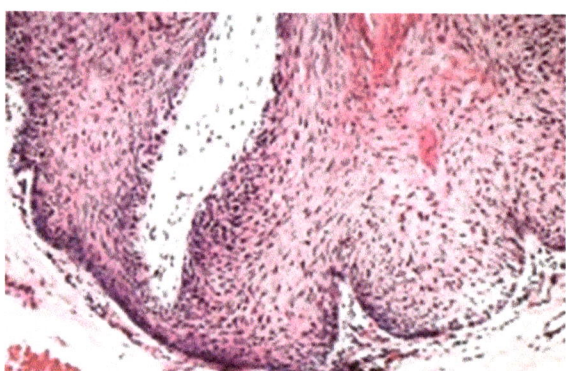

Fig. 7.16: Dysplastic epithelium demonstrates the malignant potential of an actinic keratosis.

26. A. The capillary hemangioma is a common vascular lesion of childhood and is the most common orbital tumor found in children. Usually the lesions manifest by 6 months of age with only one-third of lesions visible at birth. Treatment for visually significant lesions includes topical beta-blocker ointment. Larger and more systemic hemangiomas may require oral beta-blockers or steroids. Patients who have extensive visceral hemangiomas may develop thrombocytopenia related to entrapment of platelets within the lesion with resulting hemorrhagic diathesis known as the Kasabach–Merritt syndrome.

27. D. Xanthogranuloma tends to be diffuse in Erdheim–Chester disease (ECD) and can lead to vision loss. Despite aggressive therapies, bone involvement is common and death is frequent. Asthma is associated with adult onset asthma and periocular xanthogranuloma (AAPOX).

28. C. Often, patients have a history of sleeping prone. This can cause mechanical upper eyelid eversion and leads to the superior palpebral conjunctiva rubbing against the pillow or bed.
29 C. In patients with nevus of Ota, malignant degeneration is common particularly among Caucasians, and the choroid is the most common site of involvement.
30. E. Molluscum contagiosum is caused by a large DNA poxvirus.

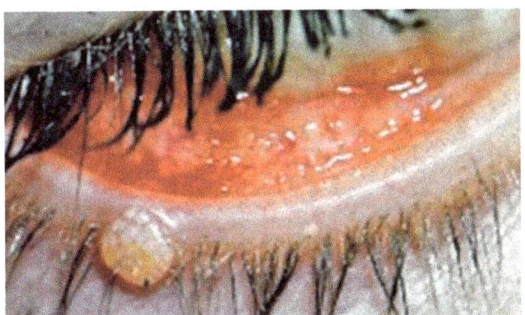

Fig. 7.17: Umbilicated lesion contains packets of material. Material is molluscum bodies as small intracytoplasmic eosinophilic bodies in the deep epithelial layers and large intracytoplasmic basophilic bodies in the superficial epithelial layers. A reactive conjunctivitis is present.

31. A. Basal cell carcinoma is locally infiltrative but rarely metastasizes.

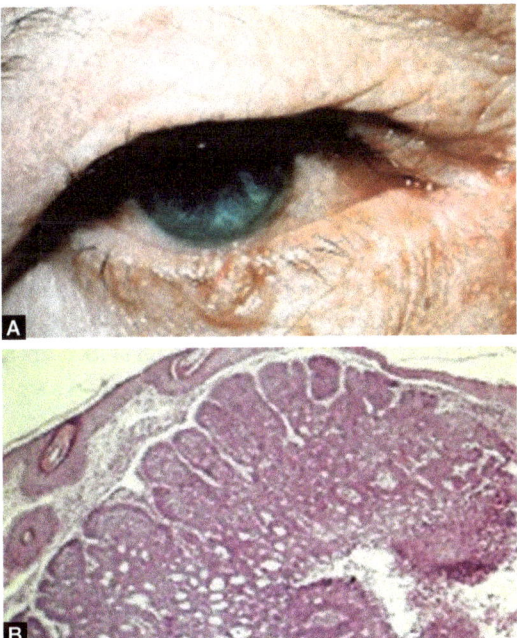

Figs. 7.18A and B: (A) Painless, slow growing lesion of lower lid; (B) Characteristic basal cell proliferation with peripheral palisading.

32. E. Basal-cell nevus syndrome (Gorlin syndrome) is a rare autosomal dominant disorder that typically presents at puberty. In additional to multiple basal cell carcinomas, manifestations of the disease include jaw cysts, skeletal abnormalities, neurological abnormalities and endocrine disorders.
33. C. Radiation therapy is generally not recommended in the initial treatment of periocular basal cell carcinoma (BCC). Surgery is the initial treatment of choice for BCC, although some surgeons also advocate cryotherapy, electrodesiccation, and laser ablation.
34. D. Most periorbital squamous cell carcinomas arise from areas of solar injury or actinic keratosis, but they may also arise *de novo*.

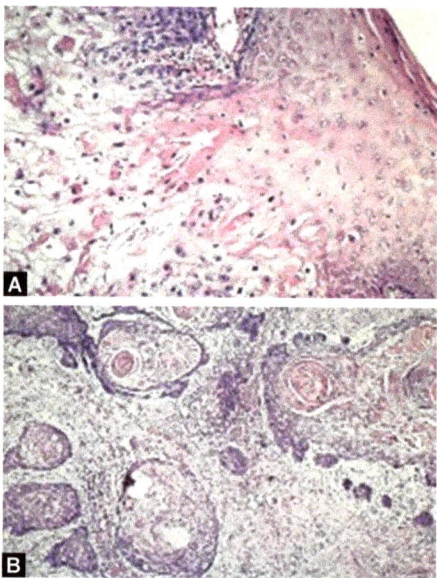

Figs. 7.19A and B: (A) Squamous cell carcinoma invading the dermis; (B) Malignant cells are forming large keratin pearls.

35. E. Sebaceous gland carcinoma is a highly malignant neoplasm that arises from the meibomian glands, glands of Zeis, and sebaceous glands of the caruncle, eyebrow or facial skin.

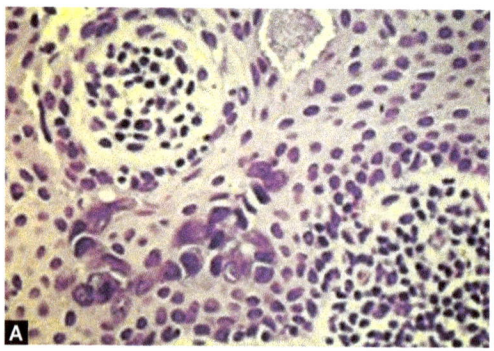

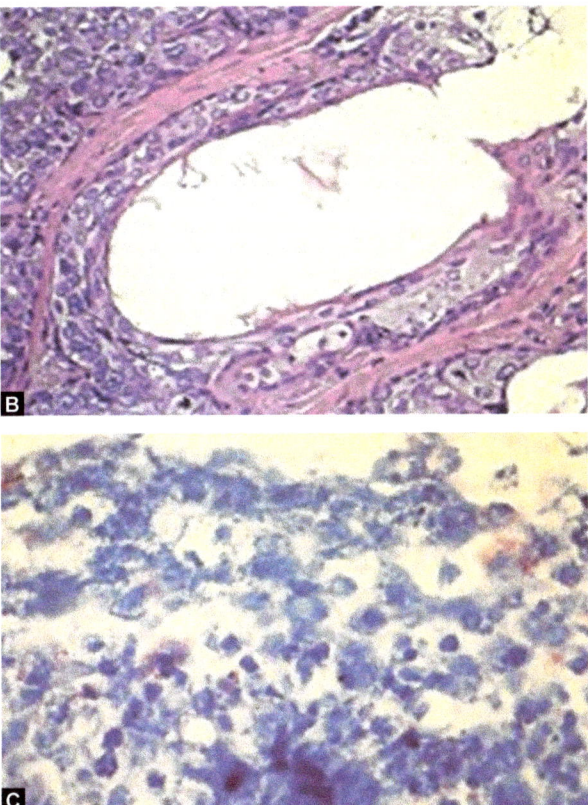

Figs. 7.20A to C: (A) Malignant sebaceous cells have invaded the epithelium (pagetoid change); (B) Cells resembling sebaceous cells have invaded the dermis; (C) Malignant cells characteristically stain positively for fat (oil red-O fat stain).

36. E. While cryotherapy may be useful in treating some conjunctival malignant melanomas, it is not an effective treatment option for cutaneous malignant melanoma of the eyelid. The procedure of choice for treatment of cutaneous malignant melanoma of the eyelid is wide surgical excision with 1 cm of skin margins (when possible) confirmed by histological monitoring. Depending on the tumor thickness (>1.5 mm), regional lymph node dissection and/or metastatic workup may also be indicated.
37. D. Actually tarsorrhaphies in eyelid burns should always be more extensive than seems to be immediately necessary.
38. E. Extraocular muscle tendons of insertion may show thickening in 50% of nonspecific orbital inflammation (NSOI) patients. In comparison, thyroid eye disease (TED) often spares the insertions. Deep-rooted, boring pain is a typical feature of this condition.
39. A. Pleomorphic adenoma (benign mixed cell tumor) occurs mainly in the orbital lobe of the lacrimal gland, and rarely in the palpebral lobe.

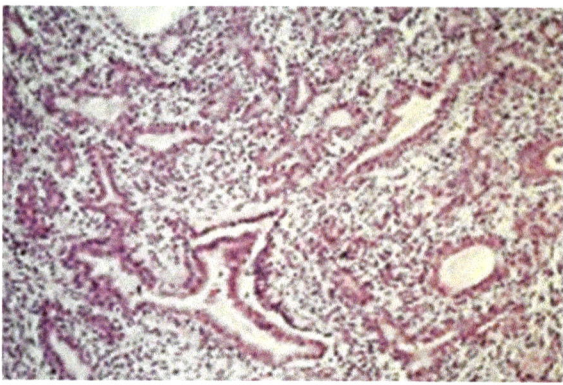

Fig. 7.21: Inner epithelium of ducts within tumor secretes mucus or undergo squamous metaplasia. Outer layer of ductal epithelium undergoes myxoid and sometimes cartilaginous metaplasia.

40. B. In patients with adenoid cystic carcinoma, orbital pain as a result of perineural spread and bone destruction is common. Other orbital symptoms include exophthalmos, downward globe displacement, ptosis, and diplopia.

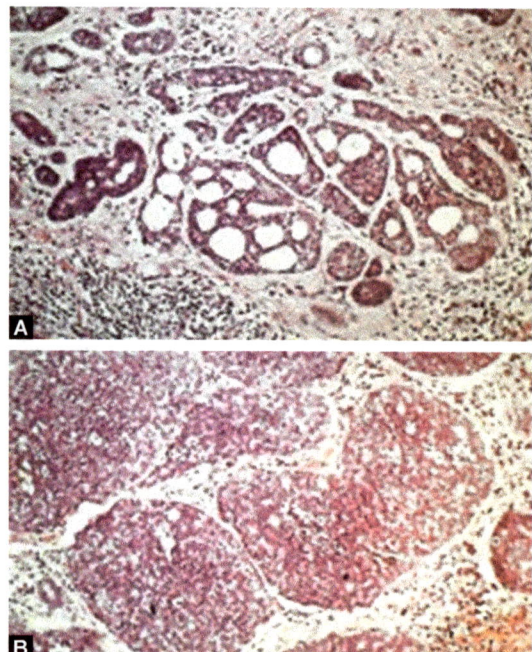

Figs. 7.22A and B: (A) Typical "Swiss-cheese" pattern of adenoid cystic carcinoma has a better prognosis than; (B) A basaloid pattern of adenoid cystic carcinoma.

41. B. Fibrous dysplasia may be monostotic or polyostotic. Magnetic resonance imaging (MRI) distinguishes this condition from

meningioma by showing lack of dural enhancement. Computed tomography (CT) shows hyperostotic bone.

42. C. The 5-year survival rate in patients with rhabdomyosarcoma is > 90% if the orbital tumor has not invaded or extended beyond the bony orbital walls. Tumors in the orbit have a favorable prognosis because of the near absence of orbital lymphatics.

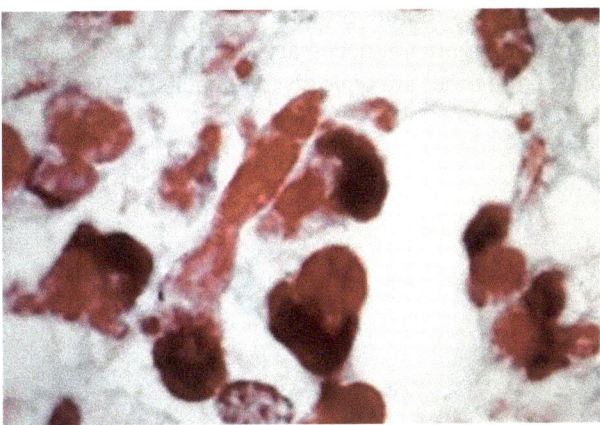

Fig. 7.23: Rhabdomyoblasts show cross-striations.

43. C. Plexiform neurofibromas are tumors within the nerve sheaths that are well-vascularized and infiltrative lesions which make complete surgical excision challenging.
44. D. Cavernous hemangioma rarely involutes spontaneously. If the lesion affects vision, leads to significant proptosis or demonstrates significant growth, then treatment consists of surgical excision.
45. C. Merkel cell carcinoma arises from the dendritic (neuroendocrine) cells of the skin.
46. A. Dermoid cysts must be completely removed en bloc. Incomplete excision or rupture of the capsule may result in recurrences of the cyst with infiltration.
47. E. A positive forced duction test and vertical diplopia in a patient with an orbital floor fracture suggest mechanical restriction. Entrapment of the fascial attachments of the inferior rectus muscle is more common than entrapment of the muscle itself. A positive forced duction test with vertical diplopia may also be seen with a contusion injury to the inferior rectus muscle.
48. D. Hydroxyapatite is a porous implant with a structure similar to that of the haversian system of cancellous bone. This microstructure allows fibrovascular ingrowth of the host tissues in the anophthalmic socket.
49. B. Based upon the surgeon's preference, the cornea may either be preserved or removed during an evisceration.
50. C. A "phantom limb" pain syndrome secondary to a severed optic nerve has not been described after exenteration surgery.

51. C. Dacryocystography is an anatomical test and does not evaluate physiological function of the lacrimal drainage system. In this procedure, injection of either a viscous oil or water-soluble contrast material into the lacrimal system demonstrates the drainage pathways and outlines any abnormalities.
52. D. Congenital amnioceles typically resolve without intervention, and therefore rarely require probing.
53. E. Silicone tubes are not necessary during a dacryocystorhinostomy. If utilized, the tubes are typically left in place for 6–12 weeks.

CHAPTER 8

Retina and Vitreous

Weiye Li, Stephanie J Weiss

QUESTIONS

Identify the correct answer for all questions (unless instructed otherwise).

1. **All of the following are located in the inner nuclear layer of the retina, *except*:**
   A. Amacrine cell nuclei.
   B. Horizontal cell nuclei.
   C. Müller cell nuclei.
   D. Bipolar cell nuclei.
   E. Rod nuclei.

2. **Phototransduction (capture of photons of light and conversion into electrical signal) takes place in:**
   A. The nuclei of the photoreceptors.
   B. The retinal pigment epithelium.
   C. Outer segments of the rods and cones.
   D. Amacrine cells.
   E. Horizontal cells.

3. **All of the following pathophysiologic roles take place in the retinal pigment epithelium, *except*:**
   A. Absorption of scattered light.
   B. Blood–retinal barrier function.
   C. Visual pigment regeneration and synthesis.
   D. Visual processing.
   E. Maintenance of retinal adhesion.

4. **All of the following pathophysiologic roles take place in the retinal pigment epithelium, *except*:**
   A. Synthesis of growth factors and other metabolites.
   B. Regulation of release of neurotransmitters.
   C. Phagocytosis and digestion of photoreceptor waste.
   D. Electrical homeostasis.
   E. Regeneration and repair after injury.

5. **Which of the following does not apply to the blood supply of the choroid?**
   A. It involves the blood–choroid barrier.
   B. It contains fenestrated capillaries.
   C. It is supplied by the anterior and posterior ciliary arteries.
   D. Each terminal choroidal artery supplies an independent lobule.
   E. The capillaries (choriocapillaris) have very large diameters (20–25 microns).

6. **Which of the following is *not* true with respect to retinal LASER photocoagulation?**
   A. Blue light is scattered less than light of longer wavelengths.
   B. Blue light is absorbed by macular xanthophyll.
   C. Green light is absorbed well by melanin and hemoglobin.
   D. Krypton red light is absorbed more deeply than argon green light.
   E. Red light is absorbed well by melanin but poorly by hemoglobin.

7. **Concerning scleral buckling, which of the following is *not* true?**
   A. Gonin first employed the concept of drainage of subretinal fluid and treatment of retinal breaks.
   B. Custodis introduced the technique of scleral buckling.
   C. Ridley introduced monocular indirect ophthalmoscopy.
   D. Schepens introduced indirect ophthalmoscopy.
   E. Licoff et at. introduced the concept of silicone sponge explants and cryotherapy.

8. **Scleral buckling surgery is best for:**
   A. Tractional retinal detachment without retinal tears.
   B. Rhegmatogenous retinal detachment.
   C. Retinal detachment in Harada's disease.
   D. Retinal detachment in eclampsia of pregnancy.
   E. Tumor-associated retinal detachment.

9. **All the following are serious complications after scleral buckling, *except*:**
   A. Infection.
   B. Macular pucker.
   C. Cystoid macular edema.
   D. Glaucoma.
   E. Choroidal detachment (choroidal edema).

10. **Which of the following statements about postoperative results of scleral buckling is *not* true?**
    A. The overall reattachment rate is at least 90%.
    B. About 10% of patients who have macula-on detachments lose two or more Snellen lines postoperatively.
    C. The overall rate for macula-off detachments is at least 90%, but only 40% of patients achieve a final vision of 20/50 or better.
    D. The anatomic results parallel the visual results.

E. The rate of anatomic success is better with macula-on detachments than with macula-off detachments.

11. The indications for vitrectomy in patients with diabetes include all the following, *except*:
    A. Nonclearing or repeat vitreous hemorrhage.
    B. Tractional retinal detachment.
    C. Macular distortion by fibrovascular proliferation.
    D. Intravitreous laser endophotocoagulation for clinically significant macular edema.
    E. Progressive fibrovascular proliferation.

12. During vitrectomy, lensectomy is indicated:
    A. As standard procedure.
    B. When vitreous traction must be dissected just posterior to the equator.
    C. When a cataract prevents visualization of the fundus or the lens is subluxated.
    D. When vitreous traction must be dissected from the posterior pole.
    E. When a nonclearing hemorrhage is being removed.

13. The indications for use of perfluorocarbon during vitreous surgery include all the following, *except*:
    A. Repositioning of giant retinal tears with large inverted posterior flaps.
    B. Expeditious removal of epiretinal macular membranes.
    C. Anterior flotation of dislocated lens fragments.
    D. Expression of liquefied blood from under the retina.
    E. Provision of intraocular homeostasis by localization of bleeding.

14. In B-scan ultrasonography, all the following apply, *except*:
    A. A 10 MHz transducer probe.
    B. Real time.
    C. Gray scale.
    D. Three-dimensional analysis.
    E. A graph-like image with vertical deflection from a baseline.

15. Which one of the following conditions is *least* well visualized with fluorescein angiography?
    A. Choroidal artery thrombosis.
    B. Diabetic retinopathy.
    C. Cystoid macular edema.
    D. Central serous chorioretinopathy.
    E. Retinal venous occlusive disease.

16. Which of the following does *not* apply to fluorescein?
    A. It has a narrow spectrum of absorption between 570 nm and 595 nm.
    B. It has the ability to fluoresce (i.e. absorb a photon of light of one wavelength and emit a photon of light at a second wavelength).
    C. About 80% of it binds to serum albumin.
    D. It is eliminated in urine within 24–36 hours after injection.
    E. It is metabolized by the liver and kidneys.

17. **All the following are causes of hyperfluorescence, *except*:**
    A. Bull's eye maculopathy.
    B. Atrophic chorioretinal hole.
    C. Subretinal hemorrhage.
    D. Retinal cavernous hemangioma.
    E. Frosted angiitis.

18. **All the following are causes of hypofluorescence, *except*:**
    A. The area supplied by branch retinal arteriole occlusion.
    B. A retinoblastoma.
    C. A choroidal nevus.
    D. Diabetic capillary nonperfusion.
    E. The posterior pole in Stargardt disease.

19. **Which one of the following known adverse reactions to fluorescein angiography is considered mild (rather than moderate to severe)?**
    A. Urticaria.
    B. Syncope.
    C. Laryngeal edema.
    D. Pruritus.
    E. Myocardial infarction.

20. **One of the greatest uses of indocyanine green angiography is to:**
    A. Detect choroidal neovascularization in presumed histoplasmosis.
    B. Delineate the ischemic area in branch retinal artery occlusion.
    C. Visualize cavernous hemangioma of the retina.
    D. Follow the response to irradiated retinoblastomas.
    E. Detect occult, poorly defined choroidal neovascularization.

21. **Which of the following does *not* apply to indocyanine green?**
    A. It is 95% bound to serum proteins.
    B. It has reduced leakage through the choriocapillaris as compared with fluorescein.
    C. It offers better visualization of choroidal circulation as compared with fluorescein.
    D. It cannot be used in patients who are allergic to fluorescein.
    E. Wavelength is near infrared.

22. **Which of the following statements concerning indocyanine green angiography is *incorrect*?**
    A. It is contraindicated in patients who have an iodide allergy.
    B. Nausea may occur with its use.
    C. The incidence of anaphylaxis is less than that which occurs with fluorescein angiography.
    D. It is contraindicated in patients with liver disease.
    E. It is contraindicated in patients who are pregnant.

23. **Which of the following statements concerning a full-field electroretinography (ERG) is incorrect?**

A. The photoreceptors generate the a-wave (initial cornea-negative component).
B. Myopia affects the ERG amplitude and implicit time.
C. Müller cells and bipolar cells generate the b-wave (later cornea-positive component).
D. Macular scarring of 4 or more disc diameters can cause a mild reduction in cone amplitude.
E. Media opacities can cause a reduction in the ERG amplitude and lengthen the implicit time.

24. Features of typical retinitis pigmentosa include all of the following, *except*:
    A. Relative preservation of midperipheral retinal pigment epithelium.
    B. Bone-spicule pigmentation of the retina.
    C. Pale, waxy optic nerve head.
    D. Posterior subcapsular cataract.
    E. Attenuation of retinal arterioles.

25. All the following are types of X-linked retinal dystrophies, *except*:
    A. Usher's syndrome.
    B. Choroideremia.
    C. Congenital stationary night blindness.
    D. Juvenile retinoschisis.
    E. Blue cone monochromatism.

26. Which of the following does *not* apply to X-linked retinitis pigmentosa?
    A. Prominent parafoveal pigmentation may be present.
    B. Usually by 20 years of age, acuity loss and field constriction are significant.
    C. Electroretinography shows a major reduction of both rod and cone responses.
    D. Dark-adapted thresholds can be elevated by as much as three log units.
    E. Bone-spicule retinal pigmentation appears between 5 years and 9 years of age.

27. The following statements about female carriers of X-linked retinitis pigmentosa are true, *except*:
    A. More than 50% of patients show one or more areas of bone-spicule pigmentation.
    B. Many carriers have myopic astigmatism at an oblique axis.
    C. Some carriers become functionally blind by late middle age.
    D. Electroretinography shows a reduction of one or more components in 80–90% of carriers.
    E. ERG amplitudes do not correlate with expected overall vision loss in later years.

28. Rod-cone dystrophy:
    A. Is the same as cone-rod dystrophy.
    B. Is more severe than cone-rod dystrophy.

C. Appears clinically as an atypical retinitis pigmentosa.
D. Has a long-term prognosis that involves loss of only peripheral vision.
E. Electroretinography shows a greater amplitude loss for cones than for rods.

29. **Chloroquine retinopathy:**
    A. Is a less likely to cause retinal pigment epithelial toxicity than hydroxychloroquine.
    B. Results in a reverse Bull's eye maculopathy.
    C. Is not caused by chloroquine binding to melanin leading to an indirect retinal pigment epithelial toxicity.
    D. Can be detected earliest with visual field defects and ellipsoid zone alterations on optical coherence tomography.
    E. Fluorescein angiography is more sensitive to early changes than optical coherence tomography.

30. **Cancer-associated retinopathy:**
    A. Tends to be unilateral.
    B. Does not seem to be related to autoantigens that affect the retina.
    C. Is caused by apoptosis of retinal cells.
    D. Generally evolves slowly with mild loss of vision.
    E. Is most commonly caused by small cell carcinoma of the breast.

31. **Although clinically Stargardt disease and fundus flavimaculatus have many similarities, a few differences exist. Which of the following is true?**
    A. Both autosomal dominant Stargardt disease and fundus flavimaculatus have been mapped to the short arm of chromosome 1.
    B. Both conditions have their onsets in early adulthood.
    C. Both autosomal recessive Stargardt disease and fundus flavimaculatus have been mapped to the short arm of chromosome 1.
    D. Both conditions show a hyperfluorescent choroid on fluorescein angiography.
    E. The electrooculogram is always normal in both conditions.

32. **The differential diagnosis of Stargardt disease includes all the following, *except*:**
    A. Choroideremia.
    B. Cone-rod dystrophy.
    C. Neuronal ceroid lipofuscinosis.
    D. Pattern dystrophy.
    E. Chloroquine retinopathy.

33. **Which one of the following statements about Stargardt disease is true?**
    A. Most commonly it is inherited as an autosomal dominant condition.
    B. The recessive form has been mapped to chromosome 13q.
    C. The pisiform flecks found at the level of the retinal pigment epithelium are not present in the posterior pole.

D. It is the most prevalent inherited macular dystrophy accounting for about 7% of the total.
E. The electroretinogram is always normal with this condition.

34. Which one of the following statements about Best disease is *not* true?
    A. It is extremely rare.
    B. The gene has been mapped to chromosome 11q13.
    C. Bilateral, typically large, yellow, yolk-like (vitelliform) lesions are present in the macula.
    D. The electrooculogram is abnormal and shows a severe loss of the light rise.
    E. The electroretinogram shows a reduced b-wave.

35. Which one of the following statements about pattern dystrophy is *not* true?
    A. Some autosomal dominant forms are associated with mutations in PHPR2 (peripherin), a retinal protein encoded by a gene located on chromosome 6p.
    B. A significant percentage of patients will develop subretinal choroidal neovascularization.
    C. The pathologic evidence lies at the level of the central macular retinal pigment epithelium.
    D. The electrophysiologic testing is usually normal.
    E. In most patients, visual acuity remains normal or is only mildly reduced.

36. Which one of the following statements about North Carolina macular dystrophy is true?
    A. The gene has been mapped to chromosome 6q.
    B. It shows small, granular, corneal stromal opacities with intervening clear areas.
    C. It is related to central areolar choroidal sclerosis.
    D. The electroretinogram is diagnostic.
    E. It does not resemble geographic age-related macular degeneration.

37. Choroideremia:
    A. Has an autosomal dominant inheritance pattern.
    B. Has an autosomal recessive inheritance pattern.
    C. Has an X-linked recessive inheritance pattern.
    D. Is inherited via a point mutation.
    E. Does not have a clear inheritance pattern.

38. Which of the following is *least* true for choroideremia?
    A. Progressive nyctalopia is the presenting symptom in most patients.
    B. Female carriers typically show mild-to-moderate symptoms.
    C. It involves progressive loss of peripheral visual fields.
    D. The responsible gene encodes a subunit of Rab geranylgeranyl-transferase that modifies Rab proteins.

E. The gene is expressed both in ocular tissues and in different cells of nonocular origin.

39. Which of the following statements about choroideremia is true?
    A. Electroretinography is normal in all stages.
    B. Posterior subcapsular cataract is an early finding.
    C. Loss of visual field greatly exceeds the clinically discernible areas of chorioretinal atrophy.
    D. Initial changes occur in the retinal pigment epithelium in the midperiphery of the fundus.
    E. The macula is affected early in the clinical course.

40. Gyrate atrophy:
    A. Has an autosomal dominant inheritance pattern.
    B. Has an autosomal recessive inheritance pattern.
    C. Has an X-linked recessive inheritance pattern.
    D. Is inherited via a point mutation.
    E. Does not have a clear inheritance pattern.

41. Which of the following is *least* true for gyrate atrophy?
    A. Hyperornithinemia is present.
    B. It is caused by a deficiency of ornithine ketoacid aminotransferase (ornithine aminotransferase).
    C. Characteristically, sharply demarcated scalloped areas of chorioretinal atrophy are noted first in the midperiphery.
    D. Ornithine aminotransferase depends on cofactor B6.
    E. Moderate to marked hyperopia is found in most patients.

42. Congenital stationary night blindness:
    A. Has its onset of nyctalopia in the third decade of life.
    B. Shows histologic evidence of rod abnormalities.
    C. Is inherited via a point mutation.
    D. Always shows an abnormal fundus.
    E. Is not treatable.

43. Which of the following is *least* true for Oguchi's disease, a form of congenital stationary night blindness?
    A. It has a characteristic yellowish metallic sheen of the posterior pole.
    B. The electroretinogram shows abnormal cone function.
    C. After prolonged dark adaptation, the posterior pole reverts to a normal appearance (Mizuo's phenomenon).
    D. The gene has been mapped to chromosome 2q probably to the region of the *arrestin* gene.
    E. The electroretinogram shows abnormal rod function.

44. Another form of congenital stationary night blindness is fundus albipunctatus. Which one of the following statements does *not* apply to this condition?
    A. Multiple tiny white fundus dots are present and characteristically extend into the fovea.

B. Monotonous deposits appearing as multiple tiny white dots in the posterior pole extend into the midperiphery.
C. A fluorescein angiographic appearance of hyperfluorescence does not correlate with the clinical picture of the fundus.
D. The electroretinogram shows abnormal scotopic response of the cone and rod function.
E. The electroretinogram shows abnormal photopic response of the cone and rod function.

45. All the following statements pertain to Stickler's syndrome *except* which one?
    A. It may be associated with a type II collagen gene mutation (COL2Al) on the long arm of chromosome 12.
    B. High myopia is very common with this condition.
    C. It usually shows an optically empty vitreous compartment that contains membranes and strands.
    D. The condition has an X-linked recessive inheritance pattern.
    E. Radial perivascular pigmentary changes are present.

46. Which of the following conditions does *not* have selective loss of electroretinogram B-wave amplitude?
    A. X-linked juvenile retinoschisis.
    B. Batten disease (neuronal ceroid lipofuscinosis).
    C. North Carolina macular dystrophy.
    D. Oguchi's disease.
    E. Myotonic dystrophy.

47. The differential diagnosis of erosive vitreoretinopathy includes all the following, *except*:
    A. Stickler syndrome.
    B. Retinitis pigmentosa.
    C. Autosomal dominant neovascular inflammatory vitreoretinopathy.
    D. Incontinentia pigmenti.
    E. Goldmann–Favre syndrome.

48. The differential diagnosis of familial exudative vitreoretinopathy includes all the following, *except*:
    A. Retinopathy of prematurity.
    B. Coats'disease.
    C. Incontinentia pigmenti.
    D. Sickle cell disease.
    E. Goldmann–Favre syndrome.

49. In X-linked juvenile retinoschisis, all the following are commonly seen, *except*:
    A. Stellate maculopathy.
    B. Bilaterality but not necessarily symmetry.
    C. A marked defect in dark adaptation.
    D. Occurrence of schisis within the nerve fiber layer of the retina.
    E. Vitreous bands.

50. All the following are key features of acute hypertensive retinopathy, *except*:
    A. Retinal arteriole copper-wire appearance.
    B. Retinal arteriolar spasm.
    C. Superficial retinal hemorrhages.
    D. Cotton wool spots.
    E. Optic disc edema.

51. Which one of the following is least characteristic of chronic hypertensive and arteriosclerotic retinopathy?
    A. Narrowing of arterioles.
    B. Arteriovenous nicking.
    C. Tortuosity of arterioles.
    D. Increase in arteriolar light reflex.
    E. Macroaneurysms.

52. All the following may be associated with acute hypertensive retinopathy, *except*:
    A. Choroidal ischemia.
    B. Rhegmatogenous retinal detachment.
    C. Optic neuropathy.
    D. Proteinuria.
    E. Retinal pigment epithelial changes.

53. All the following should be included in the differential diagnosis of hypertensive retinopathy, *except*:
    A. Diabetic retinopathy.
    B. Retinal venous obstruction.
    C. Hyperviscosity syndrome.
    D. Retinal arteriolar obstruction.
    E. Ocular ischemic syndrome.

54. Which one of the following statements is *not* true concerning central retinal artery occlusion (CRAO)?
    A. The right eye is more often affected than the left eye.
    B. Central retinal artery occlusion is rare (about 1 in 10,000 outpatient office visits to ophthalmologists).
    C. Men are more commonly affected than women.
    D. Bilateral involvement occurs in 1–2% of cases.
    E. The mean age at onset is approximately 60 years.

55. The majority of central retinal artery occlusions are thought to occur by:
    A. Thrombus formation just distal to the lamina cribrosa.
    B. Embolism just distal to the lamina cribrosa.
    C. Embolism just distal or just proximal to the lamina cribrosa.
    D. Embolism at the first branch of the central retinal artery.
    E. Thrombus formation at or just proximal to the lamina cribrosa.

Retina and Vitreous

56. In addition to central retinal artery occlusion, causes of cherry-red spots of the macula include all the following, *except*:
    A. Tay–Sachs disease.
    B. Niemann–Pick disease.
    C. Autosomal dominant neovascular inflammatory vitreoretinopathy.
    D. GM gangliosidosis type II.
    E. Farber's disease.

57. The differential diagnosis of central retinal artery occlusion includes all the following, *except*:
    A. Single- or multiple-branch retinal artery obstructions.
    B. Cilioretinal artery occlusion.
    C. Central retinal vein occlusion.
    D. Severe commotio retinae.
    E. Necrotizing herpetic retinitis.

58. Ophthalmic artery occlusion, rather than central retinal artery occlusion is suggested by all the following findings, *except*:
    A. Severe visual loss (bare to no light perception).
    B. Marked choroidal perfusion defects on fluorescein angiography.
    C. Intense ischemic retinal whitening that extends beyond the macular area.
    D. Few or no cherry-red spots.
    E. Mildly decreased amplitude of the electroretinogram.

59. Combined central retinal artery and vein occlusion is suggested by all the following findings, *except*:
    A. Severe visual loss (bare to no light perception).
    B. Few or no cherry-red spots.
    C. Features of central retinal artery occlusion and retinal hemorrhages in all four quadrants.
    D. Usually an associated systemic or local disease.
    E. Development of iris neovascularization in up to 75% of patients.

60. All the following may be associated findings after central retinal vein occlusion, *except*:
    A. Optic disc edema.
    B. Optic disc venous–venous collateral (optociliary shunt) vessels.
    C. Diffuse macular edema.
    D. Neovascular glaucoma.
    E. "Box-car" bloodstream in arterioles.

61. Which one of the following findings is usually not associated with the aftermath of central retinal vein occlusion?
    A. Rhegmatogenous retinal detachment.
    B. Cystoid macular edema.
    C. Neovascularization of iris, retina, and optic disc.
    D. Cotton wool spots.
    E. Capillary nonperfusion.

62. **All the following are associated with central retinal vein occlusion, *except*:**
    A. There is an increased risk in women.
    B. More than 90% of patients are older than 50 years.
    C. It is more likely to develop in patients who have primary open-angle glaucoma.
    D. It is probably caused by a venous thrombus at the level of the lamina cribrosa.
    E. Associated findings often include diabetes mellitus, systemic arterial hypertension, and atherosclerotic cardiovascular disease.

63. **Nonischemic and ischemic central retinal vein occlusions share common features such as dilated tortuous veins and hemorrhages in all four quadrants. It is important to distinguish between the two types for all the following reasons, *except*:**
    A. Prediction of subsequent risk of ocular neovascularization.
    B. Identification of patients who have poor visual prognosis.
    C. Determination of likelihood of spontaneous visual improvement.
    D. Risk of primary open-angle glaucoma.
    E. Decision-making as to appropriate follow-up intervals.

64. **Which one of the following is least likely to be included in the differential diagnosis of branch retinal vein occlusion?**
    A. Diabetic retinopathy.
    B. Hyperviscosity syndrome.
    C. Juxtafoveal telangiectasia.
    D. Radiation retinopathy.
    E. Ocular ischemic syndrome.

65. **Which one of the following does *not* apply to branch retinal vein occlusion?**
    A. It occurs equally in men and women.
    B. It is probably caused by underlying arteriolar disease.
    C. It almost always occurs at an arteriovenous crossing.
    D. Most instances occur superotemporally.
    E. It is about 50% as common as central retinal vein occlusion.

66. **Which one of the following statements concerning retinopathy of prematurity (ROP) is *incorrect*?**
    A. It will occur in about 47% of infants who weigh 1000–1251 g (2 lb 3 oz to 2 lb 13 oz) at birth.
    B. It will occur in about 78% of infants who weigh 750–999 g (1 lb 10 oz to 2 lb 2 oz) at birth.
    C. More than 70% of infants born between 28 weeks and 31 weeks of gestational age develop ROP.
    D. It will occur in about 90% of infants who weigh less than 750 g (1 lb 10 oz) at birth.
    E. Retinopathy of prematurity develops in more than 80% of infants born before 28 weeks of gestational age.

67. Normally, vasculogenesis transforms precursor retinal mesenchymal spindle cells to capillary networks. Which one of the following statements about this process is true?
    A. It begins at about 12 weeks of gestational age.
    B. It is not affected by hypoxia.
    C. It reaches the nasal ora serrata by the gestational age of 36 weeks.
    D. Vascular endothelial growth factor is downregulated by hypoxic tissue.
    E. Retinopathy of prematurity does not occur in low birth weight children who do not receive supplemental oxygen.

68. The international classification of retinopathy of prematurity includes five stages. Which one of the following is *incorrect*?
    A. Stage I: A thin, flat, white demarcation line develops between the vascular and avascular retina.
    B. Stage II: The demarcation line develops into an elevated thickened ridge.
    C. Stage III: Fibrovascular proliferation extends toward, but not into the ridge.
    D. Stage IV: Subtotal retinal detachment occurs with or without foveal involvement.
    E. Stage V: Total funnel-shaped retinal detachment occurs.

69. Plus disease in retinopathy of prematurity:
    A. Is the hallmark of regressing disease.
    B. Is ROP plus posterior subcapsular cataract.
    C. Is ROP plus a secondary systemic abnormality.
    D. Is vascular shunting of blood that causes posterior venous engorgement and arterial tortuosity in one or more quadrants.
    E. Occurs in the early stages of ROP.

70. The differential diagnosis of retinopathy of prematurity includes all the following, *except*:
    A. Retinoblastoma.
    B. Familial exudative vitreoretinopathy.
    C. Norrie's disease.
    D. X-linked retinoschisis.
    E. Toxocariasis.

71. All the following modalities may be indicated in the treatment of ROP, *except*:
    A. Retinal cryotherapy or laser photocoagulation.
    B. Pars plana lensectomy alone.
    C. Scleral buckling.
    D. Vitrectomy with lensectomy.
    E. Lens-sparing closed vitrectomy.

72. Which one of the following statements about adult-onset diabetic retinopathy is true?

A. It is most directly related to the duration of the disease.
B. It is not affected by tight control of blood sugar.
C. It occurs in about 25% of patients who have had diabetes for 5–10 years.
D. Diabetic renal disease cannot be used as a predictor of the presence of retinopathy.
E. Less than 5% of pregnant diabetic women without retinopathy will develop retinopathy during the course of their pregnancy.

73. **One of the earliest histologic findings in the retina of patients with diabetes is:**
    A. Death of retinal capillary endothelial cells.
    B. Budding of new capillaries from venules.
    C. Apoptosis of retinal capillary pericytes.
    D. Proliferation of retinal capillary pericytes.
    E. Proliferation of retinal capillary endothelial cells.

74. **The earliest sign of diabetic retinopathy seen clinically is:**
    A. Microaneurysms.
    B. Dilated retinal venules (venous beading).
    C. Intraretinal hemorrhages.
    D. Intraretinal exudates.
    E. Macular edema.

75. **All of the following are characteristics of severe nonproliferative (preproliferative) diabetic retinopathy, *except*:**
    A. Multiple retinal hemorrhages in all four quadrants.
    B. Large areas of capillary nonperfusion (seen on fluorescein angiography).
    C. Venous beading.
    D. Macular edema.
    E. Intraretinal microvascular abnormalities.

76. **Which of the following statements concerning diabetic retinopathy is *not* true?**
    A. Although both conditions can result in legal blindness, proliferative diabetic retinopathy can cause a more profound loss of vision than can macular edema in nonproliferative diabetic retinopathy.
    B. Most proliferative vessels arise from end arterioles or capillaries.
    C. About 50% of cases of severe nonproliferative diabetic retinopathy progress to proliferative diabetic retinopathy within a year.
    D. Retinal neovascularization almost always develops into zones of retinal ischemia.
    E. As a result of proliferative retinopathy, both traction (nonrhegmatogenous) and rhegmatogenous detachments can occur.

77. **All the following are included in the differential diagnosis of diabetic retinopathy, *except*:**
    A. Radiation retinopathy.
    B. Coats' disease.

C. Sickle cell disease.
D. Leukemia.
E. Intraocular lymphoma.

78. Generally, in terms of clinically significant macular edema, which statement is incorrect?
   A. It should not be treated until visual acuity is poorer than 20/40.
   B. It includes retinal thickening involving the central macula.
   C. It shows hard exudates within 500 μm of the center of the macula (if associated with retinal thickening).
   D. It decreases visual acuity.
   E. It consists of an area of macular edema more than 1 disc area but within 1 disc diameter of the center of the macula.

79. All the following can be considered key features of the ocular ischemic syndrome, *except*:
   A. Ocular neovascularization.
   B. Decreased ocular perfusion pressure.
   C. Nonrhegmatogenous retinal detachment.
   D. Severe ipsilateral or bilateral carotid artery obstruction.
   E. Dilated, beaded retinal venules.

80. Which of the following statements concerning ocular ischemic syndrome is *not* true?
   A. Affected men outnumber affected women by a ratio of about 2:1.
   B. The condition is most common in the 5th and 6th decades of life.
   C. Bilateral involvement is seen in approximately 20% of cases.
   D. The cause is decreased ocular arterial blood flow on a chronic basis.
   E. The incidence is estimated at 7.5 cases per one million annually.

81. The differential diagnosis of ocular ischemic syndrome includes all the following, *except*:
   A. Takayasu's arteritis.
   B. Diabetic retinopathy.
   C. Giant cell (temporal) arteritis.
   D. Nonischemic central retinal vein occlusion.
   E. Familial exudative vitreoretinopathy.

82. Which one of the following statements about the attributes of normal hemoglobin is *not* true?
   A. It is composed of a four polypeptide globin chain.
   B. Each globin chain is associated with a central heme ring (ferroprotoporphyrin).
   C. The globin chains consist of a pair of alpha and a pair of beta polypeptide chains.
   D. Normal hemoglobin confers rigidity to red blood cells.
   E. Each pair of alpha and beta chains is identical.

83. **Which statement about adult hemoglobin is *not* correct?**
    A. With two normal alpha and beta chains, it is termed hemoglobin A.
    B. A single point mutation at the sixth position is termed hemoglobin C.
    C. Qualitative errors in globin chain synthesis result in hemoglobin S.
    D. Overproduction in globin chain synthesis results in CC hemoglobin.
    E. Quantitative errors (inadequate production of either normal or abnormal globin chains) in globin chain synthesis result in thalassemia.

84. **Which one of the following statements about sickle cell (SS) disease is *not* correct?**
    A. It has the most severe ocular manifestations.
    B. Sickle cell-hemoglobin SS, especially under conditions of hypoxia or acidosis, forms a crescentic, elongated (sickled) shape.
    C. The abnormal shape causes blood cells to "stack" within vessels.
    D. The stacking exacerbates the hypoxic state.
    E. Necrosis of surrounding tissue can occur.

85. **Which of the following statements is *not* true?**
    A. SS disease has the most severe systemic manifestations.
    B. SC disease has the most severe ocular manifestations.
    C. SC disease results from the inheritance of hemoglobin S from one parent and hemoglobin C from the other.
    D. Thalassemia mutation cannot coexist with normal hemoglobin A.
    E. Thalassemia can coexist with hemoglobin S to produce S Beta-thalassemia disease.

86. **Classic findings of sickle hemoglobinopathies include all the following, *except*:**
    A. Conjunctival comma-shaped capillaries.
    B. Choroidal neovascularization.
    C. Salmon-colored retinal hemorrhages.
    D. Black subretinal sunburst lesions.
    E. Retinal neovascularization in a seafan configuration.

87. **Which of Goldberg's five stages of sickle cell retinopathy listed below is incorrect?**
    A. Stage I: Peripheral arteriolar occlusions.
    B. Stage II: Arteriovenous anastomoses.
    C. Stage III: Intraneuronal retinal microvascular abnormalities.
    D. Stage IV: Vitreous hemorrhage.
    E. Stage V: Retinal detachment.

88. **The differential diagnosis of retinal telangiectasia includes all the following, *except*:**
    A. Branch retinal vein occlusion.
    B. Eales disease.
    C. Diabetic retinopathy.
    D. Radiation retinopathy.
    E. Branch retinal artery occlusion.

89. Which of the following is *not* a cause of primary retinal telangiectasia?
    A. Coats' disease.
    B. Leber's miliary aneurysms.
    C. Radiation retinopathy.
    D. Idiopathic juxtafoveal telangiectasia.
    E. Eales disease.

90. Which of the following is *not* true concerning Coats' disease?
    A. About 20–25% of cases are bilateral.
    B. It involves retinal telangiectasia.
    C. It involves aneurysmal dilatation.
    D. Male children are affected three times more than female children.
    E. Two-third of cases first appear before the age of 10 years.

91. Histopathologic study of Coats' disease demonstrates:
    A. Sclerosed narrow vessels.
    B. Ischemic retinal atrophy.
    C. Thinning of the affected segment of retina.
    D. Preservation of photoreceptors.
    E. Periodic acid-Schiff-positive material spreading to the outer layers of the retina.

92. Idiopathic juxtafoveal retinal telangiectasia consists of all of the following features, *except*:
    A. Onset in early adulthood.
    B. Mild blurring of vision.
    C. Ectatic juxtafoveal retinal vessels.
    D. Peripheral sentinel lesion.
    E. Macular exudation.

93. Associated risk factors for the development of radiation retinopathy include all the following, *except*:
    A. Diabetes mellitus.
    B. Oat cell carcinoma of the lung.
    C. Systemic hypertension.
    D. Collagen vascular disease.
    E. Acute leukemia.

94. All the following are features of radiation retinopathy. Which one appears the earliest?
    A. Microaneurysms.
    B. Discrete foci in the posterior pole of occluded capillaries with surrounding irregular dilatation of neighboring microvasculature.
    C. Telangiectatic channels.
    D. Retinal exudation.
    E. Intraretinal microvascular abnormalities.

95. The differential diagnosis of radiation retinopathy includes all the following, *except*:

A. Papilledema.
B. Central retinal vein occlusion.
C. Branch retinal vein occlusion.
D. Nonischemic optic neuropathy.
E. Diabetic retinopathy.

96. Which of the following causes of proliferative retinopathy (retinal neovascularization) does *not* have well-defined systemic abnormalities?
    A. Sarcoidosis.
    B. Sickle cell anemia (SS) disease.
    C. Eales disease.
    D. Multiple sclerosis.
    E. Hyperviscosity syndrome.

97. Which of the following factors all of which probably are involved in retinal angiogenesis does *not* act directly on retinal vessel endothelial cells?
    A. Transforming growth factor-beta.
    B. Fibroblast growth factor.
    C. Transforming growth factor-alpha.
    D. Platelet-derived endothelial cell growth factor.
    E. Angiotropin.

98. Which of the following statements about incontinentia pigmenti is *false*?
    A. It is X-linked dominant.
    B. It includes the development of initial erythematous skin lesions that eventually become pigmented.
    C. Mental retardation is common.
    D. It is one of the causes of leukocoria.
    E. In utero, it tends to be lethal to female fetuses.

99. All the following statements concerning Eales disease are true, *except*:
    A. It occurs predominantly in young (20- to 45-year-old) patients.
    B. It occurs predominantly in men.
    C. The condition usually shows periphlebitis and peripheral (especially superotemporally) retinal capillary nonperfusion.
    D. Retinal neovascularization occurs in the region of posterior periphlebitis.
    E. The cause is unknown.

100. All the following statements concerning retinal arterial macroaneurysms are true, *except*:
    A. They tend to occur in older individuals.
    B. They are typically unilateral.
    C. They often arise at an arteriovenous crossing.
    D. Affected patients show a male preponderance.
    E. They are associated with systemic hypertension.

101. Which one of the following is *not* associated with branch retinal vein occlusion?
    A. Arterial macroaneurysms.
    B. Prearteriole macroaneurysms.
    C. Capillary macroaneurysms.
    D. Venous macroaneurysms.
    E. Collateral-associated macroaneurysms.

102. The differential diagnosis of retinal arterial macroaneurysms includes all the following, *except*:
    A. Coats' disease.
    B. Retinal capillary hemangiomas.
    C. Nonfamilial acquired retinal angioma.
    D. Branch retinal vein occlusion.
    E. Branch retinal artery occlusion.

103. Which one of the following diseases is *not* associated with choroidal neovascularization?
    A. Capillary hemangioma of optic nerve head.
    B. Angioid streak.
    C. Retinochoroidal coloboma.
    D. Myopia.
    E. Optic nerve head drusen.

104. Which of the following diseases is *not* associated with choroidal neovascularization?
    A. Sarcoidosis.
    B. Rubella.
    C. Cone-rod dystrophy.
    D. Presumed histoplasmosis.
    E. Choroidal nevus.

105. A 65-year-old black woman has presenting symptoms of choroidal neovascularization and multiple tiny lid nodules. The most likely diagnosis is:
    A. Syphilis.
    B. Tuberculosis.
    C. Sarcoidosis.
    D. Toxoplasmosis.
    E. Toxocariasis.

106. Which one of the following statements about age-related macular degeneration (AMD) is true?
    A. It is the most common cause of severe central visual loss among patients older than 50 in the United States.
    B. The visual loss results directly from retinal pigment epithelial abnormalities.
    C. The nonexudative (dry) form causes the most severe vision loss.

D. It has a direct toxic effect on the photoreceptors mediated by choroidal neovascularization.

E. Less than 25% of patients who have the exudative (wet) form of AMD can be successfully treated.

107. All the following statements concerning AMD are true, *except*:
    A. The average age at onset is 75 years.
    B. No significant difference in incidence exists between the sexes.
    C. The pathogenesis of AMD is poorly understood.
    D. The prevalence is two times higher in Caucasians than in African-Americans.
    E. Some patients probably have an inherited tendency to develop AMD.

108. Which of the following has *not* been suggested in recent literature as a risk factor for the development of age-related macular degeneration?
    A. Smoking.
    B. Systemic arterial hypertension.
    C. Hyperopia.
    D. Light iris color.
    E. Higher than normal intake of beta-carotene.

109. Which of the following statements about nonexudative (dry) age-related macular degeneration is true?
    A. Typically, in its early stage it shows large (>1 disc diameter) areas of geographic (areolar) chorioretinal atrophy.
    B. Vision loss from dry AMD is generally caused by geographic chorioretinal atrophy.
    C. In its end stage, it still can be easily differentiated from end-stage pattern dystrophy of the macula and central areolar choroidal dystrophy.
    D. It does not demonstrate drusen with geographic chorioretinal atrophy.
    E. Vision is usually moderately to severely affected (visual acuity <20/50).

110. All the following fall into the classification of drusen, *except*:
    A. Hard drusen—small, round, discrete, yellow-white.
    B. Pliable drusen—large, round, discrete, yellow, sharp borders.
    C. Soft drusen—large, poorly defined, yellow, nondiscrete borders.
    D. Basal laminar drusen—myriad, small, uniform, yellow (fluorescein angiography shows "stars-in-the-sky" pattern).
    E. Calcific drusen—glistening, secondary to dystrophic calcification.

111. At presentation, a 67-year-old man has sudden loss of vision. Examination shows soft macular drusen in one eye and a macular hemorrhage and exudation in the affected eye. The most likely diagnosis is:
    A. Neovascular (wet) age-related macular degeneration.
    B. Presumed histoplasmosis syndrome.

C. Arterial macroaneurysm.
D. Diabetic retinopathy.
E. Adult Coats' disease.

112. Detached retinal pigment epithelium (RPE) may be caused by all of the following, *except*:
    A. Fibrovascular tissue beneath the RPE.
    B. Hemorrhage beneath the RPE.
    C. Chloroquine maculopathy.
    D. Fluid beneath the RPE.
    E. Coalescence of drusen.

113. High myopia is defined as an eye that has:
    A. >9.5 diopters of myopia.
    B. >6 diopters of myopia.
    C. >8.5 diopters of myopia.
    D. >5 diopters of myopia.
    E. >7.5 diopters of myopia.

114. All the following may be seen in high myopic eyes, *except*:
    A. Tilted disc.
    B. Macular lacquer cracks.
    C. Posterior staphyloma.
    D. Vitreous syneresis.
    E. Axial length of 25 mm.

115. Which of the following does *not* occur with high myopia?
    A. Subnormal visual acuity.
    B. Suboptimal binocularity.
    C. Abnormal color vision.
    D. Image magnification.
    E. Impaired dark adaptation.

116. All of the following may be seen with central serous chorioretinopathy, *except*:
    A. Recurrences.
    B. Yellowish-white subretinal deposits.
    C. Retinal pigment epithelial detachment.
    D. Retinal hemorrhage and exudation.
    E. Retinal pigment epithelial mottling.

117. Which one of the following does *not* apply to central serous chorioretinopathy?
    A. Increased frequency in intelligent type A men especially at times of physical strain or emotional stress.
    B. A history of migraine-type headache.
    C. Systemic corticosteroid use.
    D. Prior treatment with vasoconstrictive agents.
    E. Commonly occurs in childhood.

118. **Fluorescein angiography in central serous chorioretinopathy shows:**
    A. Prominent leakage during the arterial phase.
    B. A smokestack, more characteristic of a pure RPE detachment.
    C. The area of serous retinal detachment does not fill completely and has indistinct borders.
    D. The RPE detachment component usually is about two-third of the size of the retinal detachment.
    E. The RPE detachment component "lights up" during the venous phase.

119. **A full-thickness macular hole shows all of the following features, *except*:**
    A. Yellow spots in the base of the hole.
    B. Cecocentral scotoma.
    C. A small surrounding cuff of subretinal fluid.
    D. A round central retinal tissue defect.
    E. Cystic retinal changes surrounding the hole.

120. **Most cases of full-thickness macular holes are:**
    A. Of unknown cause (idiopathic).
    B. Secondary to trauma.
    C. Caused by vitreoretinal macular traction.
    D. Proliferative diabetic retinopathy.
    E. Cystoid macular edema.

121. **In Gass' four stages of macular hole formation, stage I macular hole (premacular hole):**
    A. Is theorized to be incited by focal shrinkage of the vitreous cortex in the foveal area.
    B. Shows a very superficial hole in the inner retina.
    C. Demonstrates early degenerative changes in the photoreceptors.
    D. Shows a separation of the cortical vitreous from the internal limiting membrane.
    E. Clinically involves no visible signs on ophthalmoscopy or biomicroscopy.

122. **Which of the following is least likely to be included in the differential diagnosis of macular hole?**
    A. Epiretinal membrane.
    B. Cystoid macular edema.
    C. Retinal pigment epithelial detachment.
    D. Vitreomacular traction syndrome.
    E. Solar retinopathy.

123. **Which of the following is *not* a synonym for epiretinal membrane?**
    A. Macular pucker.
    B. Premacular fibrosis or gliosis.
    C. Cellophane maculopathy.
    D. Vitreous veil.
    E. Surface-wrinkling retinopathy.

124. Which of the following cells are *not* associated with epiretinal membranes?
    A. Retinal pigment epithelial cells.
    B. Oligodendrocytes.
    C. Fibrous astrocytes.
    D. Fibrocytes.
    E. Macrophages.

125. Patients who have an epiretinal membrane may complain of all of the following symptoms, *except*:
    A. Mild or marked metamorphopsia.
    B. Loss of visual acuity.
    C. Central photopsia.
    D. Macropsia.
    E. Delayed dark adaptation.

126. Which of the following is least likely to be included in the differential diagnosis of vitreomacular traction syndrome?
    A. Epiretinal membrane
    B. Cystoid macular edema
    C. Retinal pigment epithelial detachment
    D. Idiopathic macular hole
    E. Solar retinopathy.

127. The hallmark of vitreomacular traction syndrome is:
    A. Persistent anterior-to-posterior traction on the macula usually visible clinically.
    B. Hypofluorescent angiographic appearance in the arterial phase.
    C. Total disappearance of the beam on Watzke–Allen testing.
    D. A characteristic A-scan ultrasonic appearance.
    E. Complaint of central glare during night driving.

128. Which of the following statements about vitreomacular traction syndrome is true?
    A. If surgical treatment is performed, an improvement of visual acuity by at least four lines should be expected.
    B. Most patients do not require treatment.
    C. Treatment should be considered if the visual acuity is 20/30 or worse.
    D. In a significant percentage of cases (>10%), spontaneous resolution occurs with completion of the posterior vitreous separation.
    E. Surgical treatment offers no hope when the visual acuity drops below 20/80.

129. Cystoid macular edema has been seen with all of the following, *except*:
    A. Retinal capillary hemangioma.
    B. Topical epinephrine.
    C. Choroidal hemangioma.
    D. Oral tetracycline.
    E. Oral nicotinic acid.

130. Which of the following statements about cystoid macular edema (CME) is *not* true?
    A. It occurs in about 1% of eyes following modern cataract surgery.
    B. Inadvertent rupture of the posterior capsule confers a higher risk of CME.
    C. Persistent vitreous traction to anterior segment structures confers a higher risk of CME.
    D. Diabetic retinopathy confers a higher risk of CME.
    E. If performed 3 months or more after cataract surgery, Nd:YAG laser capsulectomy confers a higher risk of CME.

131. Cystoid macular edema may be seen in all of the following, *except*:
    A. Retinitis pigmentosa.
    B. Pars planitis.
    C. Choroidal hemangioma.
    D. Panretinal photocoagulation.
    E. GM2 gangliosidosis type II (Sandhoff's disease).

132. Treatment of cystoid macular edema includes all of the following, *except*:
    A. Corticosteroids.
    B. Cyclooxygenase inhibitors.
    C. Hydrochlorothiazide.
    D. Acetazolamide.
    E. Hyperbaric oxygen.

133. At presentation, a 33-year-old patient has a central nonrhegmatogenous retinal detachment and a peculiar gray area within the temporal portion of the optic nerve. The most likely diagnosis is:
    A. Congenital pit of the optic nerve.
    B. Rhegmatogenous retinal detachment in which the hole was not found.
    C. Central serous chorioretinopathy.
    D. Choroidal hemangioma.
    E. Malignant myopia.

134. Which one of the following statements regarding colobomas of the eye is true?
    A. Retinochoroidal and optic nerve colobomas are not associated with systemic abnormalities.
    B. Treatment of posterior nonrhegmatogenous retinal detachments is scleral buckling.
    C. Associated retinal detachments are usually nonrhegmatogenous.
    D. They can occur anywhere along the line of the fusion of the embryonic fissure.
    E. The embryonic fissure fuses completely by the 5th week of gestation.

135. CHARGE syndrome consists of all of the following, *except*:
    A. Cirrhosis.
    B. Heart disease and choanal atresia.
    C. Retarded growth.
    D. Genital hypoplasia.
    E. Ear anomalies and/or deafness

136. Which of the following is *not* part of the morning glory optic disc anomaly?
    A. Enlarged optic disc with central excavation.
    B. Rhegmatogenous retinal detachment.
    C. Central tuft of dysplastic white retina.
    D. Peripapillary subretinal fibrosis.
    E. Straightened retinal vessels, often sheathed, emanating from the edge of the optic disc.

137. All of the following can cause papillitis, macular exudation, and optic neuritis, *except*:
    A. Idiopathic optic neuritis.
    B. Diabetic optic neuropathy.
    C. Radiation optic neuropathy.
    D. Malignant hypertension.
    E. Anterior ischemic optic neuropathy.

138. Angioid streaks:
    A. Are mainly present at birth.
    B. Are caused by trauma only.
    C. Have a vascular origin.
    D. May form circumferentially around the peripapillary area.
    E. Radiate in a meridional direction from the border of the optic disc.

139. Which of the following statements concerning angioid streaks is *false*?
    A. They can be red.
    B. They can be medium to dark brown.
    C. They are surrounded by normal RPE.
    D. They can be gray.
    E. The RPE in the macula may appear mottled (peau d'orange).

140. All of the following can be associated with angioid streaks, *except*:
    A. Acromegaly.
    B. Ehlers–Danlos syndrome.
    C. Hemochromatosis.
    D. Hereditary spherocytosis.
    E. Sarcoidosis.

141. All of the following can be associated with angioid streaks, *except*:
    A. Paget's disease of bone.
    B. Tuberous sclerosis.
    C. Von Hippel–Lindau disease.
    D. Pseudoxanthoma elasticum.
    E. Abetalipoproteinemia.

142. The normal ora serrata has all of the following attributes, *except*:
   A. It is encompassed by approximately 14 dentate processes.
   B. It has more opalescent retina than is found posterior to this region.
   C. It includes small rows of microcystoid cavities.
   D. It has a darker underlying retinal pigment epithelium than is found posterior to this region.
   E. It is a continuation of the retina with the nonpigmented ciliary epithelium.

143. The vitreous base:
   A. Shows traumatic retinal breaks at its posterior aspect.
   B. Shows rhegmatogenous retinal breaks at its anterior aspect.
   C. Is more prominent in the lightly pigmented fundus, an area where the vitreous body, retina, and pigment epithelium all are loosely adherent to one another.
   D. Measures about 3.2 mm in width.
   E. Is usually wider temporally than nasally.

144. Which of the following is *incorrect* concerning degenerative adult retinoschisis?
   A. An acquired primary degenerative form exists.
   B. It is usually unilateral and temporal.
   C. An inherited X-linked form exists.
   D. An acquired secondary degenerative form exists.
   E. Large well-delineated holes often with rolled edges may develop in the inner layer of the schisis.

145. Which of the following statements about paving-stone degeneration of the peripheral retina is true?
   A. It is a prerhegmatogenous detachment lesion.
   B. It usually has an abrupt onset with symptoms of metamorphopsia.
   C. It is most commonly located superiorly just posterior to the equator.
   D. Although the lesions may extend circumferentially, they more commonly extend meridionally.
   E. Choriocapillaris is usually absent and chorioretinal scar formation occurs in the region of the lesion.

146. Which of the following statements about lattice degeneration of the retina is true?
   A. The lesions are generally oriented obliquely near the equator.
   B. Pigmentary changes within the lesion are seen in less than 40% of cases.
   C. It is so named because more than 75% of lesions contain a latticework of fine white lines.
   D. It may occur radially along vessels especially in Stickler syndrome, an autosomal dominant entity.
   E. It is located most commonly in the horizontal meridian.

147. **Which of the following statements about lattice degeneration of the retina is true?**
    A. It is present in about 20% of adult eyes.
    B. In about 5–10% of cases it will cause a detachment during the life of the patient.
    C. Prophylactic treatment is warranted in most cases.
    D. The lesion affects only the retina, not the vitreous body.
    E. Horseshoe retinal breaks usually occur on the anterior edge of the lesion.

148. **All of the following are risk factors for the development of retinal breaks, *except*:**
    A. Gender.
    B. Myopia.
    C. Lattice degeneration of the retina.
    D. Ocular nonsurgical trauma.
    E. Age of patient.

149. **Which statement about retinal tears is correct?**
    A. Uncommonly they are caused by posterior vitreous detachment.
    B. In a horseshoe tear the free-edge points toward the ora serrata.
    C. A round hole with an overlying operculum is less likely to cause a detachment than a horseshoe tear.
    D. Myopia accounts for about 25% of all retinal detachments.
    E. The most common type of retinal break after blunt trauma is a round hole with an operculum.

150. **Which of the following is *not* usually included in the differential diagnosis of retinal break?**
    A. Enclosed oral bays.
    B. White with/without pressure.
    C. Retinal erosions.
    D. Chorioretinal scars.
    E. Albinotic spots of the peripheral fundus.

151. **All of the following apply to the development of a rhegmatogenous retinal detachment, *except*:**
    A. Retinal break.
    B. Vitreous liquefaction sufficient for fluid to pass under the retina.
    C. Posterior vitreous detachment.
    D. Vitreoretinal adhesion.
    E. Epiretinal membrane formation.

152. **Retinal attachment is usually maintained by all of the following, *except*:**
    A. An adhesive-like mucopolysaccharide in the subretinal space.
    B. Oncotic pressure differences between the choroid and subretinal space.
    C. Large- and medium-sized choroidal vessel suction.

D. Hydrostatic or hydraulic forces related to intraocular pressure.
E. Metabolic transfer of ions and fluid by the retinal pigment epithelium.

153. Which of the following statements about vitreous liquefaction is true?
    A. It occurs normally in the aging retina (synchysis senilis).
    B. A single progressively enlarging pool of fluid (lacuna) is always found.
    C. Intravitreal lacunae are not optically empty but show gray fluid zones.
    D. Development of vitreous liquefaction is not affected by ocular trauma.
    E. It is independent of the development of a posterior vitreous detachment.

154. Risk factors for the development of rhegmatogenous retinal detachment include all of the following, *except*:
    A. Pseudophakia.
    B. Cytomegalovirus retinitis associated with AIDS.
    C. Penetrating nonsurgical ocular trauma.
    D. High hyperopia (>+6 diopters).
    E. High myopia (>-6 diopters).

155. Which of the following histologic criteria is *not* important in differentiating a true retinal detachment from an artifactitious one?
    A. Fluid in the subretinal space.
    B. Retinal pigment epithelium degeneration.
    C. Photoreceptor degeneration.
    D. Pigment adherent to the photoreceptors.
    E. Outer nuclear degeneration.

156. Of the following, which is the least used option for managing a primary rhegmatogenous retinal detachment?
    A. Observation.
    B. Laser demarcation.
    C. Permanent scleral buckle.
    D. Temporary scleral buckle (e.g. Lincoff balloon).
    E. Pneumatic retinopexy.

157. In a serous retinal detachment, all of the following are key features, *except*:
    A. Elevation of the retina.
    B. Shifting, dependent subretinal fluid.
    C. Presence of a retinal break or traction.
    D. Universal decrease in central vision.
    E. Being secondary to local ocular or systemic problems.

158. Coats' disease, a cause of serous retinal detachment:
    A. Is a condition of male patients that peaks in incidence toward the end of the second decade of life.
    B. Is a condition of abnormal telangiectatic vessels that occur only in the periphery.
    C. Never causes a bullous detachment of the retina.

D. Is characterized by fluid that is low in lipid and high in protein when intraretinal or subretinal leakage occurs.
E. Is an idiopathic disorder of the retina that causes the vessels to become telangiectatic and leak fluid.

159. Which one of the following conditions is *not* associated with serous retinal detachment?
    A. Vogt–Koyanagi–Harada syndrome.
    B. Lattice degeneration of the retina.
    C. Nanophthalmos.
    D. Uveal effusion syndrome.
    E. Optic nerve pit.

160. All of the following are helpful in ruling out long-standing serous retinal detachment, *except*:
    A. A retinal break.
    B. Normal retinal pigment epithelium.
    C. A demarcation line.
    D. Vitreoretinal traction.
    E. A smooth and convex internal surface.

161. The differential diagnosis of serous retinal detachment includes all of the following, *except*:
    A. Retinoschisis.
    B. Rhegmatogenous retinal detachment.
    C. Central serous chorioretinopathy.
    D. Retinal or subretinal cyst.
    E. Choroidal tumor.

162. Marked choroidal hemorrhage is:
    A. Spontaneous in most cases.
    B. Treated well with modern vitreoretinal surgery, yet most patients eventually have visual loss.
    C. Present to some degree in more than 25% of patients after extracapsular cataract extraction and lens implantation.
    D. Not affected by systemic conditions.
    E. Independent of the placement of a scleral buckle at the time of vitrectomy.

163. Which one of the following is *not* an associated feature of significant choroidal hemorrhage?
    A. One or more dome-shaped choroidal protrusions.
    B. Darkening of the red reflex.
    C. Breakthrough vitreous hemorrhage.
    D. Absence of pain even in the face of a massive choroidal hemorrhage.
    E. Rhegmatogenous retinal detachment.

164. Which statement concerning massive choroidal hemorrhage during cataract surgery is *false*?

A. It complicates more than 0.9% of cataract surgeries.
B. Severe intraoperative pain occurs at the time of onset.
C. Sudden iris prolapse occurs.
D. Forward movement of the cataract and vitreous body occurs.
E. Darkening of the red reflex is noted.

165. Proliferative vitreoretinopathy is:
A. An increase in avascular tissue associated with a rhegmatogenous retinal detachment.
B. Fibrovascular tissue on the internal surface of the retina.
C. Always associated with diabetic retinopathy.
D. A rare cause of secondary failure of a previously successful retinal reattachment procedure.
E. Usually associated with glaucoma.

166. All of the following are key features of proliferative vitreoretinopathy, *except*:
A. Flattening of the retina.
B. Epiretinal or subretinal fibrous proliferation.
C. Membrane contracture.
D. Retinal shortening.
E. Formation of new retinal breaks.

167. Which of the following is *not* a usual ocular manifestation of proliferative vitreoretinopathy?
A. Macular pucker.
B. Marked vitreous flare.
C. Increased stiffness of the detached retina.
D. Increased undulation of the detached retina.
E. Star folds.

168. The differential diagnosis of proliferative vitreoretinopathy includes all of the following, *except*:
A. Proliferative diabetic retinopathy with tractional retinal detachment.
B. Severe preproliferative diabetic retinopathy.
C. Severe choroidal detachments.
D. Severe ocular hypotony.
E. Vitreoretinal traction syndrome with retinal detachment.

169. Posterior segment ocular trauma can occur after all of the following, *except*:
A. Blunt trauma with globe perforation.
B. Blunt trauma without globe perforation.
C. A sharp penetrating injury of the globe.
D. Glaucoma surgery.
E. High-velocity injury of the orbit by a foreign object.

170. Which of the following is *not* usually an associated finding after posterior segment trauma?

A. Retinal hemorrhage.
   B. Choroidal rupture.
   C. Serous retinal detachment.
   D. Cataract.
   E. Proliferative vitreoretinopathy.

171. Blunt injury to the globe is usually associated with all of the following, *except*:
   A. Giant retinal tear.
   B. Retinal dialysis.
   C. Macular hole.
   D. Avulsion of the vitreous base.
   E. Avulsion of the medial rectus tendon.

172. General principles in dealing with penetrating ocular trauma include all of the following, *except*:
   A. Primary closure of the penetrating wound.
   B. Removal of foreign material.
   C. Preferred use of topical anesthesia during surgery.
   D. Anatomic and visual rehabilitation of the eye.
   E. Prevention of further or secondary injury to the involved eye.

173. Which one of the following statements about Terson's syndrome is correct?
   A. It includes any type of intraocular hemorrhage that follows spontaneous or trauma-induced intracranial bleeding.
   B. It occurs in less than 10% of cases of intracranial bleeding.
   C. It is usually unilateral.
   D. It generally results in irreversible visual loss.
   E. The rare associated retinal detachment requires surgical intervention.

174. The differential diagnosis of Purtscher's retinopathy includes all of the following, *except*:
   A. Terson's syndrome.
   B. Shaken baby syndrome.
   C. Valsalva retinopathy.
   D. Commotio retinae.
   E. Blood dyscrasia.

175. All of the following systemic diseases can be associated with Purtscher's retinopathy, *except*:
   A. Severe head, chest, or long bone trauma.
   B. Acute pancreatitis.
   C. Fat embolism syndrome.
   D. Systemic lupus erythematosus.
   E. Chronic lung disease.

176. Which of the following does *not* apply to shaken baby syndrome?
   A. It involves intracranial or ocular bleeding without external signs of head trauma.

B. Permanent vision loss is uncommon.
C. It occurs mainly in children younger than 12 months.
D. The pathogenesis of the ocular hemorrhage is not well understood.
E. The intraretinal hemorrhages tend to be concentrated in the posterior pole.

177. The visible light (optical spectrum) that the eye primarily perceives is between:
    A. 400 nm and 760 nm.
    B. 200 nm and 577 nm.
    C. 390 nm and 590 nm.
    D. 455 nm and 680 nm.
    E. 420 nm and 597 nm.

178. Protective mechanisms within and around the eye include all of the following, *except*:
    A. The cornea absorbs most UV-B (280–315 nm) and UV-C (<280 nm) wavelengths as well as some infrared radiation.
    B. The lens absorbs most UV-A (315–400 nm) and visible blue light wavelengths.
    C. The aqueous humor absorbs near infrared (760–820 nm) light.
    D. The eyebrows, squint and blink reflexes have protective functions.
    E. Macular xanthophyll absorbs near UV and blue light wavelengths.

179. Solar retinopathy includes all of the following events, *except*:
    A. It is induced by direct or indirect solar viewing.
    B. Visual acuity is initially reduced to 20/40 to 20/200.
    C. A small yellow spot is surrounded by a gray margin in the central fovea.
    D. In the late stage, focal depression in the retinal region or retinal pigment epithelial mottling occurs.
    E. Usually a return to 20/30 to 20/50 vision occurs without scotoma or metamorphopsia.

180. A 65-year-old welder comes to the emergency department directly from work and complains of bilateral pain and photophobia. The most likely cause is:
    A. Infrared burn to the eyes.
    B. Acute photic keratitis.
    C. Ultraviolet absorption by the lens.
    D. Secondary anterior uveitis.
    E. Retinal toxicity and secondary choroiditis.

181. Which one of the following statements concerning chloroquine/hydroxychloroquine toxicity is *not* true?
    A. Patients who have retinopathy may be asymptotic.
    B. A chloroquine regimen that includes a daily dose of 250 mg, a cumulative dose of less than 100 g, and a duration of treatment of less than 1 year is associated with a low risk of retinopathy.

C. A daily dose of 400 mg of hydroxychloroquine has a low risk of retinopathy.
D. Central visual fields and color fundus photography are not valuable as baseline studies.
E. The most important factor in avoiding retinal toxicity appears to be the daily dose.

182. All of the following statements concerning niacin (nicotinic acid, vitamin B6) are true, *except*:
    A. Patients who take 1.5 g or more are at high-risk for maculopathy.
    B. The maculopathy resembles cystoid macular edema.
    C. Visual symptoms when they occur usually develop weeks to months after the initial administration of niacin.
    D. Fluorescein angiography shows dye accumulation in the macula in middle to late phases.
    E. After drug withdrawal, the subjective and objective findings are partially or completely reversible.

183. All of the following can occur with excessive (1–2 g per day) doses of thioridazine, *except*:
    A. Withdrawal of the drug soon after the onset of visual symptoms does not reverse vision loss.
    B. Onset of symptoms when they occur is noted 2 or more weeks after the initial administration of thioridazine.
    C. Symptoms include nyctalopia and a brownish discoloration of vision.
    D. An early sign is pigment granularity posterior to the equator.
    E. Geographic areas of depigmentation and loss of choriocapillaris are noted.

184. Which of the following statements concerning the vitreous body is *false*?
    A. It contains type II collagen.
    B. It contains type IX collagen.
    C. It contains type VI collagen.
    D. It contains a hybrid of types V and Xl collagen.
    E. It has considerable similarities to the nucleus pulposus of the spine.

185. All of the following statements concerning the hyaluronan (hyaluronic acid) constituent of the vitreous body are true, *except*:
    A. It may be synthesized initially by the hyalocytes of the vitreous body, Müller cells, or ciliary epithelium.
    B. The degree of hydration of hyaluronan has no effect on the size and configuration of the molecular network.
    C. Hyaluronan, through steric exclusion, resists penetration into its molecular network of other molecules (depending on their size and shape).
    D. Changes in the ionic milieu of the vitreous can cause extension or contraction of the hyaluronan molecule.
    E. Hyaluronan was first isolated from bovine vitreous.

186. Which of the following statements about the vitreous is *false*?
   A. The hyaloideocapsular ligament of Wieger is where the vitreous body is attached to the posterior aspect of the lens.
   B. Erggelet's (Berger's) space is at the center of the hyaloideocapsular ligament.
   C. The canal of Cloquet arises from Erggelet's space and courses posteriorly.
   D. The area of Martegiani is a funnel-shaped region anterior to the optic disc.
   E. Vogt's (Weiss') ring surrounds and is attached to the optic disc.

187. All of the following statements concerning posterior vitreous detachment (PVD) are true except which one?
   A. Posterior vitreous detachment is a separation between the posterior vitreous cortex and the internal limiting membrane of the retina.
   B. Posterior vitreous detachment occurs in 63% of individuals by the eighth decade.
   C. Moore's "light flashes" occur in about 25% of patients at the time of PVD.
   D. On average, PVD occurs 10 years earlier in myopic eyes than in normal eyes.
   E. The most common patient complaint with PVD is "floaters."

188. Which one of the following statements about synchysis scintillans (cholesterolosis of the vitreous) is true?
   A. It is usually a result of vitreous hemorrhage.
   B. The vitreous opacities are attached to the collagen framework.
   C. The vitreous opacities tend to remain in the same plane moving in concert with movement of the vitreous body.
   D. The opacities appear as rounded white bodies.
   E. Erythrocytes are often associated with the opacities.

189. Which of the following statements about asteroid hyalosis is true?
   A. It is more prevalent in women.
   B. It is unilateral in 50% of cases.
   C. The opacities tend to settle to the most dependent part of the vitreous compartment.
   D. Calcium and phosphorus are the main elements in asteroid bodies.
   E. Histologic staining is positive for elastin and negative for lipids and mucopolysaccharides.

190. Which of the following statements about bilateral amyloidosis is true?
   A. Nonfamilial amyloidosis is always unilateral.
   B. It can be an early manifestation of the dominant form of amyloidosis.

C. The opacities first appear in the vitreous in the midperipheral vitreous body.
D. The early opacities appear thick and ropy.
E. Histochemical stains for amyloid cannot differentiate the amyloid fibrils from 10 to 15 nm vitreous fibrils.

191. Which of the following is *not* usually a key feature of persistent hyperplastic primary vitreous?
    A. Leukokoria.
    B. Cataract.
    C. Microphthalmos.
    D. Retrolenticular fibrovascular membrane.
    E. Retinal dysplasia.

192. A male child who is otherwise completely normal has leukokoria and a small eye (present at birth). The condition is probably caused by:
    A. Retinoblastoma.
    B. Persistent fetal vasculature.
    C. Retinopathy of prematurity.
    D. Toxocariasis.
    E. Coats' disease.

193. Which one of the following statements concerning persistent fetal vasculature is *false*?
    A. It may occur in a posterior form.
    B. It may occur in an anterior form.
    C. It usually is unilateral.
    D. It may show stubby, shrunken ciliary processes.
    E. It may cause late-onset angle-closure glaucoma.

ANSWERS

1. E. Müller cells, bipolar cells, horizontal and amacrine cells are located in the inner nuclear layer.
2. C. Phototransduction takes place in the outer segments of the photoreceptors, i.e. the rods and cones.
3. D. Visual processing consisting of phototransduction and higher-order processing is accomplished mainly by neurons in the retina, not by RPE cells.
4. B. Regulation of release of neurotransmitters is not a function of the RPE cells.
5. A. The blood supply of the choroid is from branches of the anterior and posterior ciliary arteries. Each terminal choroidal artery supplies an independent polygonal segment of the choriocapillaris referred to as a lobule which is in turn drained by a venule. The choriocapillaris

contains fenestrations and has a large diameter (20–25 microns) which allows the passage of multiple red blood cells at any moment in time.

6. A. LASER is an acronym for *light amplification by stimulated emission of radiation*. Blue light is scattered more than (not less than) light of longer wavelengths and is absorbed well by macular xanthophylls. Green light is absorbed well by melanin and hemoglobin. Red light is absorbed well by melanin but poorly by hemoglobin. Krypton red light is absorbed more deeply than argon green.

7. C. In 1968, a completely new approach to ophthalmoscopy was taken by the American Optical Company with its monocular indirect ophthalmoscope. This instrument produced an erect image and a larger field of view than the conventional direct ophthalmoscope. Its further claim was the ability to examine eyes through a small pupil.

8. B. The primary surgical procedure for the repair of rhegmatogenous retinal detachment is scleral buckling.

9. E. Although choroidal detachment or choroidal edema is relatively common after scleral buckling, it is not considered a complication, and it may actually be associated with a better prognosis with/without medical treatment.

10. D. The anatomic results do not usually parallel the visual results. Other factors are much more strongly predictive of visual outcome including whether the retinal detachment is a macula-on or macula-off detachment.

11. D. For clinically significant macular edema, primary treatment options include in office procedures such as intravitreal anti-VEGF injections, focal laser or grid laser.

12. C. Lensectomy is required during vitrectomy if visualization is impaired secondary to cataract or if the lens is subluxated. It is only required for vitreoretinal traction that must be dissected if located at or just anterior to the vitreous base. There is no need to perform lensectomy for a non-clearing hemorrhage or as standard procedure.

13. B. Perfluorocarbon (PFO) may be used to stabilize the retina, thereby reducing iatrogenic retinal breaks during the procedure of epiretinal membrane removal. However, unlike procedures, such as segmentation, delamination and en bloc dissection, PFO cannot expedite the membrane removal procedure.

14. E. Interpretation of a B-scan is based on three concepts: Real time, gray scale; and three-dimensional analysis. Graphic image with vertical deflection from a baseline is the characteristic trace of A-scan ultrasonography.

15. A. Although fluorescein angiography (FA) has contributed greatly to the diagnosis of many common chorioretinal diseases, limitations exist, including the ability to image the choroidal circulation and detect choroidal artery thrombosis.

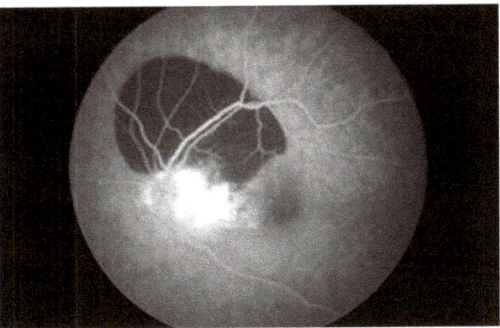

Fig. 8.1: Fluorescein angiography (FA) shows parapapillary choroidal neovascularization and a large of subretinal hemorrhage of left eye. The subretinal hemorrhage blocks the background fluorescence. By using FA per se, the choroidal circulation cannot be adequately observed.

16. A. Fluorescein has a narrow spectrum of absorption [(465–490 nm (blue)] and excitation [(520–530 (yellow-green)].
17. C. Hyperfluorescence is seen with transmission window defects and the presence of abnormal blood vessels. Subretinal hemorrhage can cause blocked choroidal fluorescence presenting as hypofluorescence on FA.
18. B. Hypofluorescence can be categorized into blockage or vascular filling defects. A retinoblastoma possesses abnormal blood vessels which present with hyperfluorescence.
19. D. Mild reactions to intravenous sodium fluorescein are defined as transient and resolve spontaneously such as nausea, vomiting, and pruritus.
20. E. Indocyanine green (ICG) angiography is an infrared-based imaging technique that is most useful for evaluating choroidal vasculature. This is particularly helpful in patients with poorly defined choroidal neovascularization (such as occult choroidal neovascular membranes or RAP lesions) in patients with polypoidal choroidal vasculopathy or in patients with central serous chorioretinopathy when FA may be of limited use.

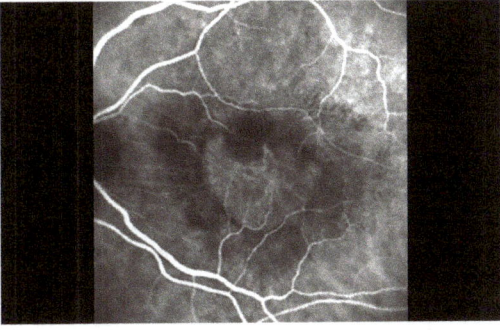

Fig. 8.2: By using indocyanine green (ICG) angiography, a choroidal neovascular net is clearly demonstrated at the macula of the left eye.

21. D. ICG does not have a cross allergic reaction with fluorescein. ICG dye contains 5% iodide and is therefore contraindicated in patients who have iodide or shellfish allergies.
22. C. The life-threatening anaphylactic reactions of ICG dyes are very rare. ICG and fluorescein anaphylactic reactions occur in equal incidence (1:1900).
23. B. Myopia affects the ERG amplitude, but implicit time appears to be unaffected.
24. A. Thinning and atrophy of the retinal pigment epithelium in the mid- and far-peripheral retina is one of the key features of typical retinitis pigmentosa.

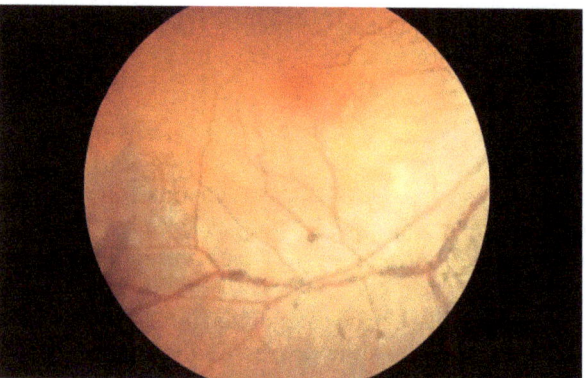

Fig. 8.3: A fundus photograph shows a case of retinitis pigmentosa of the right eye. Retinal bone-spicule pigment changes are observed in the midperipheral retina.

25. A. Usher's syndrome is nearly always autosomal recessive.
26. E. X-linked form of retinitis pigmentosa accounts for approximately 10% of cases in the United States. Affected males with this variant show subtle RPE granularity in the early years of life, but frank intraretinal bone-spicule pigmentation typically does not appear until the teenage years.
27. E. ERG amplitudes generally correlate with expected overall vision loss in later years.
28. B. Rod-cone dystrophy manifests clinically with typical retinitis pigmentosa features. In terms of visual function such as "tunnel vision", the rod-cone dystrophy is more severe than cone-rod dystrophy.
29. D. The initial changes of chloroquine retinopathy occur parafoveally and can be detected in the earliest stages by Humphrey visual field (HVF) and optical coherence tomography (OCT). On HVF, ring scotomas correspond to parafoveal RPE alterations. On OCT, photoreceptor outer segment disruptions and ellipsoid zone loss is first seen paracentrally eventually leading to the classic "flying saucer" appearance. Chloroquine and hydroxychloroquine bind to melanin in the RPE.

30. C. Cancer-associated retinopathy (CAR) involves production of autoantigens that enter the retina and cause apoptosis of retinal cells. It is typically bilateral and rapidly progressive. Common causes of CAR include small cell lung carcinoma and breast carcinoma.
31. C. Both autosomal recessive Stargardt disease and fundus flavimaculatus have been mapped to the short arm of chromosome 1. The onset of Stargardt disease is early in life, whereas the onset of fundus flavimaculatus with characteristic flecks is in adulthood.
32. A. Stargardt disease should be differentiated from cone-rod dystrophy, neuronal ceroid lipofuscinosis, pattern dystrophy, and chloroquine retinopathy. In the case of choroideremia, the macula is relatively well preserved even in the late stages of the disease.
33. D. Stargardt disease is the most prevalent inherited macular dystrophy, accounting for about 7% of the total.

It is most commonly autosomal recessive and is caused by mutations in the *ABCA4* gene. It presents with pisciform flecks at the level of the RPE surrounding an area of foveal atrophy.

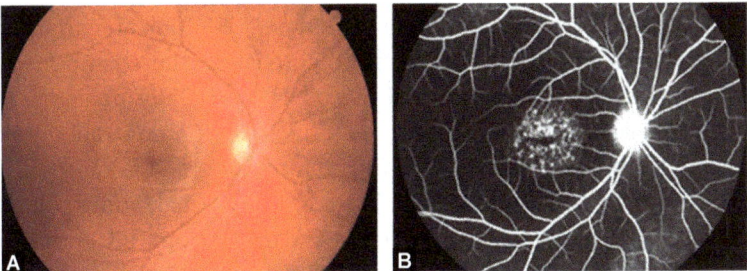

Figs. 8.4A and B: A case of Stargardt disease is viewed by (A) Color fundus photography; (B) Fluorescein Angiography (FA). The Bull's eye appearance at macula is observed.

34. E. The electroretinogram is typically normal in Best's disease. The electrooculogram is charasteristically abnormal with a severely reduced or absent light rise.

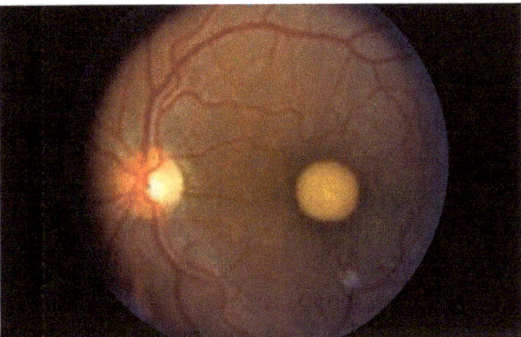

Fig. 8.5: This is a typical vitelliform (egg yolk) lesion in the left eye of a 10-year-old girl. Best disease is bilateral and symmetric in the central macula.

35. B. Pattern dystrophy is characterized by reticular pigmentation at the level of the RPE. The development of choroidal neovascularization is very rare.
36. A. Linkage analysis of a large family from North Carolina mapped the affected gene to chromosome 6q. The characteristic feature of this dystrophy is a well-demarcated area of macular atrophy at the level of the RPE and choriocapillaris, and pigment deposition in the macular region.
37. C. Choroideremia has an X-linked recessive inheritance pattern.
38. B. Female carriers of choroideremia are typically asymptomatic.
39. D. Initial changes occur in the retinal pigment epithelium in the midperipheral retina with patches of pigment mottling and hypopigmentation. Electroretinography is abnormal even in early stages of the disease.
40. B. Gyrate atrophy has an autosomal recessive inheritance pattern.
41. E. Moderate to marked myopia is found in most patients.
42. E. Congenital stationary night blindness (CSNB) is an early onset of nonprogressive difficulty with night vision. There is no histologic evidence of rod abnormalities. CSNB generally presents with a normal fundus. Inheritance patterns include autosomal dominant, autosomal recessive, and X-linked recessive.
43. B. Oguchi's disease is a form of CSNB with abnormal fundus color. Cone adaptation, final cone thresholds, and the photopic ERG response are normal in patients with Oguchi's disease.
44. A. Monotonous deposits appearing as multiple tiny white dots involve the posterior pole, spare the fovea, and extend into the midperiphery.
45. D. Stickler's syndrome has an autosomal dominant inheritance pattern.
46. C. Both electrooculography (EOG) and electroretinogram (ERG) (full field) are normal in the patients with North Carolina macular dystrophy.
47. D. Incontinentia pigmenti (IP) is an X-linked dominant disorder that has dermatological, neurological, dental, and ophthalmologic findings. In IP patients, the peripheral retinal vasculature is often poorly developed. IP should be differentiated from familial exudative vitreoretinopathy, ROP, Coats' disease, and sickle cell disease.
48. E. Goldmann-Favre disease, an autosomal recessive disorder is also known as enhanced S-cone syndrome (ESCS). Histopathology of the retina from an ESCS patient found that no rods were identified, but cones were increased two-fold, and 92% were S cones. It is a vitreoretinal dystrophy, not a type of exudative vitreoretinopathy.
49. C. Dark adaptation is normal or only minimally affected in X-linked retinoschisis.

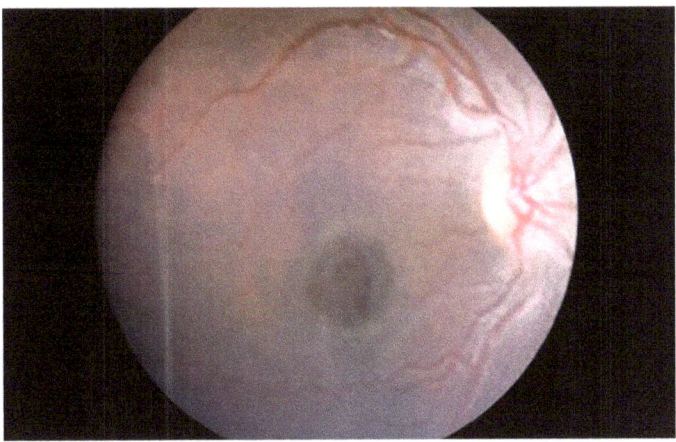

Fig. 8.6: X-linked juvenile retinoschisis shows foveal schisis which appears as small, cystoid spaces and fine striae in this color fundus photograph. Angiography shows no leakage of fluorescein associated with foveal schisis.

50. A. Retinal arteriole copper-wire appearance is caused by chronic hypertension.

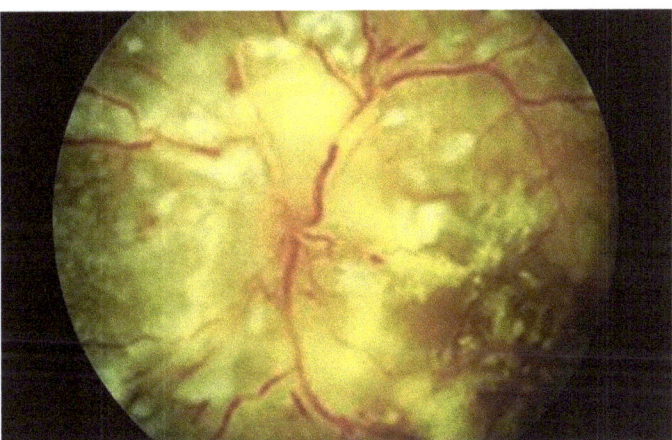

Fig. 8.7: Acute, malignant hypertensive retinopathy shows flame retinal hemorrhages, cotton wool spots, optic nerve edema, and serous retinal detachment.

51. E. Retinal arterial macroaneurysms are acquired retinal vascular abnormalities. Although they are associated with systemic arterial hypertension, macroaneurysms are not clinical characteristics of chronic hypertensive retinopathy.
52. B. Exudative retinal detachment, not rhegmatogenous retinal detachment is associated with acute hypertensive retinopathy.
53. D. Differential diagnosis of chronic hypertensive retinopathy includes diabetic retinopathy, retinal venous obstruction, hyperviscosity syndromes, congenital hereditary retinal arterial tortuosity, and ocular ischemic syndrome.

54. A. Right eyes and left eyes appear to be affected by central retinal artery occlusion (CRAO) with equal incidence.

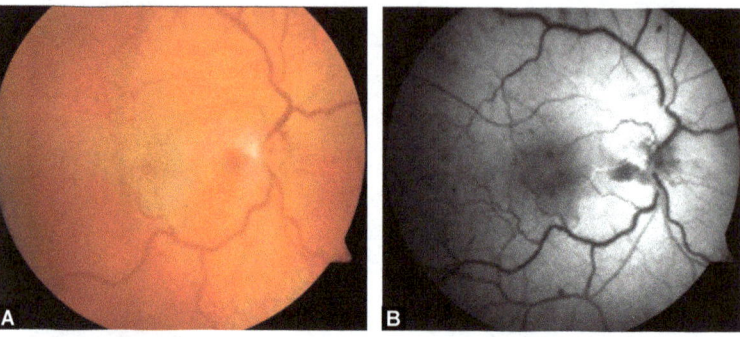

Figs. 8.8A and B: Central retinal artery occlusion (CRAO) is viewed by (A) Color fundus photography; (B) FA.

55. E. Emboli are only identified in the central retinal artery or one of its branches in 20–25% of CRAOs suggesting that an embolic cause is not frequent.
56. C. Pigmentary changes can be seen in autosomal dominant neovascular inflammatory vitreoretinopathy (ADNIV). As the disease progresses, cystoid macular edema may be seen.
57. C. Central retinal vein occlusion shows dilated tortuous retinal veins and retinal hemorrhages in all four quadrants, but does not have manifestation of retinal artery obstruction.

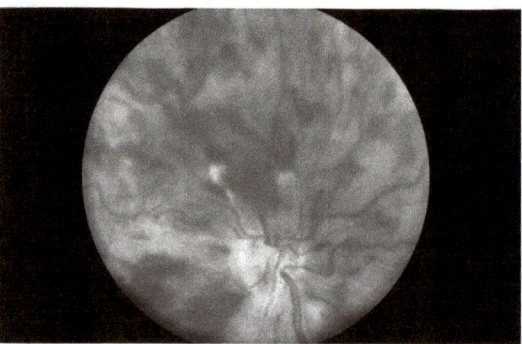

Fig. 8.9: Central retinal vein occlusion (CRVO) is viewed by red free fundus photography.

58. E. Ophthalmic artery occlusion leads to impaired function of all layers of retina (inner and outer retina layers). Therefore, severely decreased amplitude of ERG or completely extinguished ERG findings are frequently seen.
59. B. Combined artery and vein obstruction shows a cherry-red spot combined with features of a central retinal vein obstruction. Associated systemic or local disease is the rule. Collagen vascular disorders, leukemia, orbital trauma, retrobulbar injections, and mucormycosis have been implicated.

60. E. "Box-car" bloodstream pattern in arterioles may be a fluorescein angiographic sign of branch retinal artery occlusion.
61. A. There is usually no association between central retinal vein occlusion and rhegmatogenous retinal detachment.
62. A. The incidence of central retinal vein occlusion (CRVO) is slightly higher in men than in women.
63. D. The incidence of anterior segment neovascularization in ischemic CRVO is 60% or higher which may cause neovascular glaucoma. However, primary open-angle glaucoma is not a consequence of CRVO.
64. B. Hyperviscosity syndrome is a risk factor for central retinal vein occlusion but not branch retinal vein occlusion.

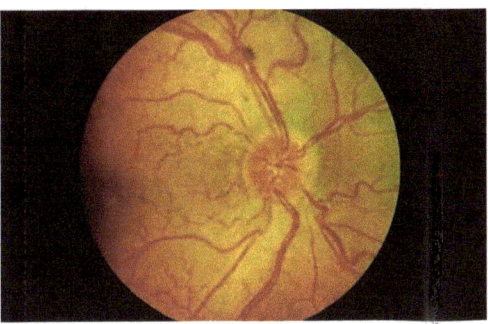

Fig. 8.10: Hyperviscosity syndrome may produce a bilateral retinopathy similar to central retinal vein occlusion.

65. E. Branch retinal vein occlusion (BRVO) occurs three times more commonly than central retinal vein occlusion (CRVO).

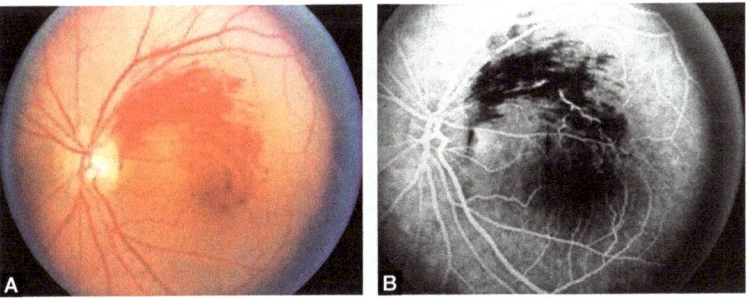

Figs. 8.11A and B: BRVO is viewed by (A) Color fundus photography; (B) FA.

66. C. Sixty percent of infants born between 28 weeks and 31 weeks gestational age develop retinopathy of prematurity (ROP).
67. C. The retinal capillary network reaches the nasal ora serrata by 36 weeks gestation and the temporal ora serrata by 40 weeks gestation.
68. C. Stage III: A ridge with extraretinal fibrovascular proliferation.
69. D. Plus disease in ROP is vascular shunting of blood that causes posterior venous engorgement and arterial tortuosity in one or more quadrants.

70. E. Toxocariasis presents as a severe unilateral intraocular inflammatory response in a child or young adult. Ocular manifestations include a severe uveitis or posterior segment granuloma often with a fibrocellular stalk extending from the disc to a posterior granuloma.
71. B. The purpose of surgery for ROP is to treat retinal detachment. For this reason, pars plana lensectomy alone would not work.
72. A. The best predictor of diabetic retinopathy is the duration of the disease.
73. C. Apoptosis of retinal capillary pericytes is responsible for selective loss of pericytes, one of the earliest pathologic findings in diabetic retinopathy.
74. A. Microaneurysms are the first ophthalmoscopically detectable change in diabetic retinopathy.
75. D. Macular edema can be seen in any stage of diabetic retinopathy.

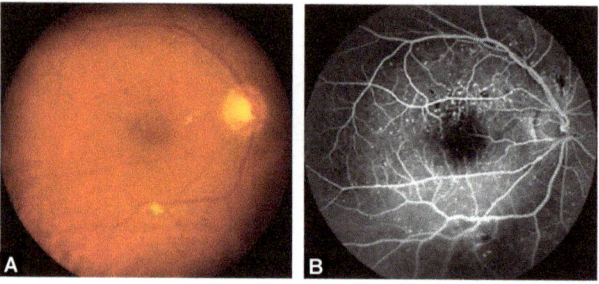

Figs. 8.12A and B: In a case of nonproliferative diabetic retinopathy, fundus photograph shows (A) Dot and blot hemorrhages, hard exudate, cotton wool spots, and microaneurysms; (B) In the FA, numerous microaneurysms are demonstrated.

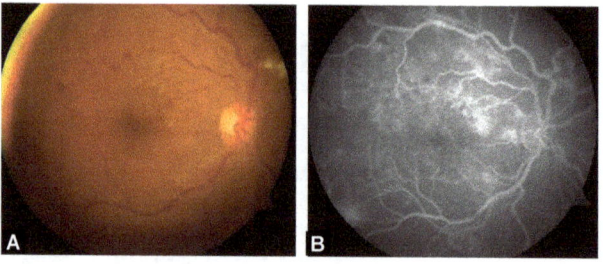

Figs. 8.13A and B: Clinically significant macular edema (CSME) is viewed by (A) Color fundus photography; (B) FA.

76. B. Proliferative vessels usually arise from retinal veins.
77. E. Intraocular lymphoma manifests with vitritis and posterior uveitis, features not typical of diabetic retinopathy.
78. A. The early treatment diabetic retinopathy study (ETDRS) defined clinically significant macular edema (CSME) for which timely laser photocoagulation is warranted. The criteria for laser treatment do not include visual acuity.

79. C. Nonrhegmatogenous retinal detachment is not a feature of ocular ischemic syndrome.
80. B. Ocular ischemic syndrome presents at a mean age of 65 years.
81. E. Familial exudative vitreoretinopathy (FEVR) is characterized by abrupt cessation of peripheral retinal vessels in a scalloped pattern at the temporal equator.

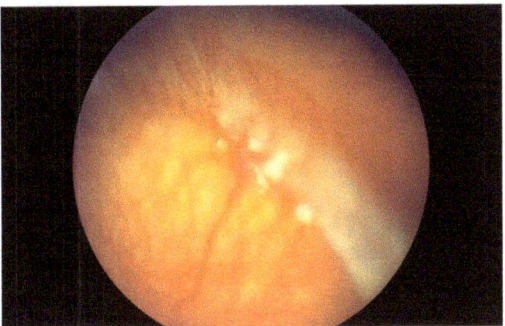

Fig. 8.14: Abrupt cessation of peripheral retinal vessels in a scalloped pattern at the temporal equator is shown in the case of FEVR.

82. D. Normal hemoglobin confers pliability (not rigidity) to the oval-shaped red blood cells which allows the red blood cells to pass easily through the microvasculature where they deliver oxygen.
83. D. The substitution of lysine for glutamic acid at this position results in hemoglobin C.
84. A. Although sickle cell (SS) disease has the most severe systemic manifestations, sickle SC and S Beta-thalassemia disease have the most severe ocular manifestations.
85. D. Thalassemia mutations can coexist with normal hemoglobin A.
86. B. Posterior segment manifestations of sickle hemoglobinopathies may be seen in the vitreous, optic disc, retina, and subretinal structures but do not typically affect the choroid.
87. C. Stage III of proliferative sickle cell retinopathy is defined as "neovascular proliferation".

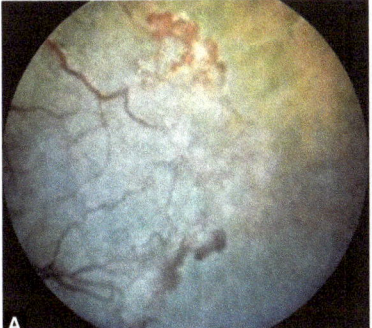 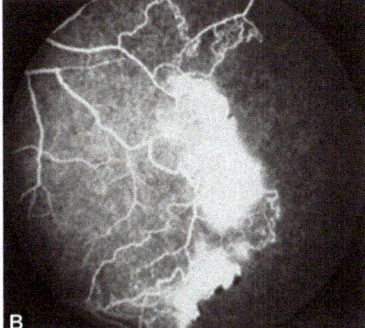

Figs. 8.15A and B: Proliferative sickle cell retinopathy is viewed by. (A) Color fundus photography; (B) Fluorescein angiography.

88. E. In most cases of branch retinal artery occlusion, there are no telangiectatic retinal vessels.

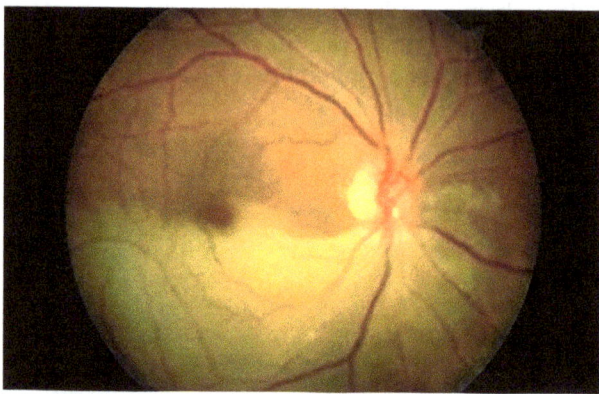

Fig. 8.16: Branch retinal artery occlusion (BRAO) (inferior) is viewed by color fundus photography.

89. C. Radiation retinopathy can cause *acquired* retinal telangiectasia.

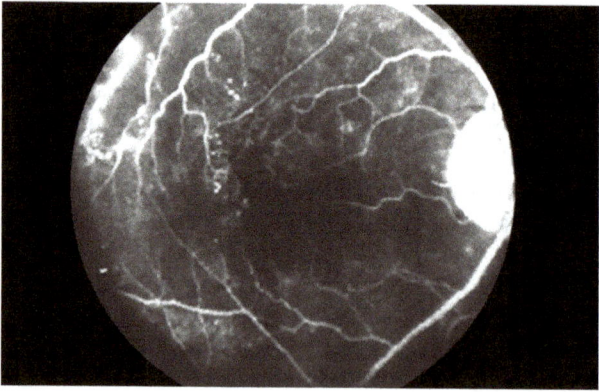

Fig. 8.17: A fluorescein angiogram shows retinal telangiectatic vessels in a case of radiation retinopathy.

90. A. In about 10–15% of cases, Coats' disease is bilateral.

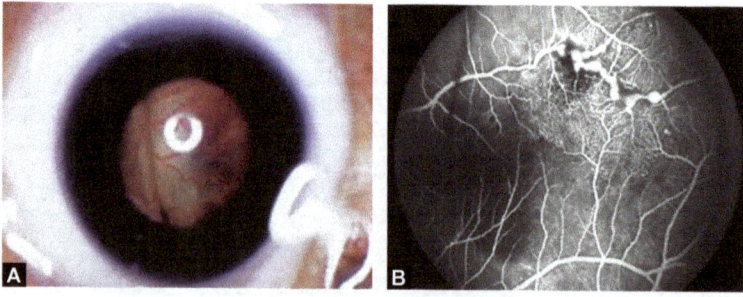

Figs. 8.18A and B: A case of Coats' disease is viewed by (A) Slit lamp; (B) Fluorescein angiography (FA), "light bulb" aneurysms are observed.

91. E. Histopathologic study of Coats' disease demonstrates irregular dilatation of intraretinal blood vessels associated with massive exudation of periodic acid-Schiff-positive material into the outer retinal layers.
92. D. Idiopathic juxtafoveal retinal telangiectasia is a disorder in the juxtafoveal region of one or both eyes. It does not typically affect the peripheral retina.
93. B. Oat cell carcinoma of the lung is not a risk factor for the development of radiation retinopathy.
94. B. The earliest fundus manifestations of radiation retinopathy are discrete foci in the posterior pole of occluded capillaries with surrounding irregular dilatation of neighboring microvasculature.
95. D. In addition, ischemic optic neuropathy, optic neuritis, and Coats' disease are also in the differential diagnosis of radiation retinopathy.
96. C. Eales disease is a bilateral disorder of young men. These patients have periphlebitis and peripheral retinal capillary nonperfusion. The cause is unknown.

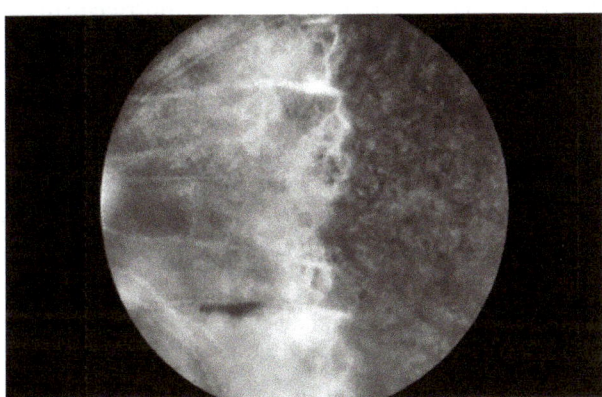

Fig. 8.19: A fluorescein angiogram shows peripheral vascular occlusion, vitreous hemorrhage, and retinal neovascularization in Eales disease.

97. A. Transforming growth factor beta does not act directly on retinal vessel endothelial cells.
98. E. Incontinentia pigmenti is an X-linked dominant disorder that tends to be lethal for male fetuses in utero.
99. D. Retinal neovascularization occurs in the region of peripheral periphlebitis.
100. D. Affected patients who have arterial macroaneurysms show a female preponderance.
101. B. Arterial macroaneurysms, capillary macroaneurysms, venous macroaneurysms, and collateral-associated macroaneurysms are often found in the area of vein occlusion. All four types are associated with hemorrhage and lipid exudation, and are found in areas of capillary nonperfusion. Prearteriole macroaneurysms are not defined.

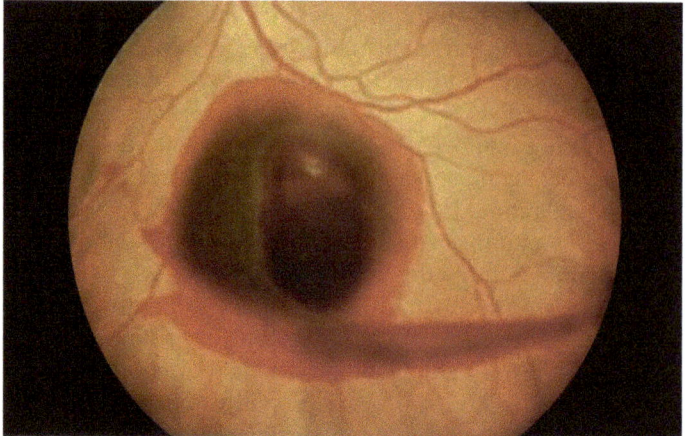

Fig. 8.20: Arterial macroaneurysm associated with subretinal, intraretinal, and preretinal hemorrhage.

102. E. Branch retinal artery occlusion is not hemorrhagic in nature.
103. A. Capillary hemangioma of the optic nerve head is also known as angiomatosis retinae, and is associated with von Hippel-Lindau syndrome.
   Retinal capillary hemangiomas are usually supplied by large feeder vessels and may occur in the optic nerve or in any part of the retina. In terms of optic nerve head drusen, hemorrhage of the optic disc is a rare complication, but peripapillary subretinal neovascularization may occur.
104. C. Fundus changes of cone-rod dystrophy are quite variable, but do not typically result in choroidal neovascularization.
105. C. Sarcoidosis is an idiopathic granulomatous disorder affecting multiple organ systems including shins. Intraocular inflammation such as uveitis and periphlebitis may stimulate neovascularization.
106. A. Age-related macular degeneration (AMD) is the most common cause of severe central visual loss among patients older than 50 years in the United States.
107. B. Female gender is a risk factor for AMD. The prevalence of AMD is 5.4% in Caucasians and 2.4% in African-Americans.
108. E. Higher than normal intake of beta-carotene has not been suggested as a risk factor for AMD. Based on AREDS, beta-carotene (15 mg daily) is one of the antioxidants that may slow the progression of AMD and the associated vision loss.
109. B. Vision loss from dry AMD is generally caused by geographic chorioretinal atrophy. This area is usually small (<1 disc area) and may surround the fovea. If the foveal center is spared, good visual acuity may be preserved.

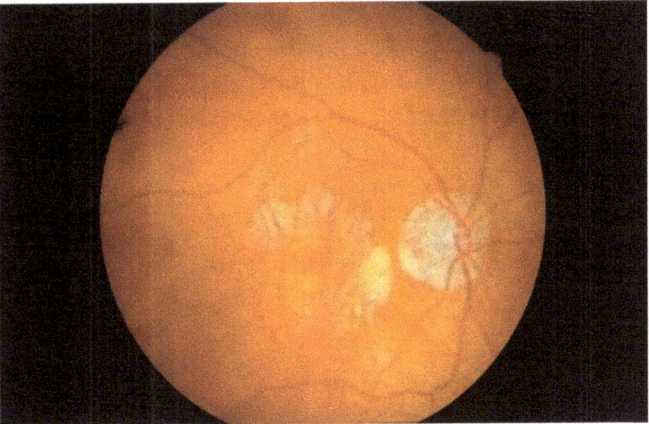

Fig. 8.21: Geographic atrophy secondary to dry AMD is viewed by color fundus photography.

110. B. Drusen consists of at least two different focal types. The first focal type, nodular drusen is hard and discrete. Basal laminar drusen are one form of nodular drusen. The second type, soft drusen, is pliable, large, round, discrete and yellow with sharp, poorly defined borders.
111. A. Neovascular (wet) age-related macular degeneration is the appropriate diagnosis.

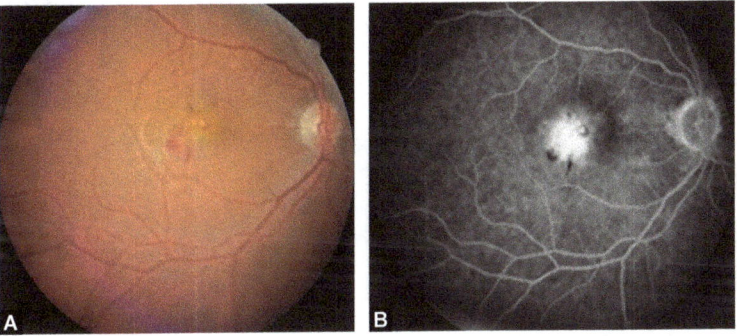

Figs. 8.22A and B: (A) Fundus photograph and (B) Fluorescein angiogram show a choroidal neovascular membrane in a case of wet age-related macular degeneration.

112. C. Chloroquine maculopathy causes atrophy of the RPE.
113. B. Myopia that is higher than –6.00 diopters is defined as high myopia.
114. E. The axial length of an eye with high myopia is generally 26.5 mm or longer.
115. D. Image minification is one of the functional defects of high myopia.
116. D. Accumulation of subretinal fluid is the key pathology of central serous retinopathy (CSR). Retinal hemorrhage and exudation are not features of CSR.
117. E. While few cases of CSR have been reported in childhood, CSR most commonly occurs in individuals aged 20–50 years.

118. C. The area of serous retinal detachment does not fill completely and has indistinct borders. On fluorescein angiography, RPE defects are hyperfluorescent in the early phase.

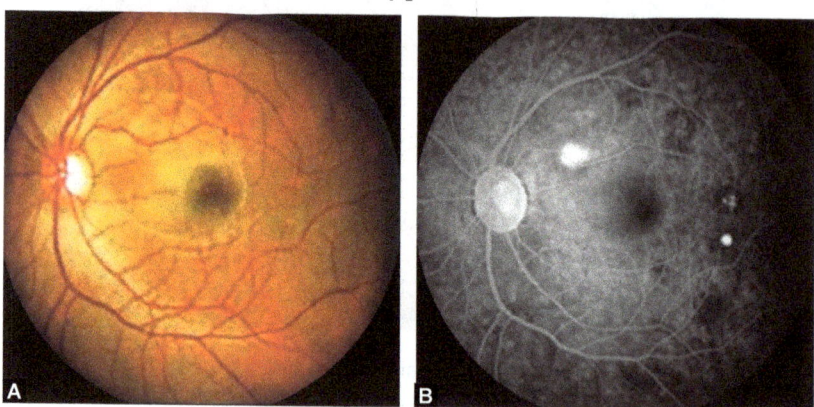

Figs. 8.23A and B: Central serous retinopathy is viewed by (A) Color fundus photography; (B) FA.

119. B. Central visual distortion or scotoma is the most common chief complaint of idiopathic macular hole.

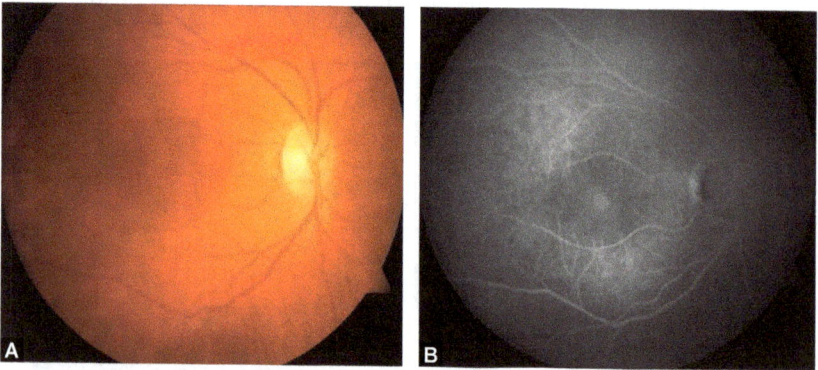

Figs. 8.24A and B: Idiopathic macular hole is viewed by (A) Color fundus photography; (B) FA. In FA, early hyperfluorescence (window defect) is noted.

120. A. The cause of most full-thickness retinal macular holes is unknown (idiopathic).
121. A. Premacular hole is theorized to be incited by focal shrinkage of the vitreous cortex in the foveal area.
122. C. In most cases, serous detachment of the RPE or pigment epithelial detachment (PED) occurs asymptomatically. Only those patients whose macula is affected will report blurred vision, metamorphopsia, micropsia, or positive scotomas. PED at the macula is slightly elevated which is different from the appearance of a macular hole or pseudohole.

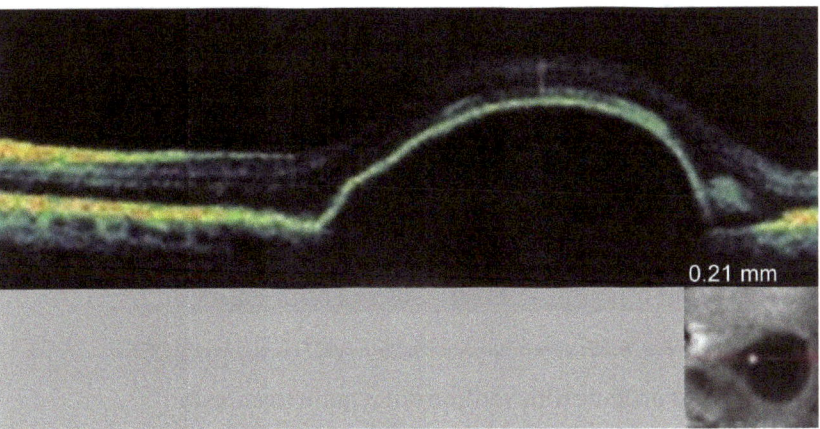

Fig. 8.25: Serous detachment of the RPE (PED) in a case of wet age-related macular degeneration is documented by OCT.

123. D. Vitreous veil is type of vitreous clouding or floater.
124. B. Oligodendrocyte is a type of glial cells in the brain, not in the retina.
125. E. Epiretinal membrane (ERM) does not cause dysfunction of rods and would therefore not affect dark adaptation.

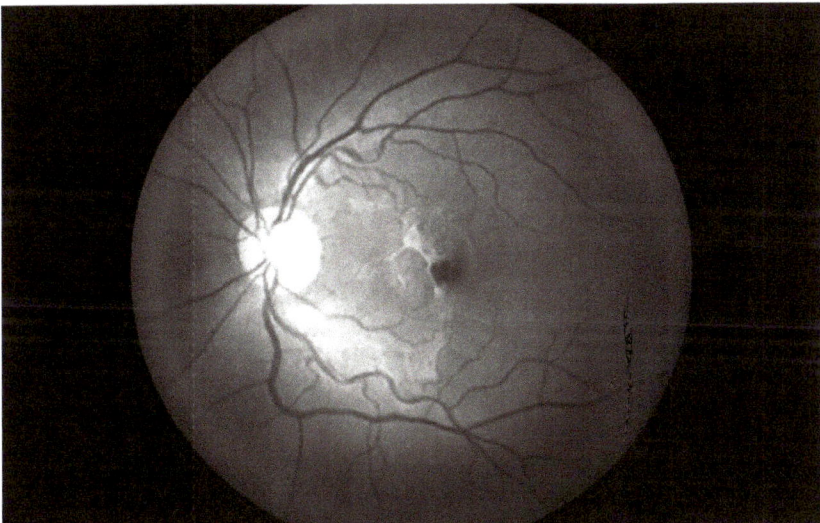

Fig. 8.26: Epiretinal membrane (macular pucker) is viewed by red-free fundus photography.

126. C. Retinal pigment epithelial detachment does not have vitreous-induced traction on the retina.
127. A. Persistent anterior-to-posterior traction on the macula is usually directly observable in vitreomacular traction (VMT) syndrome by OCT (as shown in Fig. 8.27). FA may show leakage in the macula.

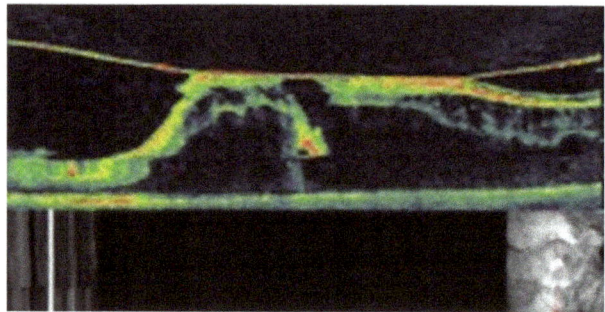

Fig. 8.27: Vitreomacular traction (VMT) is shown by OCT.

128. B. Most patients with VMT do not require treatment.
129. D. There have been no reports linking oral tetracycline to associated with cystoid macular edema.
130. E. If performed three months or more after cataract surgery, Nd:YAG laser capsulectomy does not appear to increase the incidence of CME.
131. E. GM2 gangliosidosis type II (Sandhoff's disease) has not been associated with CME.
132. C. Hydrochlorothiazide has not been found to be effective in the treatment of CME.
133. A. Congenital pit of the optic nerve can vary in color, depth, and size. Optic pits are often associated with visual field defects. A relationship between optic pits and a central serous chorioretinopathy-like presentations has been reported.

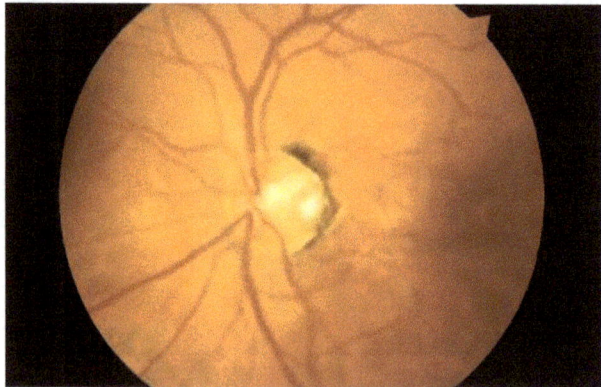

Fig. 8.28: An optic pit is seen at the temporal portion of optic disc of the left eye.

134. D. They can occur anywhere along the line of fusion of the embryonic fissure from the optic disc inferiorly to immediately posterior to the inferior pupillary frill of the iris.
135. A. CHARGE syndrome consists of coloboma, heart disease, atresia choanae, retarded growth, genital hypoplasia, ear anomalies, and/or deafness. Cirrhosis is not part of CHARGE syndrome.

136. B. One-third of reported cases of morning glory disc anomaly have an associated nonrhegmatogenous retinal detachment. Rhegmatogenous retinal detachments are not a part of this anomaly.
137. B. Diabetic optic neuropathy does not cause lipid leakage into the outer plexiform layer (Henle's fiber layer). This kind of exudation can be seen in diabetic retinopathy.
138. D. Angioid streaks typically radiate out in a cruciate pattern from an area of peripapillary pigment alterations, although they may form a circumferential ring around the peripapillary area as well.
139. C. The color of angioid streaks depends on the background coloration of the fundus and the degree of atrophy of overlying retinal pigment epithelium (RPE).

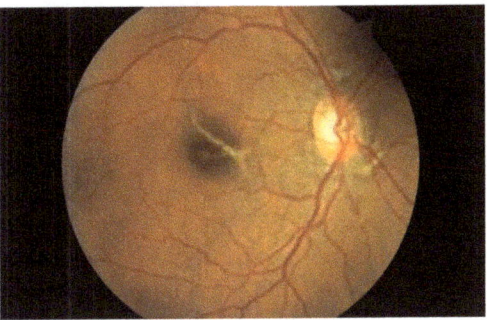

Fig. 8.29: Angioid streaks associated with pseudoxanthoma elasticum are viewed by color fundus photography.

140. E. Sarcoidosis is not associated with angioid streaks.
141. C. von Hippel–Lindau disease does not affect Bruch's membrane and is not associated with angioid streaks.
142. A. It is encompassed by approximately 20–30 dentate processes.
143. D. The vitreous base involves the full circumference of the peripheral fundus and measures approximately 3.2 mm in width. Retinal breaks frequently occur along the posterior border. In the case of traumatic detachment, breaks can occur along the anterior border as well. The description of posterior and anterior aspect is not accurate.

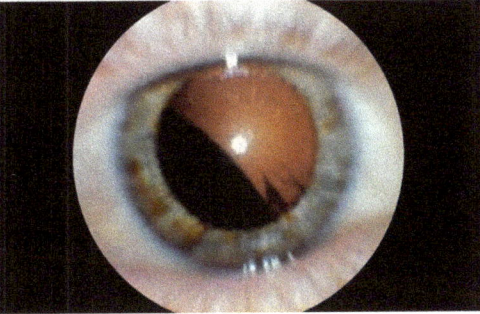

Fig. 8.30: Under a surgical microscope, the vitreous base is shown with scleral depression. The ora serrata at the peripheral retina can be observed in this photograph.

144. B. The degenerative adult retinoschisis is usually bilateral, often symmetric, and bullous.

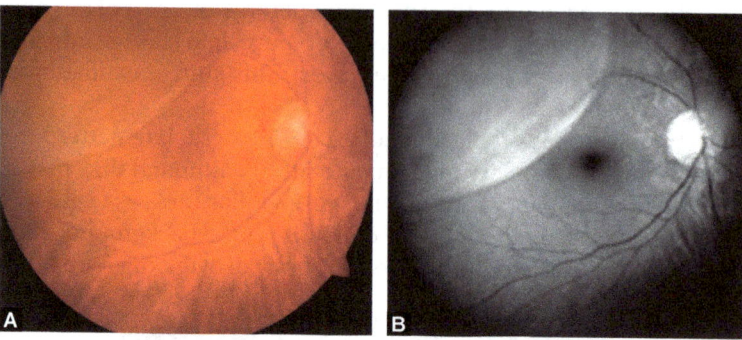

Figs. 8.31A and B: Bullous adult retinoschisis is viewed by color (A) And red-free; (B) Fundus photography.

145. E. Paving stone degeneration commonly occurs inferiorly between the equator and ora serrata, but may extend into the pars plana. Choriocapillaris is usually absent, and chorioretinal scar formation occurs in the region of the lesion.

146. D. Lattice degeneration occurs more commonly superiorly, and occurs less frequently near the inferior equator. It may occur radially along vessels especially in Stickler syndrome, an autosomal dominant entity.

147. B. About 5–10% of lattice degeneration cases will result in a detachment during the life of the patient. Approximately 20–30% of patients with rhegmatogenous retinal detachment have lattice degeneration in the same eye. This usually originates with a retinal break at the posterior margin of the lattice. Lattice degeneration is present in 6–10% of adults. Prophylactic treatment is not routinely warranted.

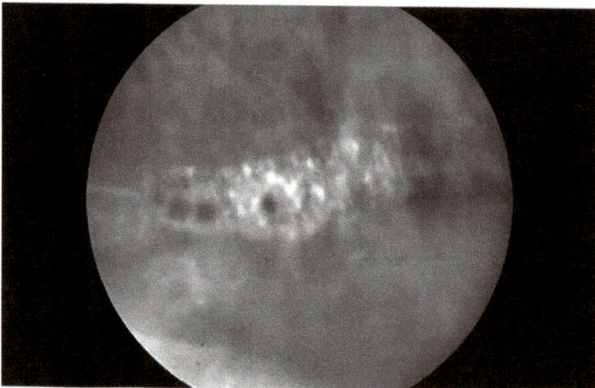

Fig. 8.32: Lattice degeneration is associated with atrophic retinal holes.

148. A. No data indicate the difference between men and women in the incidence of retinal breaks.

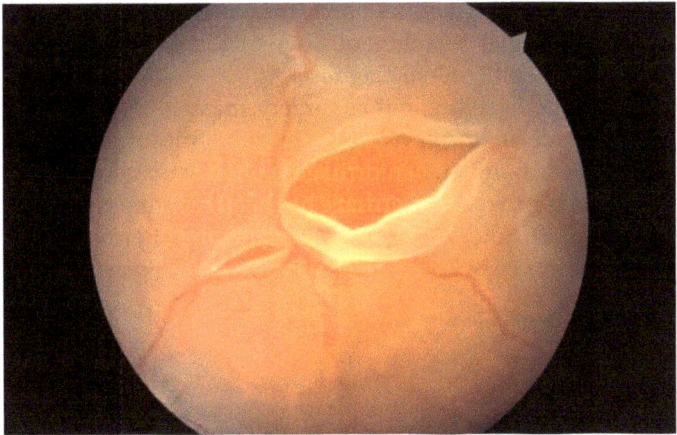

Fig. 8.33: Retinal breaks associated with shallow retinal detachment is viewed by color fundus photography.

149. C. A round hole with an overlying operculum is less likely to cause a retinal detachment than a horseshoe tear because the vitreous traction on the retina no longer exists.
150. E. Albinotic spots of the peripheral fundus are solitary lesions which do not have the appearance of retinal breaks.
151. E. Epiretinal membrane formation may be associated with nonrhegmatogenous retinal detachment.
152. C. Large- and medium-sized choroidal vessels do not have a suction function to maintain the retina in place.
153. A. Vitreous liquefaction and synchysis senilis occur normally in the aging retina.
154. D. High myopia (>−6 diopters), not high hyperopia is a risk factor for rhegmatogenous retinal detachment.
155. B. Long-standing retinal detachments are associated with atrophy of photoreceptors and cystic degeneration within the retina. These findings may be important in the differentiation of a true RD from an artifactitious one. Retinal pigment epithelium degeneration is nonspecific in many retinal diseases involving the photoreceptor-RPE-choriocapillaris complex.
156. A. Observation is not an option for treatment of a primary rhegmatogenous retinal detachment.
157. C. By definition, retinal breaks and traction are not associated features of serous retinal detachment.
158. E. Coats' disease is an idiopathic disorder of the retina that causes the vessels to become telangiectatic and leak fluid.
159. B. Lattice degeneration of the retina is associated with rhegmatogenous retinal detachment, not serous retinal detachment.
160. E. A smooth and convex internal surface is a feature of a serous retinal detachment.

161. C. One of the ocular manifestations of central serous chorioretinopathy is serous retinal detachment. Therefore, serous retinal detachment cannot be a differential diagnosis.
162. B. Despite modern vitreoretinal surgery, massive choroidal hemorrhage is still associated with vision loss in a majority of patients
163. D. A massive choroidal hemorrhage is often extremely painful.
164. A. Massive choroidal hemorrhage has been reported to complicate 0.1% of cataract extraction and 1.8% of glaucoma filtering procedures.

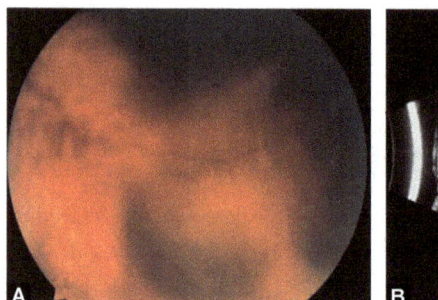
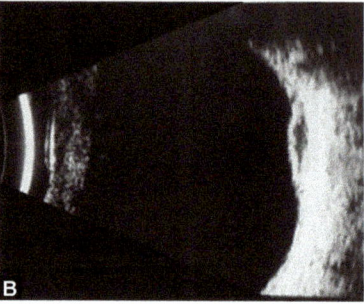

Figs. 8.34A and B: Suprachoroidal hemorrhage is associated with cataract extraction, which is demonstrated by (A) Fundus photography; (B) Ultrasonography.

165. A. An increase in avascular tissue that is independent of the vitreous is associated with a rhegmatogenous retinal detachment.
166. A. The stiffened, detached retina associated with epiretinal and subretinal membrane is the feature of proliferative vitreoretinopathy.
167. D. Decreased undulation of the detached retina is an ocular manifestation of proliferative vitreoretinopathy.
168. B. Severe preproliferative diabetic retinopathy does not have clear evidence of surface membrane formation that is a key feature of proliferative vitreoretinopathy.
169. D. Key features of posterior segment ocular trauma consist of blunt, contusive injury, with/without globe rupture; sharp, penetrating injury; and high velocity foreign body injury.
170. C. Serous detachment of the retina is usually not associated with posterior segment ocular trauma.
171. E. Avulsion of the medial rectus tendon is not usually associated with blunt injury to the globe.
172. C. In the repair of penetrating ocular wound, general anesthesia is used most commonly. This is particularly true in the case of severe lacerating injuries, pediatric patients, or patients who are uncooperative because of alcohol or drug intoxication.
173. E. Though rare, retinal detachment associated with Terson's syndrome requires surgical intervention.
174. D. Commotio retinae is associated with acute blunt eye injury and manifests as a widespread or localized whitening of the retina. Recovery of vision is common. Purtscher's retinopathy typically presents with cotton wool spots and retinal hemorrhages.

175. E. Chronic lung disease is not associated with Purtscher's retinopathy.

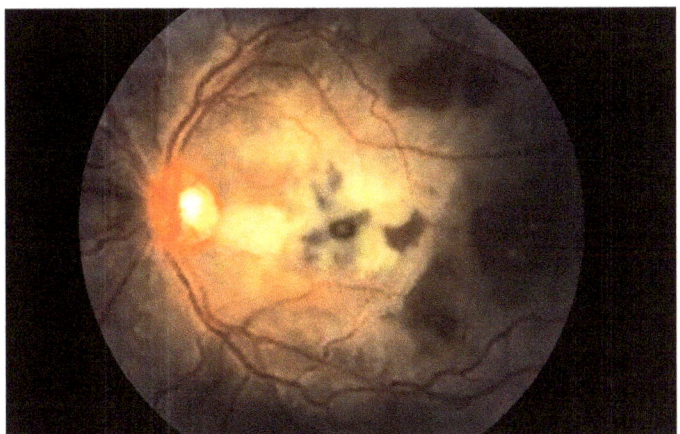

Fig. 8.35: Purtscher's retinopathy is associated with acute pancreatitis.

176. B. Some degree of permanent loss of visual acuity is common in shaken baby syndrome. Therapeutically, little can be done to alter the visual outcome.
177. A. The range of visible light is from 400 nm to 760 nm wavelengths.
178. C. Aqueous humor does not absorb near infrared (760–820 nm) light.
179. E. After several weeks, the yellow foveal lesion caused by direct or indirect solar viewing is replaced by a permanent focal depression with RPE mottling or a lamellar hole. Vision usually improves to 20/40 or better within 6 months, although scotoma and/or metamorphopsia may persist.
180. B. Acute photic keratitis is caused by ultraviolet absorption by the cornea.
181. D. Since the earliest macular changes due to hydroxychloroquine and chloroquine are nonspecific and may be indistinguishable from age-related changes, baseline central visual fields and color fundus photography are very valuable as baseline studies.
182. D. The bilateral maculopathy caused by niacin toxicity has the clinical appearance of cystoid macular edema, but there is no dye accumulation on fluorescein angiography.
183. A. With discontinuation of thioridazine soon after onset of visual symptoms, the visual loss can be reversed. However, the pigmentary changes in the fundus often progress.
184. C. The molecular constituents of vitreous do not contain type VI collagen. Type VI collagen is the major structural component of microfibrils.
185. B. The degree of hydration of hyaluronan has a significant influence on the size and configuration of the molecular network.
186. E. If peripapillary glial tissue is torn away during posterior vitreous detachment but remains attached to the vitreous cortex about the prepapillary hole, it is referred to as Vogt's or Weiss' ring.

187. C. Moore's "light flashes" occur in about 50% (not 25%) of patients at the time of posterior vitreous detachment (PVD).
188. A. Synchysis scintillans (cholesterolosis of the vitreous) is usually a result of chronic vitreous hemorrhage.
189. D. Calcium and phosphorus are the main elements in asteroid bodies.

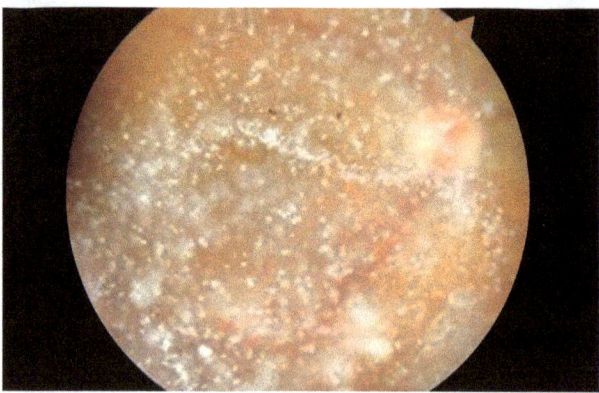

Fig. 8.36: Asteroid hyalosis is a benign condition and characterized by small yellow-white spherical opacities throughout the vitreous. In over 75% cases, asteroid hyalosis is unilateral. Asteroid bodies are associated with the vitreous gel and move with typical vitreous displacement during eye movement.

190. B. Bilateral amyloidosis in the vitreous can be an early manifestation of the dominant form of familial amyloidosis.
191. E. Although retinal dysplasia and optic nerve hypoplasia have been described, retinal dysplasia is not a key feature of persistent hyperplastic primary vitreous.
192. B. Congenital leukokoria and microphthalmia are common presenting features of persistent fetal vasculature.
193. D. In the case of persistent fetal vasculature, elongated ciliary processes are often visible readily through the dilated pupil.

CHAPTER 9

Glaucoma

Nancy Crawford, Prashanth Iyer

QUESTIONS

Identify the incorrect answer for all questions (unless instructed otherwise).

1. **The prevalence of primary open-angle glaucoma (POAG):**
   A. Is about 2% in Caucasians older than 40.
   B. Is more common in older people.
   C. Is more common in women than in men.
   D. Is about 8% in blacks older than 40.
   E. Is greater than that of angle-closure glaucoma.

2. **Significant risk factors for the development of POAG include:**
   A. Elevated intraocular pressure (IOP).
   B. Larger cup-to-disc (C/D) ratio.
   C. African descent.
   D. Cigarette smoking.
   E. Positive family history of POAG.

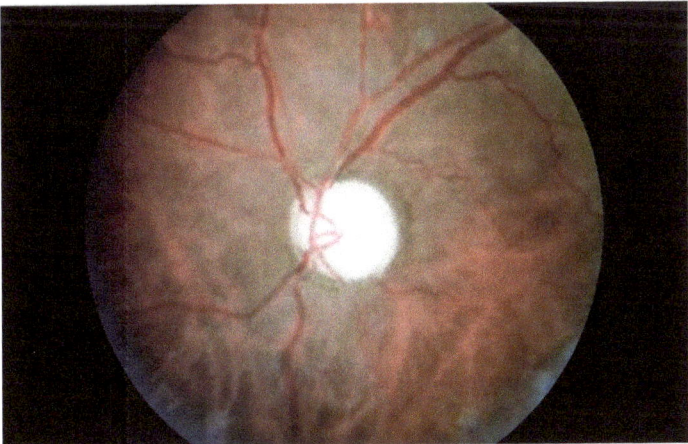

Fig. 9.1: Fundus photo of optic nerve with significant cupping.

3. According to the American Academy of Ophthalmology, preferred practice pattern, appropriate glaucoma screening includes evaluation of possible:
   A. Thinning of the optic nerve rim.
   B. Nerve fiber layer defects.
   C. Progressive change in optic nerve appearance.
   D. Intraocular pressure >21 mm Hg.
   E. Notching of the optic nerve rim.

4. Potential site(s) of internal resistance to aqueous flow is (are):
   A. Peripheral anterior synechiae.
   B. Pupillary block.
   C. The pretrabecular meshwork because of neovascular or cellular membranes.
   D. The trabecular meshwork.
   E. Increased protein and debris in the anterior chamber.

5. Juvenile onset open-angle glaucoma:
   A. Develops during the first-two decades of life.
   B. Is strongly associated with myopia.
   C. May be caused by a gene located on chromosome Iq23.
   D. Can be inherited as an autosomal recessive trait.
   E. May be caused by the gene product *TIGR*.

6. The Ocular Hypertension Treatment Study identified the following risk factors for the development of glaucoma:
   A. Elevated IOP.
   B. Increased C/D ratio.
   C. Positive family history.
   D. Thin central cornea.
   E. Older age.

7. Genetic loci for glaucoma have been identified for:
   A. Adult-onset POAG.
   B. Angle-closure glaucoma.
   C. Pseudoexfoliation syndrome (PEX).
   D. Rieger's syndrome.
   E. Congenital glaucoma.

8. The Early Manifest Glaucoma Trial (EMGT) identified the following risk factors for the progression of open-angle glaucoma:
   A. Higher IOP.
   B. The development of a disk hemorrhage.
   C. Asian ancestry.
   D. The presence of exfoliation syndrome.
   E. Thinner central cornea.

9. Errors in measurement of intraocular pressure with applanation tonometry may be caused by:

A. Excess fluorescein.
B. Extremes of corneal shape and thickness.
C. High-corneal astigmatism.
D. Deficient instrument contact time.
E. Improper instrument calibration.

10. **Intraocular pressure:**
    A. Is probably unchanged with midazolam anesthesia.
    B. Is usually elevated with general anesthesia.
    C. Tends to increase with increasing age.
    D. May increase by 9 mm Hg during the change from sitting to reclining position.
    E. Typically varies about 5 mm over the course of the day.

11. **Advantages of indirect over direct gonioscopy include:**
    A. Ability to perform indentation gonioscopy.
    B. Possible appearance of the angle as artifactitiously deep.
    C. Ability to examine the patient in an upright position.
    D. Harnessing of the slit-lamp's optics and magnification.
    E. Ease of use.

12. **Filtration angle:**
    A. Is usually narrowest superiorly.
    B. Usually forms peripheral anterior synechiae last inferiorly in patients who have angle-closure glaucoma.
    C. May exhibit a Sampaolesi line, a darkly pigmented trabecular meshwork.
    D. Usually forms peripheral anterior synechiae first inferiorly in patients who have uveitic glaucoma.
    E. May exhibit tears between the longitudinal and circular ciliary muscles after trauma.

13. **Automated perimetry with the Humphrey visual field analyzer STATPAC 2 printout:**
    A. Shows an increase in false-negative responses in patients who have glaucoma.
    B. Indicates an unreliable test when false-positive or false-negative responses exceed 10%.
    C. Global index of mean deviation is a measure of average sensitivity loss.
    D. Global index of corrected pattern standard deviation is a measure of localized nonuniformity of the surface of the hill of vision.
    E. Glaucoma hemifield test has high specificity and sensitivity for the detection of nerve fiber layer bundle defects.

14. **Artifacts of visual field testing that can produce results resembling true visual field defects include:**
    A. Cataracts.
    B. Interference from the lens holder rim.

C. Testing without correction of significant refractive errors.
D. Blepharoptosis.
E. Incorrect birthdate.

15. **Glaucomatous optic neuropathy:**
    A. Causes early nasal arcuate field defects.
    B. Affects the papillomacular bundle late in the disease.
    C. Causes wedge-shaped nerve fiber layer defects in 80% of patients.
    D. Causes pallor of the rim tissue.
    E. Usually affects the temporal areas of the superior and inferior poles of the nerve early.

16. **Patients who have glaucoma:**
    A. Suffer preferential damage to pathways from S cones (blue wavelengths).
    B. Exhibit defects with acuity perimetry testing earlier than with conventional perimetry.
    C. Have decreased pattern electroretinograms.
    D. Have normal pattern discrimination.
    E. Have decreased temporal contrast sensitivity.

17. **Nerve fiber layer defects may be evaluated by using:**
    A. Red-free light during direct fundoscopy.
    B. Nerve fiber layer planimetry.
    C. Scanning laser polarimetry.
    D. Optical coherence tomography.
    E. Retinal contour measurements.

18. **Clinical features that suggest an underlying ischemic cause for glaucoma include:**
    A. Venous trifurcations on the disc.
    B. Optic disc hemorrhage.
    C. Peripapillary choroidal sclerosis.
    D. Peripapillary vasoconstriction.
    E. Localized disc rim notching.

19. **Blood flow to the optic nerve head may be evaluated by:**
    A. Angiography.
    B. Color Doppler imaging.
    C. Laser Doppler flowmetry.
    D. Scanning laser disc polarimetry.
    E. Ocular pulse amplitude.

20. **Compared with healthy patients, patients with glaucoma have increased:**
    A. Platelet and red blood cell aggregation.
    B. Activation of the complement cascade.
    C. Incidence of migraine.
    D. Incidence of Raynaud's phenomenon.
    E. Incidence of Crohn's disease.

21. **Primary infantile glaucoma:**
    A. Appears to be familial in about 10% of cases.
    B. Is more common in girls in the United States.
    C. Has an incidence of about 1 in 12,000 in the United States.
    D. Is bilateral in 70% of cases.
    E. Is more common in Saudi Arabia and among Romany people ("gypsies") in Romania.

22. **Glaucoma in aphakic children:**
    A. Occurs in up to 40% of patients.
    B. Is associated with large corneas.
    C. May be due to trabecular blockage with pigment and synechiae.
    D. Typically occurs within 3 years of the cataract surgery.
    E. Often is unsuspected until it is very advanced.

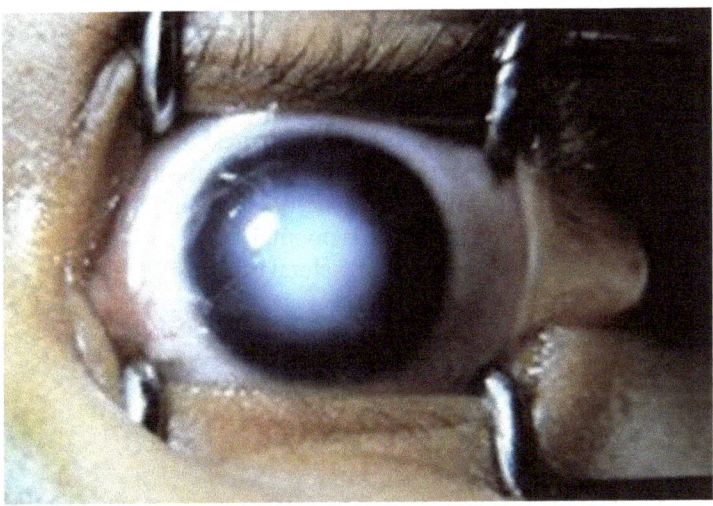

Fig. 9.2: Corneal hydrops in congenital glaucoma.

23. **Signs of congenital glaucoma include:**
    A. Epiphora, blepharospasm, and photophobia.
    B. Corneal diameter more than 10 mm horizontally.
    C. Haab's striae.
    D. Corneal hydrops.
    E. Cupping of the optic nerve.

24. **Aniridia:**
    A. Is due to a sporadic mutation in one-third of cases.
    B. Usually causes glaucoma late in the first decade of life.
    C. Is associated with mental retardation.
    D. Is associated with Wilms tumor in inherited cases.
    E. Eventually causes glaucoma in 50–75% of affected children.

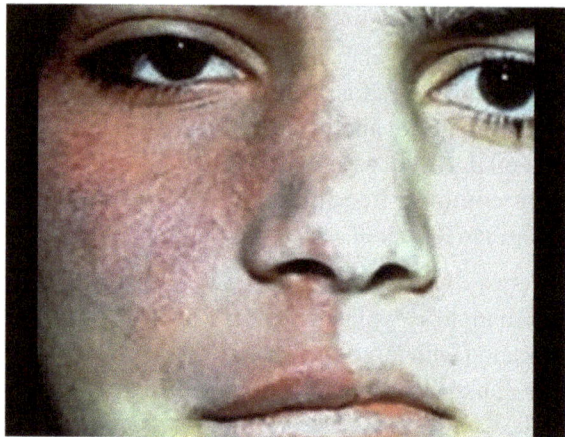

Fig. 9.3: Port-wine stain of patient with Sturge–Weber syndrome.

25. Sturge–Weber syndrome:
   A. Associated with glaucoma usually involves both lids with port-wine lesions.
   B. Is associated with glaucoma in about one-third of patients.
   C. Associated with glaucoma should be treated with goniotomy.
   D. With choroidal angioma may be associated with subretinal hemorrhage when the globe is opened.
   E. May be caused by elevated episcleral pressure.

26. Patients who have elevated intraocular pressure should be strongly considered for treatment if:
   A. They are young.
   B. Their optic nerves appear damaged from elevated IOP.
   C. They are highly myopic.
   D. They have a limited life expectancy.
   E. They have a strong family history of glaucomatous optic neuropathy.

27. Normal-tension glaucoma:
   A. Occurs in 10–30% of patients who have newly diagnosed glaucomatous optic neuropathy.
   B. Is associated with peripheral vasospasm and migraine.
   C. Is associated with nocturnal hypertension.
   D. Is associated with myopia and peripapillary choroidal atrophy.
   E. Occurs in patients who are about 10 years older on average than typical patients with POAG.

28. Normal-tension glaucoma:
   A. Affects men more frequently than women.
   B. Is associated with recurrent disc hemorrhages..
   C. Usually is ultimately bilateral.
   D. With time tends toward a higher IOP in about 8% of patients.
   E. Should be treated by lowering the IOP.

29. Potentially treatable causes of normal-tension glaucoma include:
A. Nocturnal hypotension caused by systemic hypertensive medication.
B. Carotid insufficiency.
C. Discontinuation of calcium channel blockers.
D. Lowering IOP to less than 6–8 mm Hg.
E. Systemic vasospasm.

30. Risk factors for open-angle glaucoma include:
A. Myopia.
B. Pseudoexfoliation.
C. Caucasian racial group.
D. Positive family history.
E. Age over 45 years.

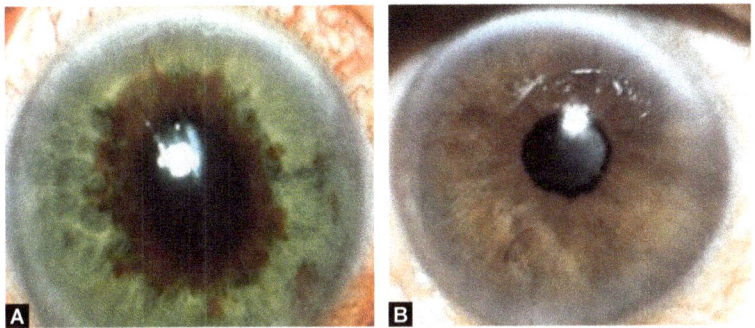

Figs. 9.4A and B: (A) Iris neovascularization, mainly around pupil; (B) More widely distributed.

31. Angle closure without pupillary block can be caused by:
A. Iris neovascularization.
B. Epithelial downgrowth.
C. Fibrous ingrowth.
D. Endothelial proliferation over the trabecular meshwork.
E. Phacomorphic glaucoma.

32. Miotics such as pilocarpine:
A. May worsen pupillary block by backward lens movement.
B. May worsen pupillary block by permitting lens thickening.
C. Are not effective if the iris sphincter is ischemic.
D. When used on a long-term basis cannot prevent angle-closure glaucoma with certainty.
E. May increase the risk of retinal detachment.

33. Argon laser iridoplasty is useful for:
A. Treatment of plateau iris syndrome or configuration if iridotomy fails to widen the angle.
B. Treatment of acute angle-closure attacks when corneal clouding prohibits iridotomy and medical treatment fails.
C. Treatment of goniosynechiae.

D. Treatment of POAG before argon laser trabeculoplasty, when the angle approach is too narrow for direct trabecular treatment.
E. Shortening iris tissue in preparation for iridotomy.

34. Pseudoexfoliation syndrome is:
A. Common among Scandinavians.
B. More common in men than in women.
C. Clinically unilateral in 50% of patients at the time of diagnosis.
D. Rarely diagnosed before 50 years of age.
E. The most common identifiable cause of secondary open-angle glaucoma.

35. In pseudoexfoliation syndrome:
A. Pigmentation of the trabecular meshwork is increased.
B. Little pigment is released after pupillary dilation.
C. Material may accumulate on intraocular surfaces.
D. Pseudoexfoliation material accumulates on the anterior lens capsule.
E. Subluxated lenses may be the initial manifestation.

36. Glaucoma in patients who have pseudoexfoliation syndrome:
A. Is more responsive to medication than is POAG.
B. Is more responsive than POAG to argon laser trabeculoplasty.
C. Develops in 10% of patients.
D. Is usually as responsive as POAG to trabeculectomy.
E. Is successfully treated with aqueous suppressants and miotics.

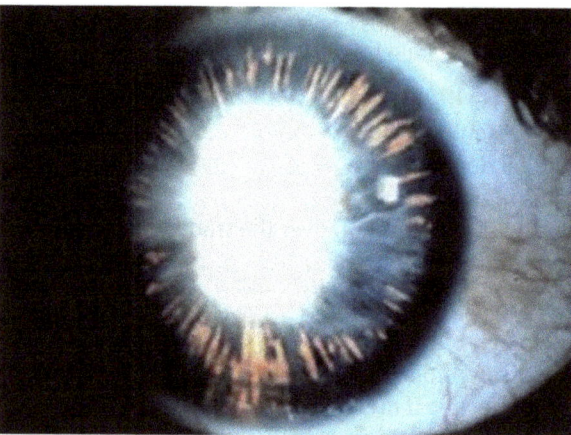

Fig. 9.5: Midperipheral iris transillumination defects.

37. Characteristics of pigmentary glaucoma include:
A. Krukenberg's spindle.
B. Heavy trabecular meshwork pigmentation.
C. Radial midperipheral iris transillumination defects.
D. Loose lens zonules.
E. Autosomal dominant transmission with gene locus on chromosome 7q35–7q36.

Glaucoma

38. Eyes that have pigmentary dispersion syndrome are likely to:
   A. Be myopic.
   B. Have a large iris.
   C. Have a posterior iris insertion.
   D. Have a relative inverse pupillary block with increased lens iris touch induced by blinking.
   E. Have a low incidence of lattice retinal degeneration.

39. The peripheral iris concavity ("backbowed iris") in pigmentary glaucoma:
   A. Is common in Asians.
   B. Is eliminated after iridotomy.
   C. Is reduced by prolonged nonblinking.
   D. Can be altered by miotics or cycloplegics.
   E. Disappears spontaneously after the age of 50 years.

40. Neovascular glaucoma can occur secondary to:
   A. Central retinal vein occlusion (CRVO).
   B. Long-standing glaucoma from any cause.
   C. Long-standing retinal detachment.
   D. Uveitis.
   E. Diabetes mellitus.

41. Neovascular proliferation of the anterior segment:
   A. Sometimes may be detected only by gonioscopy.
   B. Most often occurs with carotid artery disease.
   C. May grow over the trabecular meshwork.
   D. Is often associated with anterior chamber cell and flare.
   E. Appears first at the pupillary margin in most patients.

42. Treatment of neovascular glaucoma:
   A. With drainage valves is preferred over trabeculectomy in most cases.
   B. May involve carbonic anhydrase inhibitors.
   C. Usually causes vitritis.
   D. May involve panretinal photocoagulation.
   E. By cyclocryotherapy results in loss of light perception in 58% of patients.

43. Corticosteroid-induced elevation of intraocular pressure:
   A. Of 6–15 mm Hg occurs in 30% of patients after 6–8 weeks of topical therapy.
   B. May occur as a result of actin increase in the trabecular meshwork.
   C. Reverts to baseline about 4 weeks after discontinuation of the steroid.
   D. Occurs by enhancement of trabecular meshwork phagocytosis.
   E. May occur because of inhibition of outflow-enhancing prostaglandins.

44. Glaucomatocyclitic crisis (Posner–Schlossman syndrome):
   A. Includes marked elevation of IOP.
   B. Is rarely painful.

C. Usually responds to corticosteroid treatment.
D. Is associated with small, round keratic precipitates.
E. Includes episodic uveitis with photophobia.

45. Fuchs' heterochromic iridocyclitis is:
A. Usually unilateral.
B. Associated with cataract formation.
C. Associated with neovascular angle vessels.
D. Associated with posterior synechiae.
E. Associated with spontaneous hyphema.

46. Late-onset glaucoma after hyphema may result from:
A. Angle recession.
B. Ghost cell glaucoma.
C. Plateau iris.
D. Peripheral anterior synechiae.
E. Posterior synechiae with iris bombe.

47. Indications for surgical intervention after hyphema include:
A. Sickle cell disease and an IOP >24 mm Hg for 24 hours or >30 mm Hg.
B. Total hyphema for 9 days.
C. Corneal blood staining.
D. Rebleeding.
E. Intraocular pressure >35 mm Hg for 7 days.

48. Angle recession:
A. Is due to a tear in the ciliary body, usually between the longitudinal and circular fibers.
B. Often results in scarring of the trabecular meshwork.
C. Is usually not clinically significant unless at least 180° of angle structures are involved.
D. Associated glaucoma does not respond to argon laser trabeculoplasty.
E. Associated glaucoma is best treated with miotics.

49. Elevated episcleral venous pressure:
A. Elevates IOP by 1 mm Hg for every 1 mm Hg increase in episcleral venous pressure.
B. Can be idiopathic.
C. Occurs in ataxia-telangiectasia.
D. Measured by direct cannulation is greater than 5–12 mm Hg.
E. Has been associated with Sturge–Weber syndrome.

50. Aqueous misdirection syndrome:
A. Can occur with instillation of topical miotics.
B. Can occur after CRVO.
C. Usually occurs after intraocular surgical procedures.
D. Is more common in large myopic eyes with greater vitreous volume.
E. Can occur spontaneously.

51. Aqueous misdirection syndrome:
A. May occur weeks or months after intraocular surgery.
B. Exhibits a uniformly shallow anterior chamber without iris bombe.
C. Should not be treated with miotic drops.
D. Should initially be treated with atropine and phenylephrine drops.
E. Responds to medical therapy in 90% of cases.

52. Iridocorneal endothelial syndrome:
A. Is unilateral.
B. Occurs more frequently in women than in men.
C. Is commonly familial.
D. Is correlated with glaucoma in one-half of patients.
E. Is not associated with systemic disease.

53. Epithelial downgrowth:
A. Is rare after penetrating keratoplasty.
B. Is potentiated by wound gape or vitreous incarceration.
C. Can be identified by argon laser.
D. Often causes secondary glaucoma.
E. May be potentiated by prolonged inflammation.

54. Glaucoma after alkali chemical trauma may be due to:
A. Scleral shrinkage.
B. Trabecular damage.
C. Ciliary body damage.
D. Pupillary block.
E. prostaglandin release.

55. Aniridia:
A. Is most commonly sporadic.
B. May be associated with Wilms' tumor, mental retardation, and genitourinary anomalies.
C. May be associated with optic nerve hypoplasia.
D. May be associated with cerebellar ataxia.
E. May be inherited as an autosomal dominant trait.

56. Intraocular tumors may cause glaucoma by:
A. Clogging the trabecular meshwork with tumor- or pigment-laden macrophages.
B. Causing forward displacement of the lens-iris diaphragm.
C. Causing neovascularization of the anterior chamber.
D. Causing prostaglandin release.
E. Direct tumor cell infiltration of the trabecular meshwork.

57. Indicate the *incorrect* statement.
A. The benefit of lowering IOP in patients with glaucoma has not been proved in a prospective clinical trial.
B. Approximately 50% of patients who have glaucomatous optic neuropathy have screening IOPs of <21 mm Hg.

C. One-sixth of patients who have glaucomatous optic neuropathy never have documented IOP >21 mm Hg.
D. Even in patients who have IOP <21 mm Hg, the greater visual field loss is suffered by the eye with the higher IOP.
E. No IOP exists below which glaucomatous optic neuropathy never occurs or above which it always occurs.

58. Incisional surgery for glaucoma:
A. Generally yields an initially lower IOP than medical therapy.
B. Should be considered when maximum tolerated medical therapy fails to control IOP.
C. Is less expensive than long-term medical treatment.
D. Eliminates the need for patient compliance.
E. Is generally not considered for a blind painful glaucomatous eye.

59. Patients being considered for medical management of glaucoma should:
A. Be educated about their disease.
B. Be instructed in nasolacrimal occlusion.
C. Be informed of every local and systemic side effect of the drug being considered.
D. Undergo one-eye therapeutic trials.
E. Be instructed about techniques of drop instillation.

60. Beta-blockers:
A. May not be effective during sleep.
B. Usually lower IOP about 25%.
C. Are preferred in lower concentrations because they are about as effective as in higher ones.
D. Have increased efficacy when added to epinephrine drops.
E. Decrease aqueous production by the ciliary body.

61. Beta-blockers may cause:
A. Apnea in neonates.
B. Hypoglycemia in patients with diabetes.
C. Tachycardia.
D. Lowering of high-density lipoproteins.
E. Resuscitation after anaphylaxis to be more difficult.

62. Alpha-adrenergic agonists:
A. May cause vasoconstriction, pupillary dilation, and eyelid retraction.
B. Have peak and trough effects similar to nonselective beta-blockers.
C. Are very effective in lowering IOP after anterior segment laser surgery.
D. May be less effective overtime due to tachyphylaxis.
E. Decrease aqueous production.

63. Brimonidine 0.1%:
   A. Can cause dry mouth and lethargy.
   B. Has less incidence of ocular allergy than other concentrations.
   C. May be used with caution in infants.
   D. Increases aqueous outflow.
   E. Is administered 2–3 times daily.

64. Miotics:
   A. Lower IOP by 15–25% by increasing aqueous outflow.
   B. Are the treatment of choice for phacomorphic glaucoma.
   C. Are associated with an increased risk of retinal detachment.
   D. May cause epiphora due to punctal stenosis.
   E. Are poorly tolerated due to miosis and a myopic shift in refractive error.

65. Systemic carbonic anhydrase inhibitors:
   A. Must inhibit 50% of the enzyme in the ciliary processes to lower IOP.
   B. Commonly cause malaise, fatigue, anorexia, and depression.
   C. Can cause thrombocytopenia, agranulocytosis, and aplastic anemia.
   D. May cause an allergic reaction in patients with a sulfa allergy.
   E. Decrease aqueous production by direct antagonistic activity on ciliary epithelium carbonic anhydrase.

66. Topical carbonic anhydrase inhibitors:
   A. Have lesser systemic side effects than oral agents.
   B. Cause a bitter taste in 25% of patients.
   C. Can cause punctate keratitis.
   D. Are additive to systemic carbonic anhydrase inhibitors (CAIs).
   E. Appear to be safe for use in children.

67. Prostaglandins:
   A. Used topically result in iris pigmentation changes that are reversible once the medication is discontinued.
   B. Appear additive to the effect of beta blockers.
   C. May reduce IOP 25–35% from baseline.
   D. May result in an IOP that is less than episcleral venous pressure.
   E. Reduce IOP by increasing uveoscleral outflow.

68. Positive predictors for success after argon laser trabeculoplasty include:
   A. Aphakia.
   B. Low-tension glaucoma.
   C. Pseudoexfoliation syndrome.
   D. Pigmentary glaucoma.
   E. Age more than 65 years.

69. **Selective laser trabeculoplasty (SLT):**
   A. SLT uses a relatively large spot at 400 microns.
   B. Is generally not efficacious when repeated.
   C. Is a nonthermal laser treatment.
   D. Targets only pigmented cells without apparent damage to the surrounding structures.
   E. Ideally results in blanching without bubble formation as the endpoint.

70. **The benefits of the neodymium-doped yttrium aluminum garnet (Nd:YAG) laser over the argon laser for creation of peripheral iridectomy include:**
   A. Works well in irides of all colors.
   B. Quicker creation of opening.
   C. Lower energy requirement.
   D. Lower incidence of hemorrhage.
   E. Less likelihood of late iridectomy closure.

71. **Laser peripheral iridotomy:**
   A. Is often placed at the 3 o'clock and 9 o'clock positions to decrease the risk of linear dysphotopsias.
   B. Should be placed in iris crypts.
   C. Requires short energy pulses for light colored irides when the argon laser is being used.
   D. May cause aqueous misdirection syndrome.
   E. Is best performed with the YAG laser if active rubeosis is present.

72. **Cyclodestructive procedures may be indicated for eyes:**
   A. That have poor visual potential.
   B. That have failed multiple glaucoma surgical procedures.
   C. With shallow anterior segments.
   D. That are blind and painful.
   E. In patients unable to undergo filtration surgery.

73. **Common complications of cyclodestructive procedures include:**
   A. Pain.
   B. Uveitis.
   C. Macular edema.
   D. Sympathetic ophthalmia.
   E. Hypotony.

74. **Goniotomy:**
   A. Rarely causes bleeding.
   B. May be performed binocularly with general anesthesia if clinically indicated.
   C. Is difficult to perform if the corneal stroma is edematous.

D. Should be placed at the anterior aspect of the middle third of the trabecular meshwork.
   E. Is usually initially performed over the nasal 120° of the chamber angle.

75. **Trabeculotomy:**
    A. Requires identification of Schlemm's canal.
    B. Can be performed in eyes with cloudy corneas.
    C. Usually causes hyphema.
    D. Has less tendency to produce lens damage than goniotomy.
    E. Does not introduce instruments into the anterior chamber.

76. **Mitomycin C is:**
    A. Approximately 100 times more potent than 5-fluorouracil in current doses.
    B. Cytocidal.
    C. Reserved during filtration surgery for eyes that have a high likelihood of failure.
    D. A halogenated pyrimidine analog.
    E. One of the ten most carcinogenic substances known.

77. **Corneal traction suture is preferable to superior rectus bridle suture during filtering surgery because:**
    A. No conjunctival holes are created.
    B. It causes less distortion of the limbus.
    C. Scleral perforation is impossible.
    D. It yields better exposure during wound closure.
    E. The globe can be inferiorly rotated more easily.

78. **Factors associated with a high-risk of failure of filtering surgery include:**
    A. Neovascularization of the anterior segment.
    B. Chronic uveitis.
    C. Failure of previous filtration surgery.
    D. Older age.
    E. Previous conjunctival surgery.

79. **Complications of antimetabolites used during glaucoma filtering surgery include:**
    A. Retinal damage.
    B. Development of malignant conjunctival tumors.
    C. Scleritis and scleromalacia.
    D. Epithelial erosions.
    E. Hypotony.

80. Drainage implants have increased usefulness in patients who have:
A. Glaucoma caused by intraocular tumors.
B. Extensive anterior conjunctival scarring.
C. Extensive filtration angle scarring.
D. Aphakic glaucoma.
E. Neovascular glaucoma.

81. Common complications associated with drainage implants include:
A. Hypotony.
B. Tube occlusion.
C. Tube-corneal contact.
D. Plate migration.
E. Erosion of the tube through the sclera.

82. Buttonholed conjunctiva during glaucoma filtering surgery:
A. At the limbus can be closed with a 10-0 mattress suture.
B. Must be repaired and determined to be watertight before the end of the procedure.
C. Does not affect antimetabolite use.
D. Is often caused by toothed forceps.
E. Away from the limbus is best closed in two layers.

83. Intraoperative bleeding from the iris root or ciliary body after surgical iridectomy may be treated by:
A. Placement of cold balanced salt solution with epinephrine in the wound.
B. Wet-field cautery.
C. Viscoelastic material.
D. Intravenous mannitol.
E. Tight wound closure.

84. A shallow anterior chamber after glaucoma filtering surgery:
A. Is always associated with hypotony.
B. May be caused by aqueous misdirection.
C. May be caused by pupillary block.
D. May be due to choroidal effusions.
E. May be due to a leaking bleb.

85. Treatment for a leaking bleb may include:
A. Patching the eye.
B. A bandage soft contact lens.
C. Laser iridoplasty.
D. Autologous fibrin tissue glue.
E. Autologous blood injection into the bleb.

86. Tenon cyst formation after filtering surgery:

A. Seems less common in eyes receiving 5-fluorouracil or mitomycin C.
B. May lead to sudden pressure elevation.
C. Usually requires surgical removal.
D. May remodel with time.
E. Limits aqueous percolation through the bleb.

ANSWERS

1. C. The effect of gender on glaucoma prevalence is not certain. Studies such as the Baltimore, Beaver Dam and Roscommon showed no significant difference in prevalence between sexes. Over the age of 40 years the prevalence of glaucoma in African, Americans is four times that of Caucasians.

2. D. Studies have investigated cigarette smoking as a proposed risk factor of glaucoma but no significant association has been found.

3. D. Intraocular pressure alone has been unacceptably poor in screening for glaucoma. The American Academy of Ophthalmology defines primary open-angle glaucoma (POAG) as a multifactorial optic neuropathy in which there is acquired loss of optic nerve fibers.

4. E. When proteins and debris fill the anterior chamber aqueous is still able to travel through the trabecular meshwork as long as it is clear.

5. D. Juvenile onset open-angle glaucoma is inherited as an autosomal dominant trait.

6. C. Ocular Hypertension Treatment Study (OHTS) identified elevated intraocular pressure (IOP), older age, thinner cornea, larger C/D ratio, and increased pattern standard deviation (PSD) as risk factors for the development of glaucoma. Although a positive family history has been identified as a risk factor in epidemiologic studies, it was not reported in OHTS.

7. B. Genetic loci that harbor genes responsible for angle-closure glaucoma have not been found on the human genome. Currently mapped glaucoma genetic associations include *TIGR/MYOC* with POAG (juvenile and adult-onset), *LOXL1* with pseudoexfoliation syndrome (PEX), *PITX2* with Rieger syndrome, and *CYP1B1* with congenital glaucoma.

8. C. Asian ancestry is a risk factor for the development of angle-closure glaucoma. The Early Manifest Glaucoma Trial (EMGT) identified higher IOP, thin central corneal thickness (CCT), older age, presence of exfoliation syndrome, and development of disk hemorrhage as risk factors for the progression of open-angle glaucoma.

9. D. Contact time is not a variable in the calculation of intraocular pressure with an applanation tonometer. Excess fluorescein results in over estimation of IOP. Extremes in corneal thickness and shape may result in errors in measurement of IOP. Error measurements are also caused by astigmatism and improperly calibrated tonometer.
10. B. Intraocular pressure generally decreases with general anesthesia. Exceptions are ketamine and succinylcholine which usually cause an increase in IOP.
11. B. Direct gonioscopy is useful in that a real image of the angle is visualized. The benefits of indirect gonioscopy include the ability to perform indentation gonioscopy, examine the patient in the upright position and harnessing the slit-lamp's optics and magnification.
12. C. A Sampaolesi line is commonly seen with pseudoexfoliation glaucoma and not normally seen in the angle.
13. B. The Humphrey visual field analyzer printout shows false-positive and false-negative answers. A false-positive rate >20% or false-negative rate >33% suggests an unreliable test.
14. A. Generalized depression of the visual field that is caused by a cataract is not an artifact; it is a nonglaucomatous visual field defect.
15. D. Pallor of the rim tissue suggests a nonglaucomatous optic neuropathy.
16. C. Patients with glaucoma have loss of the second negative wave on pattern electroretinograms or an overall increase in pattern ERG.
17. B. Optic nerve head planimetry was formerly used to quantify optic nerve head parameters.
18. A. Optic disc hemorrhage, peripapillary atrophy, peripapillary vasoconstriction and rim notching are signs of ischemic optic nerve damage.
19. D. Scanning laser polarimetry provides information about the relative thickness of the nerve fiber layer, not optic nerve head blood flow.
20. E. Patients with glaucoma have a higher prevalence of concomitant vascular abnormalities such as migraines and Raynaud's phenomenon. There is no association with Crohn's disease.
21. B. Primary infantile glaucoma is more common in boys in North America and Europe; but more common in girls in Japan.
22. B. There is no known association with secondary aphakic glaucoma in children and large corneas.
23. B. The hallmark of glaucoma in infants and young children is ocular enlargement. A horizontal corneal diameter >12 mm is associated with glaucoma.
24. D. Aniridia is associated with Wilms tumor in 20% of sporadic cases.
25. C. Treatment of secondary glaucoma associated with Sturge–Weber syndrome is not clear cut. When the glaucoma is due to elevated

episcleral venous pressure, a trabeculectomy or drainage device may be a better option.
26. D. Patients with ocular hypertension and not optic nerve damage may be best served by observation in the case of limited life expectancy.
27. C. Normal tension glaucoma (NTG) is associated with nocturnal hypotension.
28. A. Reports reveal that women are affected twice as frequently as men with NTG.
29. D. In NTG, the IOP should be lowered by 30% from say a starting IOP of 17 mm Hg. IOP in the range of less than 6–8 mm Hg can result in hypotony.
30. C. African, Americans have a prevalence of POAG four times that of Caucasians.
31. E. Phacomorphic glaucoma is caused by a mature large cataract that blocks the pupillary border.
32. A. Miotics may worsen papillary block by forward lens movement.
33. C. Argon laser iridoplasty is not indicated for goniosynechialysis.
34. B. Pseudoexfoliation glaucoma is more common in women than men. 50% of cases present unilateral at diagnosis.
35. B. Often a significant amount of pigment is released with pupillary dilation in patients with PEX.
36. A. Pseudoexfoliation syndrome is more refractive to medical treatment than POAG. PEX is more responsive to laser trabeculoplasty.

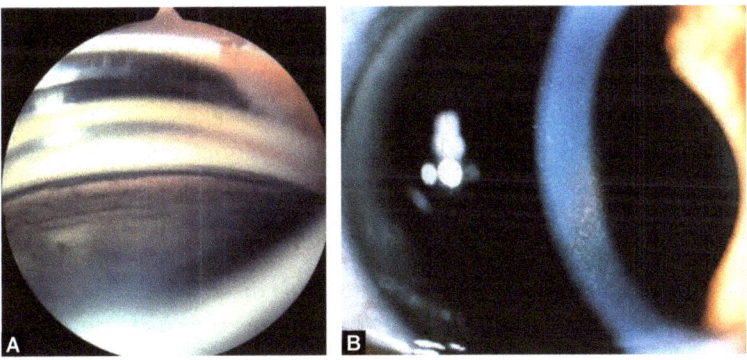

Figs. 9.6A and B: (A) Pigmentary glaucoma angle with heavily pigmented trabecular meshwork; (B) Krukenberg spindle.

37. D. Loose lens zonules are not part of the clinical manifestation of pigmentary glaucoma.
38. E. There is a higher incidence of myopia and lattice degeneration in eyes with pigmentary dispersion and pigmentary glaucoma.
39. A. Africans, Americans and Asians rarely manifest pigmentary glaucoma. This is likely because of a thicker and denser iris stroma in these eyes.

40. B. Long-standing glaucoma is not a cause of neovascular glaucoma (NVG). Diabetic retinopathy and central retinal vein occlusion (CRVO) are the most common causes.
41. B. Neovascularization of the anterior chamber usually occurs with proliferative diabetic retinopathy or central retinal vein occlusion.
42. C. There is no association of the treatment of NVG and vitritis.
43. D. Corticosteroid-induced elevation of IOP may occur by inhibition of trabecular meshwork phagocytosis.
44. C. In Posner-Schlossman syndrome, there is no evidence that corticosteroids shorten the duration or prevent reccurrences.
45. D. There is no association of Fuchs' heterochromic iridocyclitis with post synechiae. There is often only a mild amount of anterior chamber inflammation which is asymptomatic.
46. C. Plateau iris syndrome is not a cause of late-onset glaucoma after a hyphema.
47. D. Rebleeding is not an indication for surgical intervention after a hyphema.
48. E. Angle-recession glaucoma does not always respond to miotics. In angle recession, the trabecular meshwork is damaged and there is a dependence on uveoscleral outflow. Miotics cause a decrease in uveoscleral outflow.
49. C. Ataxia-telangiectasia is not associated with elevated episcleral venous pressure.
50. D. Aqueous misdirection is more common in small hyperopic eyes.
51. E. In aqueous misdirection syndrome, medical treatment is successful approximately 50% of the time.
52. C. Iridocorneal endothelial (ICE) is rarely familial.
53. A. Epithelial downgrowth is commonly associated with penetrating keratoplasty.
54. C. Ciliary body damage after alkali chemical trauma may cause intermediate hypotony.
55. A. Aniridia is most commonly autosomal dominant.
56. D. Release of prostaglandin by intraocular tumors is not a cause of glaucoma.
57. A. The benefit of lowering IOP in patients with glaucoma has been proven in multiple prospective multicenter trials.
58. D. Surgical treatment for glaucoma still requires compliance with postoperative care.
59. D. There is no evidence that monocular trials are effective in assessing the efficacy of a particular topical glaucoma medication. IOP fluctuation between the two eyes and possible systemic absorption of the medication are two factors that complicate monocular trials.

Glaucoma

60. D. Nonselective adrenergic agonists such as epinephrine and dipivefrin are generally not used concomitantly with beta-blockers because of lack of additional efficacy. Beta-blockers are only additive to alpha-2 adrenergic agonists.
61. C. Beta-blockers may cause bradycardia.
62. B. Alpha-adrenergic agonists lower IOP by 14–15% at trough which is less than that with nonselective beta-blockers.
63. C. Brimonidine should never be used in infants and young children because of the risk of respiratory arrest and central nervous system depression.
64. B. Contraction of the ciliary muscle by miotics causes a forward movement of the lens–iris diaphragm which may exacerbate pupillary block in an eye with a large lens.
65. A. Carbonic anhydrase inhibitors must inhibit 90% of the enzyme in the ciliary processes to lower IOP.
66. D. For patients taking an oral carbonic anhydrase inhibitors (CAIs), there is no further advantage or additional IOP lowering by adding a topical CAI.
67. A. Increased iris pigmentation is permanent and is due to an increased number of melanosomes within the melanocytes. The frequency of this effect depends on the eye color at baseline.
68. A. Aphakia is a negative predictor of argon laser trabeculoplasty (ALT) success.
69. B. Repeat selective laser trabeculoplasty (SLT) is generally effective.
70. D. YAG laser has a higher incidence of hemorrhage than argon laser because there is no coagulation of the iris blood vessels.
71. E. The risk of bleeding is increased in patients with active rubeosis or those on anticoagulants. In these patients, the argon laser may be more appropriate since it can cauterize vessels and minimize bleeding.
72. C. Cyclodestructive procedures are reserved for eyes with abnormal anterior segments, i.e. with neovascularization and inflammation, or those with poor visual potential.
73. D. Sympathetic ophthalmia is a rare complication of cyclodestructive procedures.
74. A. It is common to have a small amount of bleeding with a goniotomy.
75. E. The trabeculotomy does introduce instruments into the anterior chamber.
76. D. Mitomycin C is an alkylating agent that results in DNA crosslinking.
77. B. A corneal traction suture may distort the limbus but does not complicate the filtering surgery.
78. D. The success rate of filtering surgery is decreased in younger patients.

79. B. Development of malignant conjunctival tumors is not a risk of antimetabolites.
80. A. A drainage implant is not useful for glaucoma caused by intraocular tumors.
81. D. Plate migration is unlikely with drainage implants due to encapsulation of the plate.
82. C. Antimetabolites should be avoided if a button holed conjunctiva is found during filtering surgery.
83. D. IV mannitol is not a treatment of intraocular bleeding from a surgical iridectomy.
84. A. A shallow anterior chamber after glaucoma filtering surgery is not always associated with hypotony. IOPs may be low, normal or even high such as in aqueous misdirection syndrome.
85. C. Laser iridoplasty is not a treatment for a leaky bleb.
86. C. Tenon's cyst after filtering surgery usually resolves on its own.

CHAPTER

10

Intraocular Tumors

Myron Yanoff, Nicole Pumariega

QUESTIONS

Identify the correct answer for all questions (unless instructed otherwise).

1. **A neoplasm:**
   A. Is composed of cells that stop responding to a normal growth-restraining mechanism.
   B. Is a malignant tumor.
   C. Has the ability to metastasize.
   D. Shows cells containing mitotic figures and pleomorphism.
   E. Tends to grow expansively rather than to infiltrate.

2. **Which of the following statements is *false*?**
   A. Hamartoma is a neoplasm composed of cells and tissues that are normally found in the area of growth.
   B. Choristoma is a neoplasm composed of cells and tissues that are not normally found in the area of growth.
   C. Carcinoma is a neoplasm derived from cells of epithelial origin (endoderm or ectoderm).
   D. Sarcoma is a neoplasm derived from cells of mesenchymal origin (e.g. muscle, bone, blood vessels, and blood-forming tissue).
   E. Teratoma is a neoplasm derived from cells of both mesodermal and endodermal origin.

3. **All the following statements concerning retinoblastoma are true *except* which one?**
   A. It is the most common primary intraocular malignancy of childhood.
   B. It arises from immature retinoblasts.
   C. About 20% of treated patients die of the disease within 2–4 years of onset of symptoms.
   D. It occurs in about 1 in 14,000–20,000 individuals.
   E. The vast majority of cases occur in children younger than 6 years.

4. **Identify the incorrect answer concerning retinoblastoma.**
   A. The yearly incidence is highest in the 3rd year of life.
   B. About 20–35% of cases are bilateral.
   C. In bilateral cases, unlike unilateral cases, usually more than 1 tumor is present in each eye.
   D. The majority of cases are sporadic (i.e. not inherited).
   E. Inherited cases seem to follow the genetic rules of autosomal dominance.

5. **Which one of the following statements about retinoblastoma is true?**
   A. It appears to result from loss or inactivation of one of the two alleles of the "retinoblastoma gene".
   B. The retinoblastoma gene is localized to a small segment of the long arm (q14 region) of chromosome 13.
   C. The loss or inactivation of one of the two alleles takes place only in a germinal cell.
   D. At a gene level the genetic rules of autosomal dominance are followed.
   E. If both alleles at q14 are affected in a somatic cell, the affected child can pass on the condition to his/her offspring.

6. **A mother brings in her 11-month-old child because of a "funny" reflex in one eye, described as a cat's eye reflex. Retinoblastoma is suspected. Which of the following is the most common presentation of retinoblastoma?**
   A. Pseudohypopyon.
   B. Neovascular glaucoma.
   C. A red eye.
   D. Photophobia and tearing.
   E. Leukokoria (white pupil).

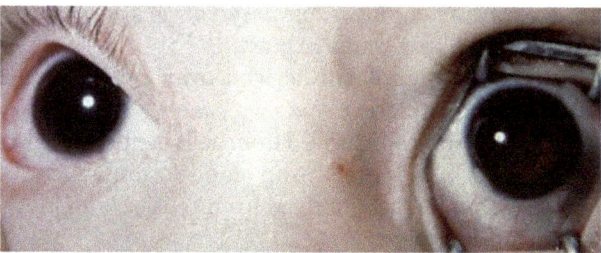

Fig. 10.1: Left eye has a "cat's eye" reflex.

7. **A tumor resembling an irradiated retinoblastoma is found during a routine ophthalmoscopic examination of a 6-year-old child who had an esotropia. No other ocular findings were noted. The child had never had a known ocular tumor and was otherwise healthy and normal. The most likely diagnosis is:**
   A. Medulloepithelioma.
   B. Incorrect history from the mother.
   C. Coats' disease.

D. Retinocytoma (retinoma).
E. Unsuspected prior ocular trauma.

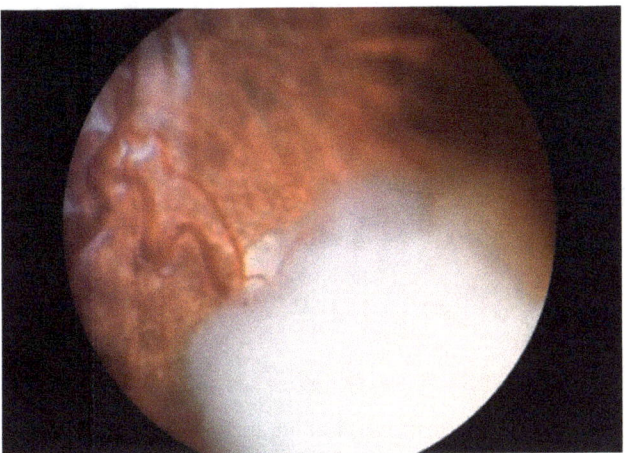

Fig. 10.2: Fish-flesh, large lesion inferiorly in a young child.

8. **A child has unilateral leukokoria. Which of the following is *least* likely?**
    A. Coats' disease.
    B. Persistent hyperplastic primary vitreous.
    C. Ocular onchocerciasis.
    D. Ocular toxocariasis.
    E. Medulloepithelioma.

9. **Histologically, all of the following, *except* one, is characteristic of retinoblastoma?**
    A. Lack of necrosis.
    B. Malignant neuroepithelial cells (retinoblasts).
    C. Flexner–Wintersteiner rosette.
    D. Homer Wright rosette.
    E. Fleurette.

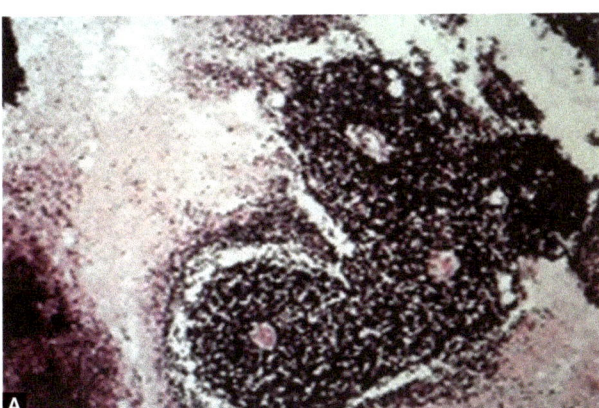

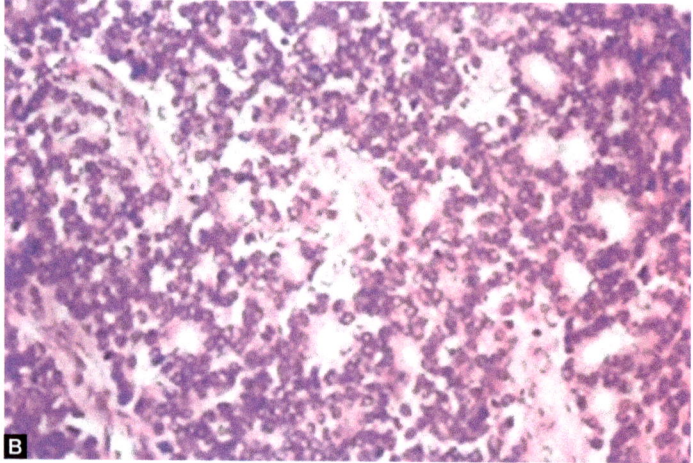

Figs. 10.3A and B: (A) Necrosis, calcification, and undifferentiated small, blue cells; (B) Undifferentiated cells form multiple, small rosette.

10. **A uveal malignant melanoma:**
    A. Most commonly metastases to the brain.
    B. Most commonly arises from the ciliary body.
    C. Arises from iris and ciliary body at an equal frequency.
    D. Spreads mainly via the lymphatics.
    E. Is the most common primary intraocular malignant neoplasm in adults.

11. **Which one of the following statements about uveal malignant melanoma is true?**
    A. It has a cumulative lifetime incidence of about 1 in 20,000–30,000 Caucasian individuals.
    B. It is about 10% more common in Caucasians than in blacks.
    C. After the age of 65 years the annual incidence plateaus.
    D. The average age at detection is about 60 years.
    E. The average age at detection is the same for melanomas of the iris, ciliary body, and choroid.

12. **All *but* one of the following is considered a risk factor for the development of uveal melanoma?**
    A. Intense, sustained, and recurrent exposure to sunlight.
    B. Congenital ocular melanocytosis.
    C. Smoking.
    D. Choroidal nevi.
    E. A strong familial history of uveal melanoma spanning more than one generation.

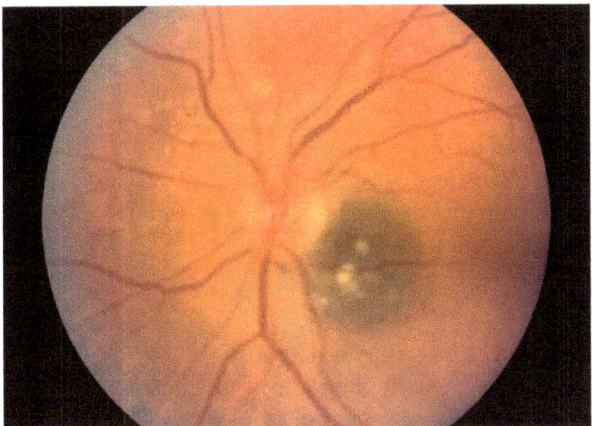

Fig. 10.4: Dark, flat area inferior temporal to the optic nerve is a choroidal nevus. The yellow areas are drusen which often develop in these nevi.

13. All the following gross and histological features are helpful in assessing the malignant potential of an iris melanoma, *except*:
    A. Size of lesion.
    B. Color of neoplasm.
    C. Apparent cohesiveness.
    D. Intrinsic vascularity.
    E. Effects on adjacent ocular tissue.

14. Which is the *least* likely way that a ciliary body or choroidal melanoma may appear clinically?
    A. Asymptomatic, discovered on routine ocular examination.
    B. Blurred vision.
    C. Ocular pain.
    D. Sentinel episcleral blood vessels overlying the region of the uveal melanoma.
    E. Heterochromia.

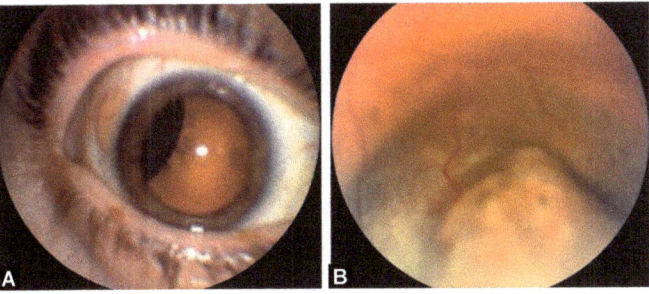

Figs. 10.5A and B: (A) Dark mass in region of ciliary body seen behind dilated pupil. Pink subconjunctival lesion on left is an epibulbar extension of the ciliary body melanoma; (B) Mushroom-shaped, solid mass noted in posterior fundus.

15. **B-scan ultrasonography of a dome-shaped choroidal melanoma shows:**
    A. A cystic sonolucent mass.
    B. A solid, biconvex cross-sectional shape with internal acoustic darkness in its base.
    C. A solid, acoustically bright mass.
    D. A significant mushroom like, cross-sectional component.
    E. Increasing brightness toward the base.

16. **Which one of the following statements about choroidal melanoma is true?**
    A. A-scan ultrasonography is diagnostic.
    B. Indocyanine green angiography is diagnostic.
    C. Fluorescein angiography is diagnostic.
    D. Computed tomographic scanning is diagnostic.
    E. Magnetic resonance imaging is highly suggestive.

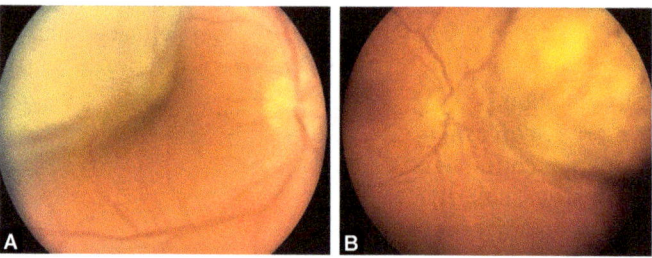

Figs. 10.6A and B: (A and B) Different presentations of choroidal melanomas.

17. **Commonly used histological criteria for the prognosis of ciliary body and choroidal melanomas include all the following, *except*:**
    A. Callender classification (spindle A and B cells, epithelioid cells, and mixed-cell type).
    B. Cytomorphometric parameters of the nuclei.
    C. Invasion of Bruch's membrane.
    D. Vortex vein invasion.
    E. Extraocular extension.

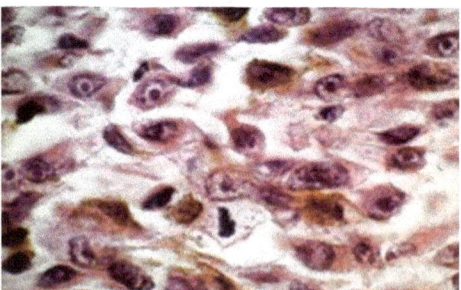

Fig. 10.7: Malignant cells showing prominent nucleoli and a mitotic figure.

18. Which one of the following is *not* an acceptable mode of ocular therapy of a presumed choroidal melanoma?
    A. Observation.
    B. Chemotherapy.
    C. Enucleation.
    D. Radiation therapy.
    E. Microsurgical resection.

19. Which one of the following ocular structures is *least* involved by metastatic cancer to the eyes?
    A. Retina.
    B. Choroid.
    C. Optic disc or nerve.
    D. Iris.
    E. Ciliary body.

20. A 60-year-old woman with a history of a primary cancer (surgical removal within the prior 5 months) complains of blurred vision. A golden yellow lesion, presumably metastatic is noted in the choroid. The most likely primary site is the:
    A. Cervix.
    B. Kidney.
    C. Lung.
    D. Ovary.
    E. Colon.

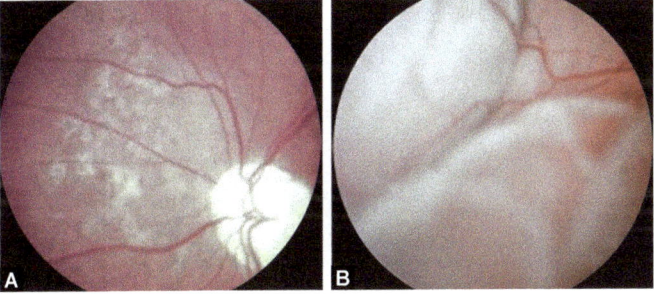

Figs. 10.8A and B: (A) A slightly elevated, amelanotic lesion of the choroid. Patient had a history of breast carcinoma; (B) An amelanotic choroidal lesion has caused a secondary retinal detachment. Patient had a history of lung carcinoma.

21. Which one of the following is *least* likely to be confused with a metastatic choroidal tumor?
    A. Amelanotic melanoma.
    B. Syphilitic granuloma.
    C. Choroidal hemangioma.
    D. Primary intraocular lymphoma.
    E. Choroidal osteoma.

22. Lymphoma and leukemia:
   A. Are linked by their common leukocytic basis.
   B. Occur with equal frequency in the eye.
   C. Never involve the conjunctiva.
   D. Most commonly involve the vitreous.
   E. When associated with central nervous system malignancy, most commonly arise from reticulum cells.

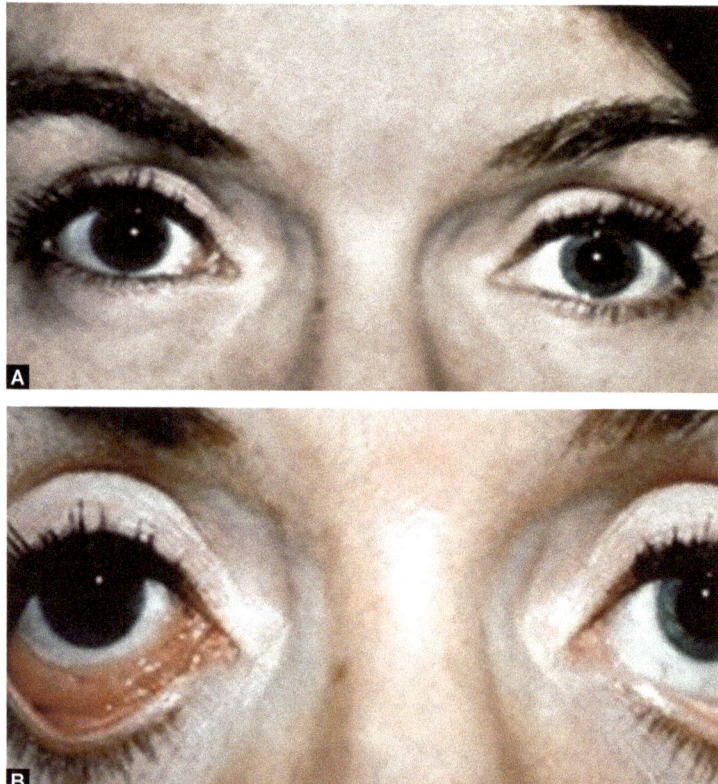

Figs. 9A and B: (A) Fullness is present mainly around the right lower lid; (B) Salmon-pink, smooth mass present in inferior cul-de-sac.

23. Primary intraocular lymphoma has all the following characteristics *except* which one?
   A. It may arise within the neural retina.
   B. It may arise within the uvea.
   C. It does not present as a uveitis.
   D. It may be diffuse within the eye.
   E. It may be multicentric within the eye.

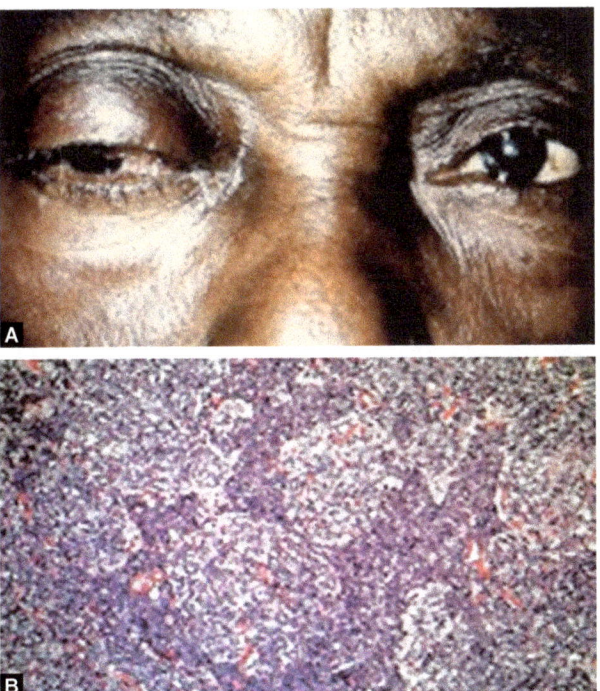

Figs. 10.10A and B: (A) Lymphomas may present wholly within the eye or in the orbit; (B) Sheets of malignant B-cell lymphocytes are present.

24. **Intraocular leukemia has all the following characteristics *except* which one?**
    A. Leukemic cells may accumulate in the neural retina.
    B. It protects against concurrent microbial infection.
    C. Less than 5% of affected patients have infiltrative fundus lesions at the time of initial leukemia diagnosis.
    D. Leukemic cells may accumulate in the optic nerve.
    E. Leukemic cells may accumulate in the uvea.

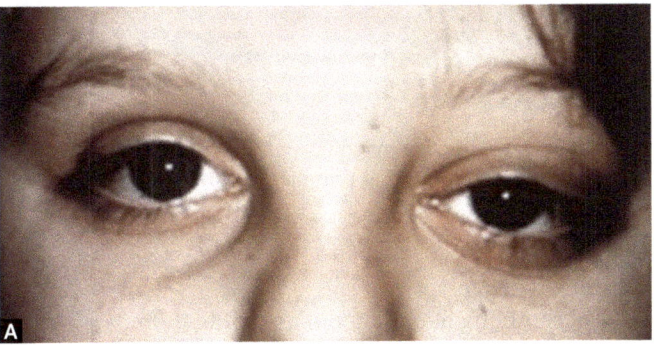

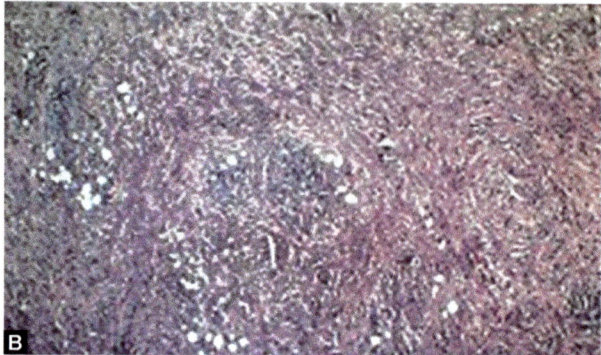

Figs. 10.11A and B: (A) Child has mass involving left upper lid; (B) Biopsy shows an infiltrate of immature leukocytes. Leukemia can involve the inside of the eye or the orbit.

25. A 6-year-old child has a 2-months history of a red eye, a visible tan-to-white iris mass, and glaucoma. The child is otherwise normal and healthy. The most probable diagnosis is:
   A. Amelanotic melanoma.
   B. Juvenile xanthogranuloma.
   C. Nematode granuloma.
   D. Medulloepithelioma.
   E. Leiomyoma.

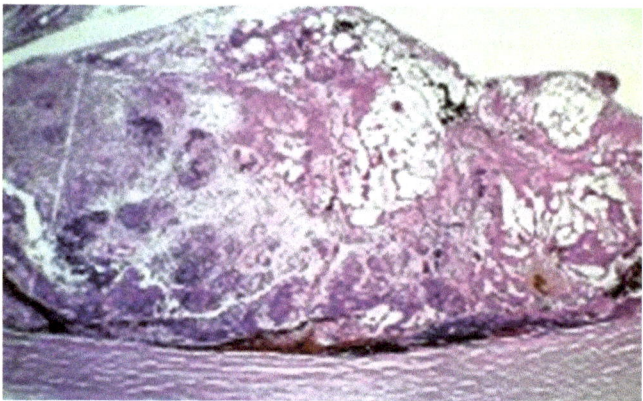

Fig. 10.12: Low-power magnification shows a tumor that looks somewhat primitive in nature.

26. A nonteratoid medulloepithelioma has all the following histologic features, *except*:
   A. Hyaline cartilage.
   B. Cells resembling neural medullary epithelium.
   C. Cystic spaces filled with hyaluronic acid.
   D. Primitive cells with a malignant potential.
   E. Rosette and tube-like structures.

27. **Which one of the following statements is *least* true of uveal nevus?**
    A. It is the most common primary intraocular tumor.
    B. About 20% of persons over age 50 years have at least one choroidal nevus.
    C. Although nevi are congenital, they may not be detectable clinically until they become pigmented after puberty.
    D. It is more common in darkly pigmented races.
    E. About 1 in 4,000–5,000 of such tumors may become malignant (melanoma).

28. **All the following are typical clinical findings of choroidal nevi *except* which one?**
    A. Most are less than 5 mm in diameter.
    B. Most have irregular edges and a stippled surface.
    C. Most are less than 1.0 µ thick.
    D. Many show overlying drusen.
    E. An occasional halo appearance is caused by a golden-orange marginal zone surrounding the brown to gray central zone.

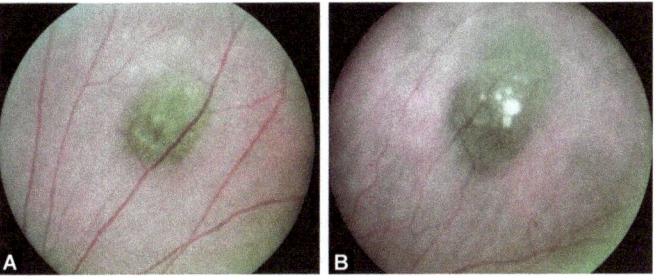

Figs. 10.13A and B: (A) Choroidal nevi are small usually with regular borders; (B) It may acquire drusen.

29. **A choroidal nevus has been followed for a number of years. Which one of the following features *most* strongly suggests malignant change?**
    A. Development of surface drusen.
    B. Accumulation of overlying serous subretinal fluid.
    C. A thickness of 1.5 mm.
    D. Accompanying choroidal neovascularization.
    E. Substantial tumor enlargement over a 6-months period.

30. **A solitary red-orange, ill-defined, disc-shaped choroidal tumor, and 2.8 mm in greatest diameter, is noted on routine ophthalmoscopy in the posterior pole of an otherwise healthy 26-year-old man. The most likely diagnosis is:**
    A. Metastatic carcinoma.
    B. Amelanotic melanoma.
    C. Nodular posterior scleritis.
    D. Harada's disease.
    E. Circumscribed form of choroidal hemangioma.

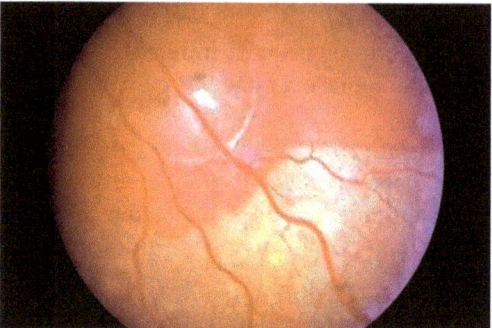

Fig. 10.14: Sharp demarcation from superior bright, red fundus to inferior, and normal-appearing fundus.

31. **The main entities to be differentiated from a diffuse choroidal hemangioma, the type generally associated with Sturge–Weber syndrome, include all the following *except* which one?**
    A. Primary lymphoma of the uvea.
    B. Presumed ocular histoplasmosis.
    C. Leukemic or secondary lymphomatous uveal infiltrate.
    D. Diffuse posterior scleritis.
    E. Uveal effusion syndrome.

32. **Diffuse choroidal hemangiomas, the type generally associated with Sturge–Weber syndrome, have all of the following histopathological features *except* which one?**
    A. They are composed of cavernous vascular channels lined by endothelial cells separated by thin fibrous septa.
    B. They have an orange or bright red appearance.
    C. They are composed of capillary-size vascular channels lined by endothelial cells separated by thin fibrous septa.
    D. They are diffuse, and it is difficult to determine the end of the tumor and the beginning of normal choroid.
    E. The overlying neural retina and retinal pigment epithelium may show cystic changes.

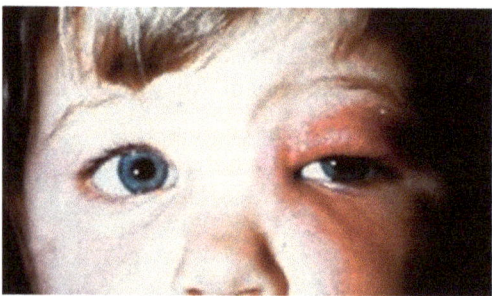

Fig. 10.15: Left eyelids enlarged and reddened in color.

33. On routine examination, a 27-year-old woman is found to have a slightly irregular, yellow-white, and juxtapapillary choroidal tumor. The tumor is dense ultrasonographically with the posterior tissues silent. Although all of the following can be mistaken for the tumor, which is most likely?
    A. Circumscribed choroidal hemangioma.
    B. Metastatic choroidal carcinoma.
    C. Choroidal osteoma.
    D. Amelanotic melanoma.
    E. Fundus lesions in Aicardi's syndrome.

34. Multiple astrocytomas of the neural retina most likely are associated with:
    A. Tuberous sclerosis.
    B. von Recklinghausen's disease.
    C. Sturge–Weber syndrome.
    D. Von Hippel–Lindau syndrome.
    E. A sporadic, nonsyndromic disorder.

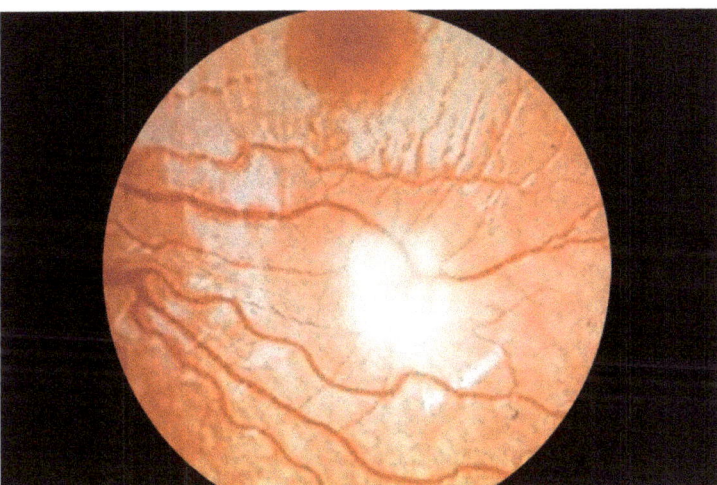

Fig. 10.16: "Young" retinal lesion inferiorly in child.

35. Which one of the following is not usually included in the differential diagnosis of astrocytoma of the retina?
    A. Retinoblastoma.
    B. Toxocariasis.
    C. Amelanotic choroidal melanoma.
    D. Retinopathy of prematurity.
    E. Massive gliosis of the retina.

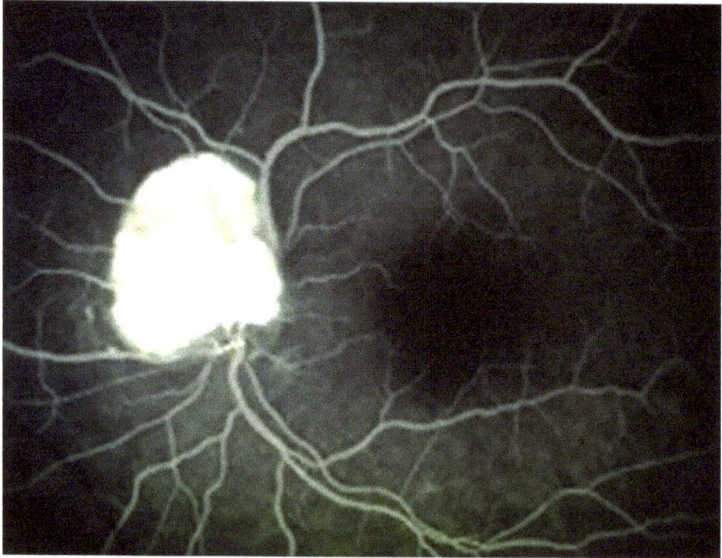

Fig. 10.17: "Mulberry" lesion of optic nerve head.

36. **A retinal lesion is noted on routine examination of a 55-year-old woman. Fluorescein angiography shows slow filling of multiple tiny saccules that remain brightly fluorescent long after the normal intravascular fluorescence has faded. The lesion probably is:**
    A. Neural retinal astrocytoma.
    B. Retinoblastoma.
    C. Neural retinal capillary hemangioma.
    D. Cavernous hemangioma of the retina.
    E. Idiopathic juxtafoveal retinal telangiectasia.

37. **The combined hamartoma of the retina is composed of neural retina, retinal pigment epithelium, retinal blood vessels, and vitreoretinal membranes. All of the following statements are true, *except*:**
    A. It has malignant potential.
    B. It tends to be unilateral and unifocal.
    C. It can have a familial pattern.
    D. It is usually located in the posterior pole.
    E. It is a congenital lesion.

38. **Which of the following is *not* a histopathologic characteristic of combined hamartoma of the retina?**
    A. Interlacing cords of hyperplastic retinal pigment epithelium.
    B. Disorganized and thickened neural retina.
    C. Proliferation of benign glial cells on the vitreal surface of the lesion.
    D. Neural rosette formation.
    E. Abnormal intraneuronal retinal blood vessels.

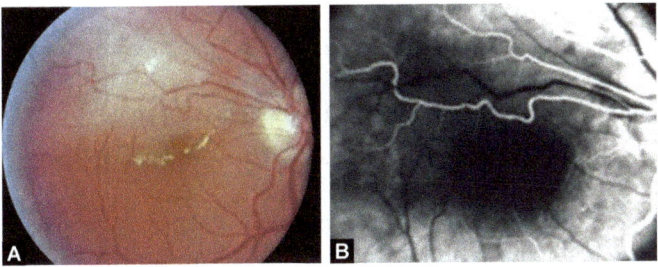

Figs. 10.18A and B: (A) Thickened retina superior to macula in young woman; (B) Early fluorescein shows abnormal retinal vessel.

39. **Which one of the following statements concerning congenital hypertrophy of the retinal pigment epithelium (CHRPE) is false?**
    A. It is congenital.
    B. It is always smooth and velvety black.
    C. It has a unifocal, uniocular variety.
    D. It has a multifocal, uniocular variety (grouped pigmentation; *bear tracks*).
    E. It has rare malignant potential.

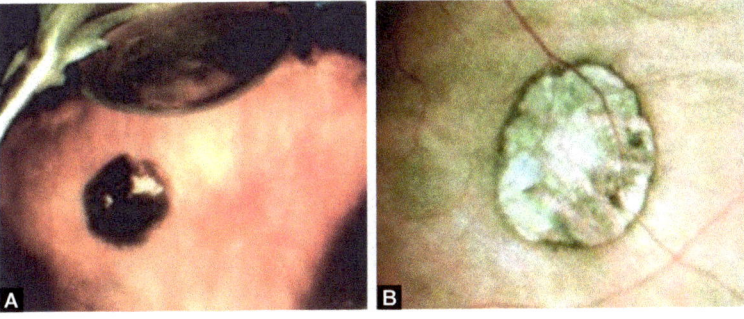

Figs. 10.19A and B: (A) The smooth, velvety surface, often surrounded by a halo is characteristic; (B) With time the lesion can loose pigment.

40. **A patient with multifocal, bilateral, and atypical congenital hypertrophy of the retinal pigment epithelium probably:**
    A. Has colonic adenomatous polyps and Gardner's syndrome.
    B. Has Turcot's syndrome if additional neuroepithelial central nervous system tumors are present.
    C. Also has Farmer's syndrome if bone cysts and soft tissue tumors are present.
    D. Has a virtual 100% chance of developing colon carcinoma during adult life if prophylactic removal of colonic polyps is not performed.
    E. Has an abnormality in chromosome 5q21-q22.

41. **All the following are very rare primary intraocular neoplasms, *except*:**
    A. Leiomyoma.
    B. Neurilemoma.

C. Glioneuroma.
D. Adenoma and adenocarcinoma of the neuroepithelium (e.g. ciliary epithelium).
E. Intraocular extension of conjunctival carcinoma.

42. Which one of the following does *not* apply to neurofibromatosis type 1 (NF-1)?
   A. It has been localized to chromosome 17qII.
   B. The incidence is about 1 per 3,500–4,000 persons.
   C. All features of the syndrome are manifest by early childhood.
   D. Along with neurofibromatosis type 2 (NF-2), it is the most common phakomatosis.
   E. It affects men and women equally.

43. A young patient is seen to have findings suggestive of neurofibromatosis type 1 (NF-1). Which of the following would you *not* expect to see?
   A. Intellectual disability.
   B. Cutaneous café-au-lait spots.
   C. Axillary and inguinal freckling.
   D. Iris (Lisch) nodules.
   E. Optic nerve gliomas.

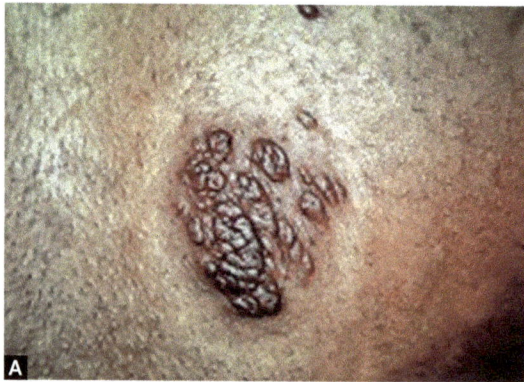

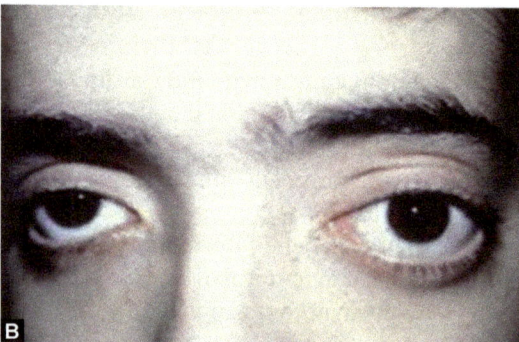

Figs. 10.20A and B: (A) Patient has multiple, elevated, skin lesions; (B) Plexiform neurofibroma present in the patient's left orbit.

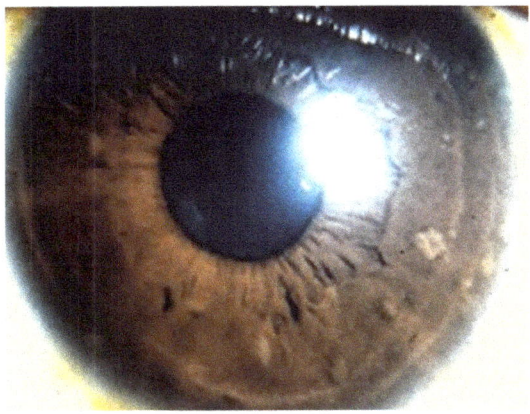

Fig. 10.21: Spider-like, small lesions on the anterior iris surface.

44. A patient has bilateral acoustic neuromas. Testing shows an abnormality of the 22 band on the chromosome 22q12. Which of the following findings does *not* fit the suspected diagnosis?
    A. Schwannoma.
    B. Multiple meningiomas.
    C. Sensorineural deafness.
    D. Juvenile posterior subcapsular and cortical lens opacities.
    E. Renal adenomas.

45. Which of the following statements about tuberous sclerosis (TS) is *not* correct?
    A. Its prevalence in the general population is about 1 in 10,000.
    B. About one-third of cases are familial, and two-third are sporadic.
    C. Tuberous sclerosis genes are located on the long arm of chromosome 9 (9q32–34), the long arm of chromosome 11, the short arm of chromosome 16 (16pI3), and the arm of chromosome 12 (l2q22–24).
    D. Hamartomas of the stomach.
    E. Its most consistent chromosomal abnormality is 9q32–34.

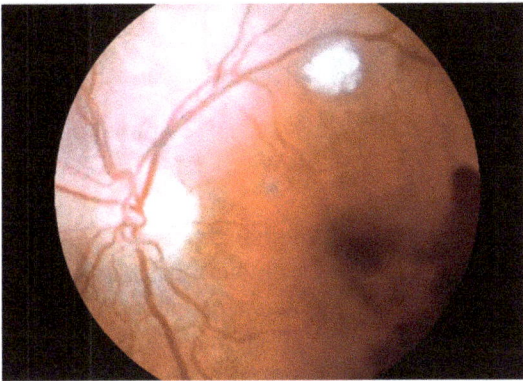

Fig. 10.22: "Old" mulberry retinal lesion in child.

46. A young patient is suspected of having tuberous sclerosis. All *but* one of the following findings are consistent with that diagnosis:
   A. Low-grade astrocytomas of the central nervous system
   B. Rhabdomyosarcoma of the liver.
   C. Neural retinal astrocytoma.
   D. Adenoma sebaceum.
   E. Angiomyolipoma of the kidney.

47. A patient presents with poor vision in one eye. Macular edema and a peripheral retinal vascular lesion that contains feeder vessels are found in the periphery. Tests show an abnormality in the 3p25–26 gene. Which of the following would you *not* expect to find?
   A. Retinal capillary hemangioma.
   B. Central nervous system hemangioblastoma.
   C. Cardiac rhabdomyoma.
   D. Renal cell carcinoma.
   E. Pheochromocytoma.

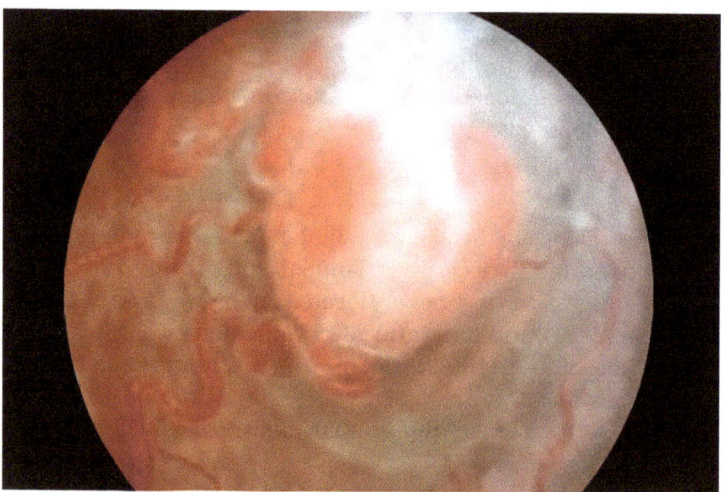

Fig. 10.23: Large, peripheral, vascular lesion has feeder vessels.

48. A patient is seen with a port-wine, facial birthmark, and congenital glaucoma on the same side. Which of the following would you *not* expect to find?
   A. Neural retinal cavernous hemangiomas.
   B. Cutaneous facial nevus flammeus move to left.
   C. Ipsilateral diffuse, cavernous hemangioma of the choroid.
   D. Ipsilateral meningeal hemangiomatosis.
   E. Cutaneous, ocular, and central nervous system lesions present at birth.

Intraocular Tumors

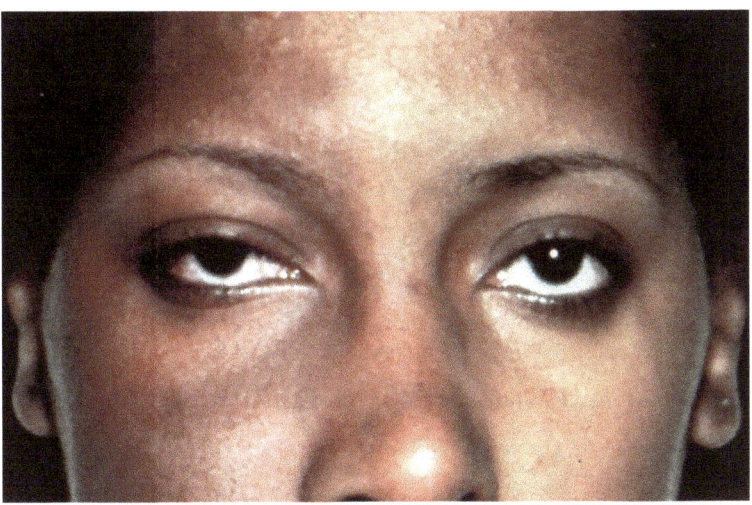

Fig. 10.24: Right side of face reddened and thickened.

ANSWERS

1. A. A neoplasm is a continuous increase in the number of cells in a tissue caused by unregulated proliferation. It differs from hyperplasia in that its growth never reaches equilibrium.
2. E. A teratoma is a neoplasm derived from cells of all three germ layers, ectoderm, mesoderm, and endoderm.
3. C. Less than 5% of treated cases in the United States of America (USA) die from the disease.
4. A. The average age of diagnosis of retinoblastoma is 13 months. About 90% of cases are diagnosed before the age of 3 years.
5. B. Chromosomal region 13q14 (*RB1* gene) regulates the development of normality. If both 13q14 chromosome regions are normal, no retinoblastoma will develop. If one of the two 13 chromosomes has a 13q14 deletion, duplication, or point mutation, no retinoblastoma will develop. If both 13 chromosomes have a 13q14 deletion, duplication, or point mutation, a retinoblastoma will develop.
6. E. Leukokoria and strabismus (esotropia or exotropia) are the most common presenting signs of retinoblastoma.
7. D. Medulloepithelioma usually presents with glaucoma, Coats' disease with an exudative retinal detachment, and ocular trauma would show other findings. Typically, a retinocytoma (retinoma) appears as a radiated tumor or has a fish-flesh appearance.
8. C. Onchocerciasis almost never causes leukokoria and usually presents as a chronic, bilateral closed-angle glaucoma.

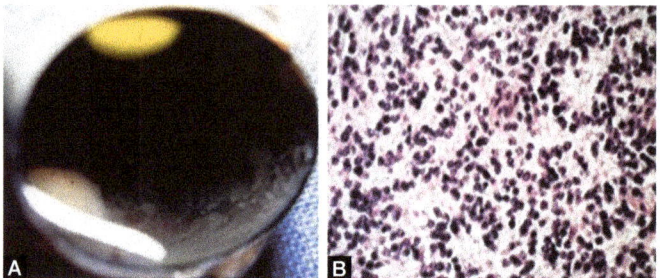

Figs. 10.25A and B: (A) Sectioned gross eye that contained mostly differentiated retinomas; (B) Differentiated retinoma cells are forming fleurette.

9. A. An extensive, bland necrosis is characteristic of retinoblastoma.

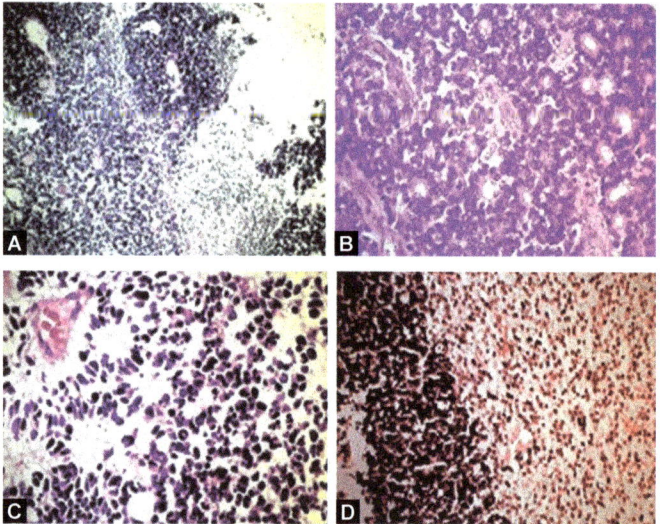

Figs. 10.26A to D: (A) Necrosis and undifferentiated retinoblastoma blue cells; (B) Retinoblastoma cells are more differentiated and are forming tubular-like structures (Flexner–Wintersteiner rosette); (C) Cells are lining up around acellular areas containing cobweb-like material (Homer Wright rosette); (D) Deep blue undifferentiated retinoblastoma cells (on left) abruptly change to differentiated retinoma cells (on right) forming fleurettes.

10. E. Uveal melanomas are most commonly metastasize to the liver, arise mainly from the choroid, spread hematogenously (not via lymphatics), and are the most common primary intraocular malignant neoplasm in adults.
11. D. Iris melanomas are detected at a slightly earlier age than ciliary body and choroidal melanomas. White patients have intraocular melanomas more frequently than black patients in a ratio of 15:1. The median age at diagnosis is 60 years, but the frequency does not plateau.
12. C. Smoking does not seem to be a risk factor for the development of melanoma.

13. B. Iris melanomas range in color from maximally pigmented to amelanotic. The color of the tumor does not correlate with prognosis.
14. E. If a melanoma causes a hemorrhage into the vitreous body (Knapp-Ronne type), heterochromia may develop (an extremely rare event).
15. B. B-scan ultrasonography of a dome-shaped choroidal melanoma characteristically shows a solid, biconvex cross-sectional shape with internal acoustic darkness in its base.
16. E. No test is diagnostic of choroidal melanoma. Indirect ophthalmoscopy and a wide variety of ancillary testing including wide-field fundus photography and ultrasonography are necessary for clinical evaluation. Ultrasonography is helpful for monitoring growth and regression.
17. C. Invasion of Bruch's membrane is not a prognostic indicator.

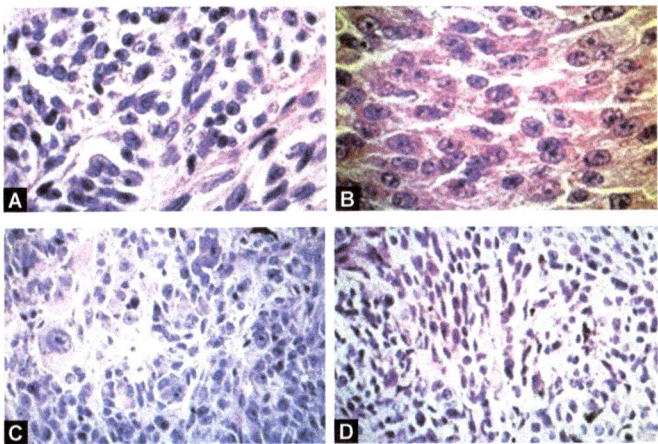

Figs. 10.27A to D: (A) Small, spindled melanoma cells without nucleoli and often with stripe down nucleus (spindle A cells—best prognosis); (B) Moderate size, spindled melanoma cells with nucleoli (spindle B cells—second best prognosis); (C) Large, round size, melanoma cells with very prominent nucleoli (epithelioid cells—worst prognosis); (D) Epithelioid cells surround spindle B cells in middle (mixed cell type—bad prognosis).

18. B. Although chemotherapy may be used if there is metastatic ocular malignant melanoma, it has no benefit in the "pure" ocular form.
19. A. Commonly, metastatic carcinoma metastasizes to the eye, particularly the posterior choroid due to the rich vascular supply. It rarely metastasizes to the retina and optic disc or nerve supplied solely by the central retinal artery.
20. C. Breast and lung are the two most frequent primary sites of metastatic carcinoma to the eye in women (frequency of 70% and 10%, respectively). The most common primary site for males being lung (40%).
21. B. Syphilitic granulomas of the choroid usually present in the tertiary stage show signs of inflammation that distinguish it from neoplasms.
22. A. Leukemia frequently involves ocular structures with ophthalmic findings in approximately 40% of patients at diagnosis. Lymphomas rarely involve ocular structures such as conjunctiva. Central nervous system (CNS) lymphomas which can also involve the vitreous, arise from B-cell lymphocytes.

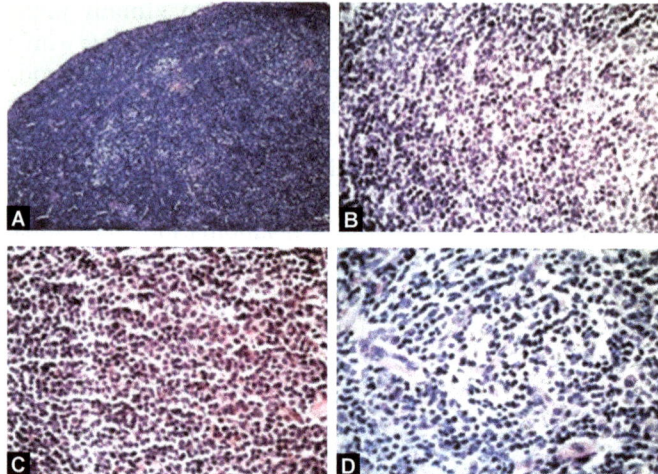

Figs. 10.28A to D: (A) Conjunctival biopsy of salmon-pink smooth mass shows sheets of dark cells; (B) Cells are almost all lymphocytes; (C) Occasional mitotic figure is seen. These lesions usually are low-grade small B-cell lymphomas; (D) If the infiltrate contains plasma cells, histiocytes, and proliferating vascular endothelial cells along with the lymphocytes; the lesions are inflammatory pseudotumors.

23. C. Primary intraocular lymphoma may arise within the neural retina, the uvea, and may be solitary, diffuse, or multifocal. Occasionally, non-Hodgkin's lymphoma may involve the eye primarily and simulate a chronic uveitis.

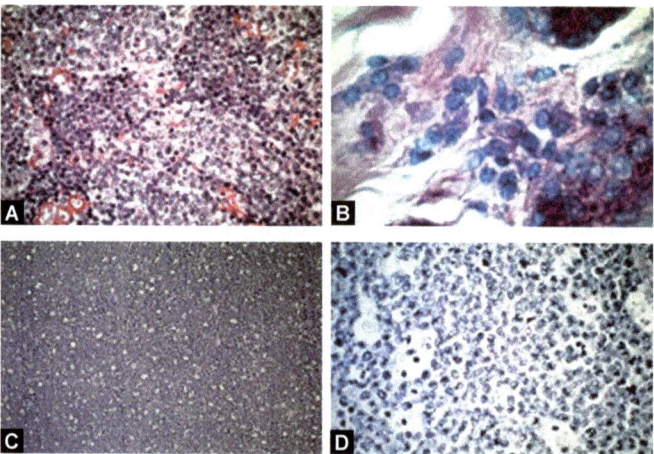

Figs. 10.29A to D: (A) The malignant lymphocytes are a mixture of small and larger B-cell lymphocytes; (B) Periodic acid-Schiff-positive, eosinophilic, intraocular inclusions, Dutcher bodies are indicative of malignancy; (C) Another tumor shows a "starry-sky" appearance under low magnification; (D) Interspersed among the large, undifferentiated, malignant B cells are clear-cell histiocytes containing cellular debris accounting for the low power appearance (Burkitt's lymphoma).

24. B. Leukemic cells do not protect against concurrent microbial infection.

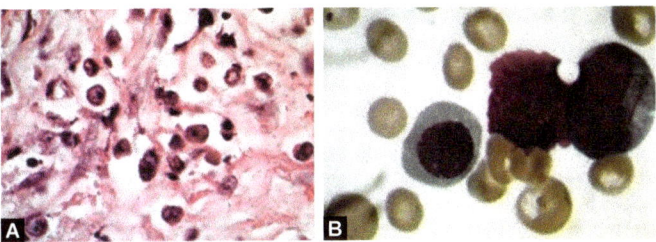

Figs. 10.30A and B: (A) High magnification of infiltrate of immature leukocytes; (B) Bone marrow biopsy demonstrates immature leukocytes in this case of acute, myelogenous leukemia.

25. D. Melanoma and leiomyoma are extremely rare in a 6-year-old child. Juvenile xanthogranuloma is usually accompanied with orange skin lesions. Nematode granulomas affect the posterior part of the eye. Often, medulloepitheliomas present as anterior lesions accompanied by glaucoma.

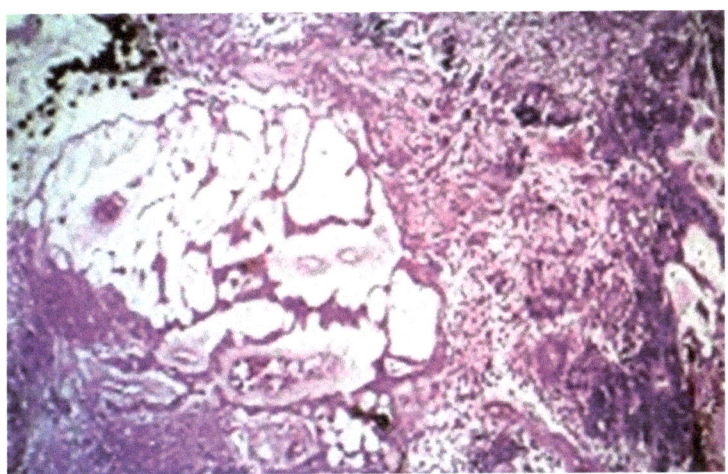

Fig. 10.31: Medulloepithelioma. Increased magnification shows cell tubules forming lumina in some areas and in other areas simulating primitive vitreous.

26. A. The presence of cartilage is characteristic of a teratoid medulloepithelioma.
27. D. Nevi are extremely common uveal tumors. Their numbers are underestimated because only the pigmented nevi are visible. Nevi are much more common in lightly pigmented people than in darkly pigmented people.
28. B. Choroidal nevi generally have sharp edges and a smooth surface. Even though they tend to accumulate drusen, the surface remains smooth. Irregular edges and surface (*lumpy*) are suggestive of malignant change.

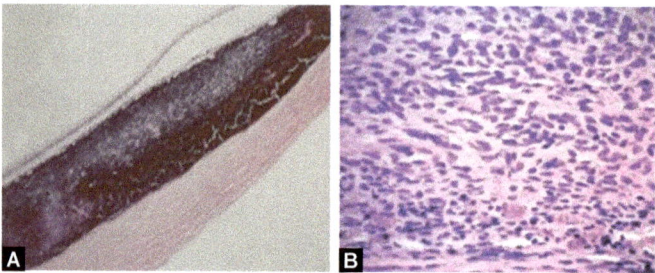

Figs. 10.32: (A) Heavily pigmented choroidal tumor; (B) Bleached section shows innocuous spindle, nevus cells.

29. E. Choroidal nevi often develop drusen, may reach a thickness greater than 1.5 mm, and occasionally develop subretinal fluid and even choroidal neovascularization. Substantial tumor enlargement, however, is suggestive of malignant transformation.
30. E. The red-orange color is most suggestive of choroidal hemangioma.

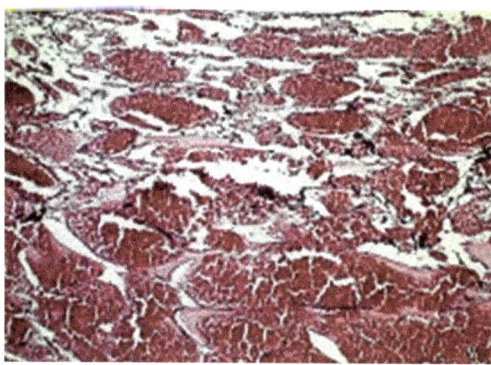

Fig. 10.33: Choroidal hemangioma is of the cavernous type typical both of Sturge–Weber choroidal hemangioma and of the incidental type of choroidal hemangioma.

31. B. Primary lymphoma of the uvea, leukemic or secondary lymphomatous uveal infiltrate, diffuse posterior scleritis, and uveal effusion syndrome can all simulate a diffuse choroidal hemangioma.
32. C. The choroidal hemangiomas appear like cavernous hemangiomas, not capillary hemangiomas. In Sturge–Weber syndrome, the hemangioma tends to be large and diffuse, blending subtly into the contiguous choroid.
33. C. Although the most likely diagnosis is choroidal osteoma, a similar lesion can be seen in Aicardi's syndrome. Aicardi's syndrome shows chorioretinopathy with lacunar defects that may resemble choroidal osteoma. The margins of the lesion are usually smooth without localized extensions.
34. A. Sturge–Weber syndrome and von Recklinghausen's disease causes diffuse choroidal thickening and von Hippel–Lindau syndrome cause retinal angiomas.

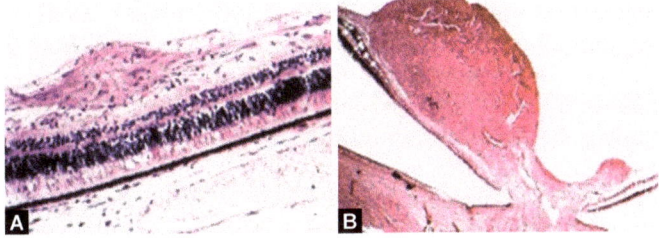

Figs. 10.34A and B: (A) "Young" astrocytoma of the retina composed of spindle astrocytes; (B) Large, astrocytoma of middle and inner layers of retina.

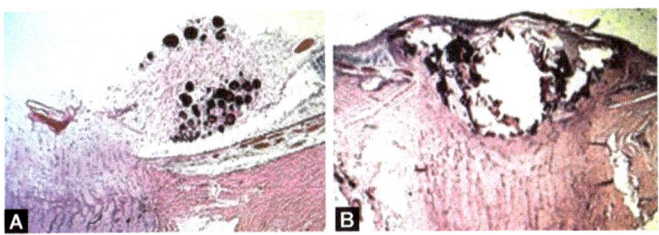

Figs. 10.35A and B: (A) "Mature" retinal astrocytoma containing calcified spherules; (B) Large astrocytoma of optic nerve head (mulberry configuration).

35. D. All except retinopathy of prematurity can cause discrete retinal tumors.
36. D. Cavernous hemangioma of the retina is quite rare, congenital, stationary, and most frequent in women. An overlying serous retinal detachment may develop.
37. A. It is a congenital, benign lesion that has no malignant potential. Because of the common posterior location, the patient may present with amblyopia and strabismus.
38. D. Neural rosette formation does not occur in this lesion. Combined hamartoma is mostly seen in young men between the ages of 20 years and 45 years. Growth has rarely been documented.

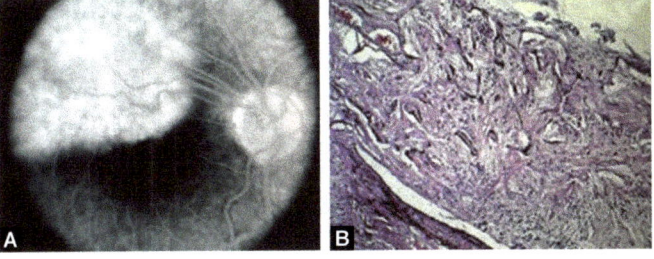

Figs. 10.36A and B: (A) Late stage of fluorescein shows abnormal vessels leaking into retina; (B) Histologically, retinal pigment epithelium and abnormal blood vessels present in retina.

39. B. Often, depigmented areas (lacunae) develop in the congenital hypertrophy of the retinal pigment epithelium (CHRPE) lesions,

giving the appearance of "punched-out" lesions. CHRPE lesions may enlarge overtime, and only rarely malignant lesions have developed such as adenocarcinoma. Multiple CHRPE-like lesions may represent Gardner's syndrome associated with an increased risk of colon polyps, benign tumors, and cancer.

40. C. Farmer's syndrome, a hypersensitivity pneumonitis induced by the inhalation of biologic dusts coming from hay dust or mold spores or other agricultural products is not associated with congenital hypertrophy of the retinal pigment epithelium. It is important to know the relationship between CHRPE and familial polyposis (Gardner's syndrome) because the ophthalmoscopic examination may for the first time yield findings suggestive of the potentially deadly disease.

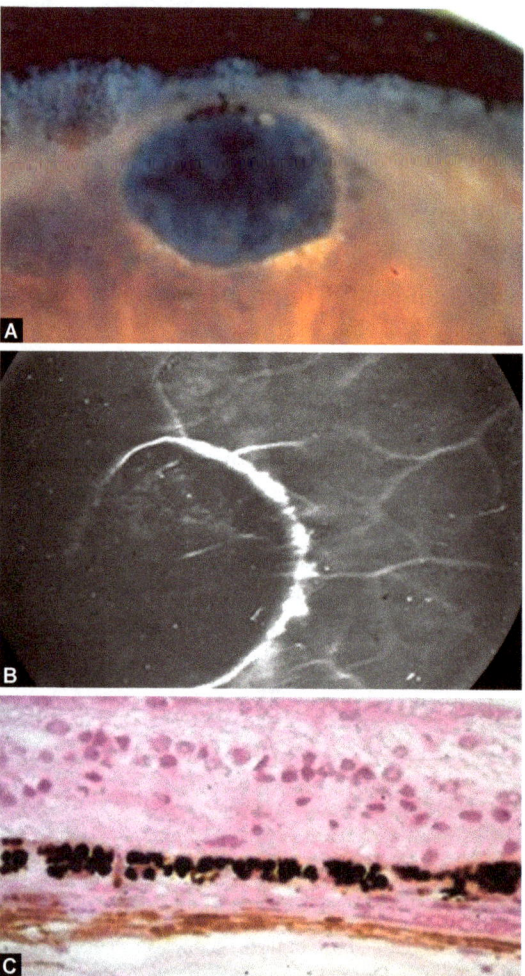

Figs. 10.37A to C: (A) The surrounding halo is easily visualized; (B) The halo is caused by a lack of pigment in the retinal pigment epithelium (RPE), which is viewed as a round hypofluorescent area with fluorescence; (C) Histologically, the RPE is hypertrophic (enlarged) except at the edge (halo) where it is atrophic.

41. D. Although all five entities are uncommon, adenoma and adenocarcinoma of the neuroepithelium are much less rare than the other 4.

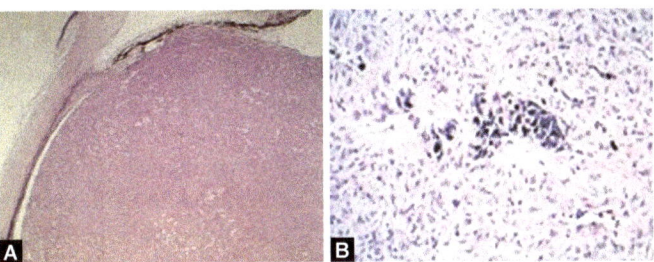

Figs. 10.38A and B: (A) Large tumor occupies ciliary body (CB); (B) Increased magnification shows the CB adenoma is composed of a papillary proliferation of cords of benign epithelial cells some of which are pigmented.

42. C. Some of the findings of neurofibromatosis type 1 (NF-1) especially the neoplastic changes may not occur until adulthood. Lisch nodules (iris, melanocytic, and spider-like lesions) are the most common clinical findings.

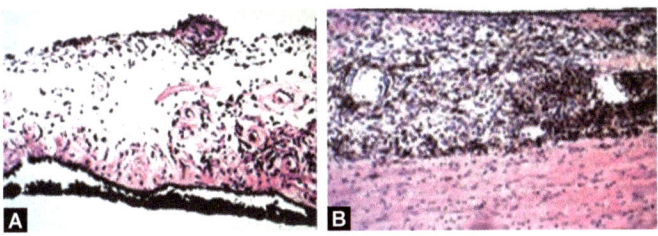

Figs. 10.39A and B: (A) Melanocytic accumulation on the anterior surface of iris noted clinically as Lisch nodules; (B) Choroid markedly thickened by neurofibromatosis hamartoma.

43. A. Intellectual disability is not one of the characteristics of NF-1. Tuberous sclerosis is associated with high rates of intellectual disability and autism.

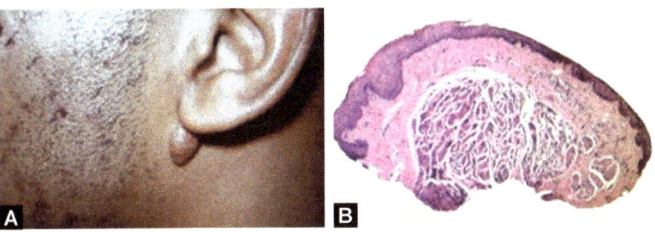

Figs. 10.40A and B: (A) Neurofibroma present under left earlobe; (B) Schwann cells forming dermal neurofibroma.

44. E. Renal adenomas are not part of neurofibromatosis type 2 (NF-2). NF-2 has much less ocular involvement than NF-1.

45. D. Hamartomas occur in the cerebrum, skin (adenoma sebaceum), lung, heart, and kidney, but usually are not found in the stomach.
46. B. Rhabdomyosarcoma of the liver has not been reported in tuberous sclerosis. Because of the many findings in this condition, the prognosis is poor and most patients die by 20 years of age.
47. C. Cardiac rhabdomyoma is not associated with von Hippel–Lindau syndrome.
48. A. Neural retinal cavernous hemangiomas do not occur in the Sturge–Weber syndrome. Cavernous hemangioma of the choroid is the most common intraocular finding. Almost always, the congenital glaucoma, when present, is seen on the same side as the port-wine stain, usually accompanied by ipsilateral lid hemangiomas.

CHAPTER 11

Neuro-ophthalmology

Stephanie J Weiss, Robert T Spector

QUESTIONS

Identify the **INCORRECT** answer for all questions (unless instructed otherwise).

1. **In magnetic resonance imaging:**
   A. Long time to echo (TE) and short time to repetition (TR) yield a poor signal-to-noise ratio.
   B. Long TE and long TR yield a T2-weighted scan.
   C. Short TE and short TR yield a T1-weighted scan.
   D. Short TE and long TR give an intermediate or proton-density scan.
   E. Short TR are 600–1,000 ms.

2. **In magnetic resonance imaging:**
   A. Orbital fat yields a bright T1 and dark T2 image.
   B. Air yields a dark T1 and T2 image.
   C. Vitreous yields a bright T1 and dark T2 image.
   D. Gadolinium yields a bright T1 and dark T2 image.
   E. Flowing blood yields a dark T1 and T2 image.

3. **Gadolinium:**
   A. Lengthens T1 relaxation time.
   B. Is a toxic metallic ion.
   C. Has biodistribution characteristics similar to those of iodinated contrast materials.
   D. Is typically used for T1-weighted imaging and yields a bright signal.
   E. Is relatively contraindicated in patients who have hemolytic anemia.

4. **Magnetic resonance imaging is contraindicated in patients who have:**
   A. Cochlear implants.
   B. Cardiac pacemakers.
   C. Metallic cardiac valves.
   D. Intraocular metallic foreign bodies.
   E. Psychiatric disorders.

5. Magnetic resonance angiography:
A. Tends to overdiagnose vascular stenosis.
B. Exhibits vessels larger than noted in conventional angiography.
C. May miss aneurysms, plaques, and ulcerations.
D. Is a form of noninvasive imaging.
E. Is as effective as contrast-enhanced computed tomographic angiography for detection of aneurysms.

6. Conventional angiography:
A. Is relatively expensive.
B. Is accompanied by systemic morbidity in 2.5% of cases.
C. Remains the definitive method for diagnosis of vascular disease and intracranial aneurysms.
D. Is performed by placing a catheter intravenously.
E. Is performed by using iodinated contrast dye.

7. Computed tomographic scanning of the globe is preferred over magnetic resonance imaging for:
A. Suspected calcification.
B. Acute hemorrhage.
C. Radiopaque intraocular foreign bodies.
D. Trauma.
E. Uveal melanoma.

8. The optic nerve:
A. Is about 25-30 mm long in the orbit.
B. Is about 25-30 mm long in the optic canal.
C. Contains both M and P cells.
D. Is about 55 mm long from globe to chiasm.
E. Carries approximately 1.2 million axons.

9. The ophthalmic artery:
A. Enters the orbit along with the optic nerve through the optic canal.
B. Gives off branches that feed the radial pial circulation to the optic nerve.
C. Runs superior to the optic nerve.
D. Becomes the central retinal artery.
E. Does not contribute directly to the circle of Zinn–Haller.

10. Optic neuropathies:
A. Are associated with an afferent pupillary defect.
B. Are associated with reduced brightness sense.
C. Are associated with metamorphopsia.
D. Are associated with reduced color vision.
E. Rarely change the eye's refractive error.

11. Macular disease is usually associated with:
A. Slow recovery from photostress.
B. Loss of contrast sensitivity at 18 cycles/degree.

C. No latency delay on visual-evoked response testing.
D. Absence of scotoma on Amsler grid testing.
E. Absence of Pulfrich phenomenon.

12. **Optic nerve hypoplasia:**
    A. Is incompatible with 20/20 (6/6) acuity.
    B. Often appears with a double-ring sign.
    C. Is associated with midline brain defects.
    D. May be demonstrated with magnetic resonance imaging.
    E. Is often associated with endocrine abnormalities.

13. **Morning glory disc anomaly:**
    A. Contains a white tuft of glial tissue.
    B. Is not associated with iris or choroidal colobomas.
    C. Is not associated with retinal detachment.
    D. May be associated with transsphenoidal encephalocoele.
    E. May be associated with panhypopituitarism.

14. **Optic disc coloboma is associated with:**
    A. Transsphenoidal encephalocele.
    B. Linear sebaceous nevus syndrome.
    C. Acardi syndrome
    D. CHARGE syndrome.
    E. Walker–Warburg syndrome.

15. **Optic nerve pits:**
    A. Can be located in any sector of the nerve.
    B. Never produce visual field defects.
    C. Are of unknown cause.
    D. Are not associated with brain malformations.
    E. Are associated with serous retinal detachments in 45% of cases.

16. **Megalopapilla:**
    A. Can be unilateral or bilateral.
    B. Is most commonly sporadic.
    C. Can be associated with enlarged blind spot on visual field testing.
    D. Requires neuroimaging because of associated brain anomalies.
    E. Is never acquired.

17. **Congenital tilted disc syndrome:**
    A. Is usually bilateral.
    B. Is usually autosomal dominant.
    C. Is accompanied by nasalization of the retinal vessels.
    D. Is associated with high myopia.
    E. May have superior bitemporal visual field defects that improve with refractive correction.

18. **Aicardi syndrome:**
    A. Is inherited as an X-linked dominant trait that is lethal in hemizygous males.

B. Is associated with choroid plexus papillomas.
C. Features infantile spasms and vertebral anomalies.
D. Rarely involves both eyes.
E. Can be confused with infectious chorioretinitis.

19. **Pseudotumor cerebri (idiopathic intracranial hypertension):**
    A. Is associated with permanent visual loss in 50% of cases.
    B. May be caused by drugs such as corticosteroids or tetracycline.
    C. Has an identifiable cause in almost all patients.
    D. Often first presents with headache.
    E. Is more common in patients who have hypoparathyroidism and adrenal adenomas.

20. **Axoplasmic transport:**
    A. Is impaired in optic disc swelling.
    B. If anterograde, is always rapid.
    C. Is oxygen dependent.
    D. May be retrograde.
    E. Occurs along the entire length of the optic nerve.

21. **Clinical signs of optic disc edema include:**
    A. Blurring of the optic disc margin.
    B. Obliteration of the optic cup.
    C. Anterior extension of the nerve head into the vitreous.
    D. Retinal or choroidal folds.
    E. Attenuation of retinal veins.

22. **Headaches associated with increased intracranial pressure are often:**
    A. Worse when the patient is recumbent.
    B. Associated with pulsatile tinnitus.
    C. Associated with nausea and/or vomiting.
    D. Frontal in location.
    E. Associated with transient visual obscurations.

23. **Treatment options for idiopathic intracranial hypertension (pseudotumor cerebri) include:**
    A. Oral carbonic anhydrase inhibitors.
    B. Beta-blockers.
    C. Optic nerve sheath fenestration.
    D. Ventriculoperitoneal shunt.
    E. Weight loss.

24. **Optic neuritis:**
    A. Is most common in patients between 20 years and 50 years of age.
    B. Affects women more often than men.
    C. Is commonly associated with an afferent pupillary defect.
    D. Causes gradual visual loss over months to years.
    E. Is associated with pain in or around the eye.

25. Neuroretinitis:
A. Can be caused by sarcoidosis.
B. Can be associated with cat-scratch fever.
C. Presents with optic disc edema and macular exudation in a stellate pattern.
D. Can be caused by toxoplasmosis.
E. Is associated with an increased risk of developing multiple sclerosis.

26. Parainfectious optic neuritis:
A. Typically follows onset of viral infection by 1–2 months.
B. Is more common in children than in adults.
C. Is often bilateral.
D. May be associated with meningoencephalitis.
E. Is associated with excellent visual recovery.

27. According to the Optic Neuritis Treatment Trial, optic neuritis progresses to multiple sclerosis:
A. In 56% of patients within 10 years of developing optic neuritis in patients with 1 or more white matter lesions on MRI at the time of optic neuritis.
B. In 16% of patients within 5 years of developing optic neuritis in patients with a normal MRI at the time of optic neuritis.
C. In 22% of patients within 10 years of developing optic neuritis in patients with a normal MRI at the time of optic neuritis.
D. With increased certainty if optic neuritis occurred in the other eye.
E. With increased certainty if optic disc edema was present.

28. The Optic Neuritis Treatment Trial found that:
A. Patients treated with oral corticosteroids alone recovered visual acuity faster than those treated with placebo.
B. Patients treated with oral corticosteroids alone had increased risk of new attacks of optic neuritis.
C. Patients treated with intravenous corticosteroids followed by oral corticosteroids recovered visual acuity faster than those treated with placebo.
D. Patients treated with intravenous corticosteroids followed by oral corticosteroids had a decreased incidence of multiple sclerosis at 2 years.
E. Patients with at least one white matter lesion on MRI at the time of optic neuritis were at increased risk for developing multiple sclerosis.

29. Visual recovery in patients who have optic neuritis:
A. Is 20/40 or better in 92% of patients according to the optic neuritis treatment trial.
B. May occur up to 1 year after disease onset.
C. Occurs more rapidly in patients treated with intravenous steroids.
D. Is always associated with complete recovery of color vision and brightness.
E. May be incomplete with regard to color vision and brightness.

30. Anterior ischemic optic neuropathy:
A. Always presents with optic disc swelling in the acute phase.
B. Is more commonly nonarteritic than arteritic in origin.
C. Is most common in Caucasians patients.
D. Usually occurs in patients between 30 years and 50 years of age.
E. Most commonly produces an altitudinal or arcuate visual field defect.

31. Arteritic anterior ischemic optic neuropathy:
A. Results from long ciliary artery vasculitis.
B. Is associated with delayed choroidal filling on fluorescein angiography.
C. Is more common in women than in men.
D. Is usually associated with a pale (chalky white) disc.
E. Is associated with a poor visual prognosis.

32. Nonarteritic anterior ischemic optic neuropathy:
A. Produces a normal appearing optic nerve on magnetic resonance imaging including gadolinium enhanced images.
B. Tends to occur in a "disc at risk" with structural crowding of disc.
C. Is more common in men than in women.
D. Produces an optic disc that may be hyperemic or pale.
E. Is rarely associated with systemic symptoms such as headache or jaw claudication.

33. Nonarteritic anterior ischemic optic neuropathy is associated with:
A. An altitudinal visual field defect.
B. A relative afferent pupillary field defect.
C. Optic disc edema.
D. Rare improvement in visual acuity during the recovery period.
E. Delayed optic disc filling on fluorescein angiography.

34. Arteritic anterior ischemic optic neuropathy is associated with:
A. Headache.
B. Jaw claudication.
C. Scalp tenderness.
D. Fever.
E. Joint pain.

35. Erythrocyte sedimentation rate:
A. Is more commonly elevated in arteritic than nonarteritic anterior ischemic optic neuropathy.
B. Is normal in about 15% of biopsy-proven cases of arteritic anterior ischemic optic neuropathy.
C. May be elevated in diabetic patients who do not have arteritis.
D. Always reverts to normal after one dose of systemic corticosteroids.
E. May be elevated in older patients who do not have arteritis.

36. Superficial temporal artery biopsy in patients who have temporal arteritis:

A. May be normal.
   B. May show intimal thickening.
   C. Must be performed before corticosteroid therapy is begun.
   D. In some cases, should be performed bilaterally.
   E. May show internal elastic lamina fragmentation.

37. **Nonarteritic anterior ischemic optic neuropathy may be associated with:**
    A. Systemic hypertension.
    B. Diabetes mellitus.
    C. Carotid occlusive disease.
    D. Hyperlipidemia.
    E. Sleep apnea.

38. **Arteritic anterior ischemic optic neuropathy may be treated with:**
    A. High-dose intravenous methylprednisolone.
    B. Daily oral prednisone.
    C. Alternate-day oral prednisone.
    D. Intravenous methylprednisolone followed by oral prednisone.
    E. Daily intravenous methylprednisolone and daily aspirin.

39. **Treatment of nonarteritic anterior ischemic optic neuropathy by:**
    A. Oral corticosteroids are of unproven benefit.
    B. Optic nerve sheath fenestration may possibly be harmful.
    C. Hyperbaric oxygen is of unproven benefit.
    D. Optic nerve sheath fenestration has been proved beneficial by the ischemic optic neuropathy decompression trial.
    E. Intravenous methylprednisolone is of unproven benefit.

40. **Diabetic papillopathy:**
    A. Presents with optic nerve edema and hyperemia.
    B. Manifests prominent and dilated disc surface microvasculature.
    C. Occurs in patients with type 1 or type 2 diabetes mellitus.
    D. Always occurs in the setting of diabetic retinopathy.
    E. Is associated with variable visual acuity.

41. **Papillophlebitis:**
    A. Is often bilateral.
    B. Is a subset of central retinal vein occlusion.
    C. Is usually associated with normal visual acuity.
    D. Appears with marked retinal venous engorgement and hemorrhage.
    E. Tends to resolve spontaneously within 1 year without significant visual sequelae.

42. **Leber's hereditary optic neuropathy:**
    A. Is inherited as an X-linked recessive trait.
    B. Typically is monocular at onset.
    C. Involves the second eye within weeks or months of involvement of the first eye.

D. Typically leads to visual acuity of 20/200 or worse.
E. In early stages, has a peripapillary telangiectasia.

43. **Toxic optic neuropathy may develop from a deficiency in:**
    A. Vitamin B_{12}.
    B. Folic acid.
    C. Thiamine.
    D. Sulfur-containing amino acids.
    E. Methanol.

44. **Toxic optic neuropathy will result from exposure to toxic doses of:**
    A. Carbon monoxide.
    B. Ethambutol.
    C. Isoniazid.
    D. Folic acid.
    E. Methanol.

Prechiasmal Pathways Compression by Optic Nerve and Sheath Tumors

45. **Gliomas of the anterior visual pathway:**
    A. Commonly present with exophthalmos.
    B. Are rarely malignant.
    C. Rarely involve the chiasm.
    D. Occur most commonly in the first decade of life.
    E. Is the most common primary tumor of the optic nerve.

46. **Optic nerve gliomas:**
    A. Are more commonly found in patients who have neurofibromatosis type 2 than those with type 1.
    B. Are found in approximately 15% of patients who have neurofibromatosis type 1.
    C. May be bilateral in patients with neurofibromatosis.
    D. In patients with neurofibromatosis type 1 typically occur in the first decade of life
    E. Are more commonly found in patients who have neurofibromatosis type 1 than those with type 2.

47. **Optic nerve sheath meningiomas:**
    A. Primarily affect middle-aged women.
    B. Are usually benign.
    C. Are characterized by slowly progressive vision loss.
    D. Often present with optociliary shunt vessels.
    E. Have a tumor-related mortality of 25%.

48. **Traumatic optic neuropathy:**
    A. If unilateral, will not appear with an afferent pupillary defect.
    B. Is most commonly caused by indirect trauma.
    C. May occur after a minor head injury.

D. Usually affects the intracanalicular portion of the nerve.
E. Has no proven treatment.

49. **The optic chiasm:**
    A. Is usually situated directly over the pituitary fossa of the sella turcica.
    B. Is flanked laterally by the carotid arteries.
    C. Contains macular fibers that cross in the anterior chiasm.
    D. Receives its blood supply from branches of the anterior communicating arteries.
    E. Sits anterior to and below the third ventricle.

50. **Pituitary adenomas:**
    A. Cause most chiasmatic dysfunction.
    B. Comprise 40% of symptomatic intracranial tumors.
    C. Are uncommon before age of 20 years.
    D. That cause chiasmatic compression is usually quite large.
    E. That are asymptomatic may represent 25% of all adenomas.

51. **Suprasellar meningiomas:**
    A. Represent approximately 15% of all primary intracranial tumors.
    B. Increase in incidence with age.
    C. Are more common in women than in men.
    D. Are occasionally familial.
    E. Are not associated with neurofibromatosis.

52. **Craniopharyngiomas:**
    A. Are histologically benign.
    B. Are derived from Rathke's pouch.
    C. Have a bimodal incidence occurring before age of 20 years and between age of 50 years and 70 years.
    D. Most commonly produce a superior bitemporal visual field defect.
    E. Frequently cause see-saw nystagmus.

53. **Chiasmatic lesions may cause a:**
    A. Unilateral temporal hemianopia.
    B. Bitemporal hemianopia.
    C. Junctional scotoma.
    D. Paracentral temporal hemianopic scotoma.
    E. Homonymous scotoma.

54. **Meningiomas of the chiasm:**
    A. Are usually malignant.
    B. May contain psammoma bodies.
    C. May contain concentrically organized spindle cells that form whorls.
    D. May histologically appear as syncytial tumors with intertwined cell membranes.
    E. Probably derive from cap cells that line the outer arachnoid surface.

55. Management of pituitary adenomas:
  A. That secrete prolactin is initially pharmacologic.
  B. That secrete growth hormone is initially surgical.
  C. Surgically is usually via a transsphenoidal approach.
  D. Should include serial visual field testing.
  E. May include radiation.

56. Treatment of craniopharyngiomas:
  A. Is associated with visual recovery 90% of patients.
  B. May include placement of chemotherapeutic agents in the tumor cavity.
  C. Is particularly difficult if the tumor is cystic.
  D. Is often associated with recurrence within 2 years.
  E. May require adjunctive radiation therapy.

57. The lateral geniculate body:
  A. Contains axons from the contralateral eye that synapse in layers 2, 3, and 5.
  B. Is located in the posterior portion of the thalamus.
  C. Has 6 total layers.
  D. Contains large M cells in layers 1 and 2.
  E. Contains small P cells in layers 3–6.

58. The primary visual cortex:
  A. Is arranged in hypercolumn.
  B. Contains fibers from the temporal crescent of the contralateral eye that lie most anteriorly.
  C. Is also known as V2.
  D. Straddles the calcarine fissure.
  E. Contains macular fibers that lie most posteriorly.

59. Patients with non-organic vision loss:
  A. Includes malingering but not hysteria.
  B. May have spiraling or crossing isopters on Goldmann visual fields.
  C. May have a tunnel configuration to visual fields.
  D. May perform normally on stereoscopic testing.
  E. Will not have an afferent pupillary defect.

60. Horizontal saccades:
  A. Are fast eye movements.
  B. Are triggered by the ipsilateral frontal lobe.
  C. Are termed dysfunctional if they overshoot or undershoot.
  D. May be tested by asking the patient to alternate gaze rapidly between two targets separated in space.
  E. Are controlled by the paramedian pontine reticular formation.

61. Smooth pursuit eye movements:
  A. Are slow eye movements.
  B. Allow the eyes to reach velocities of up to 70° per second.

C. Allow the eyes to follow a target when the target, the head, or both are moving.
D. Requires catch-up saccades to follow faster moving targets.
E. Are conjugate.

62. Vertical eye movements:
A. Require involvement of the rostral interstitial nucleus of the medial longitudinal fasciculus.
B. Require involvement of the interstitial nucleus of Cajal.
C. If saccadic, require simultaneous activation of both frontal eye fields.
D. May be affected by brainstem tumors.
E. Are never affected by pituitary adenomas.

63. The oculocephalic reflex:
A. Helps distinguish supranuclear from infranuclear lesions.
B. Ideally should be performed with the patient's head erect.
C. Cannot overcome gaze palsies caused by supranuclear lesions.
D. Cannot overcome gaze palsies caused by infranuclear lesions.
E. Should not be performed if the neck is unstable.

64. Vestibular caloric testing:
A. Tests the vestibulo-ocular reflex.
B. Should be preceded by examination of the tympanic membranes.
C. With cold water, causes a fast-beating eye movements to the opposite side.
D. In a comatose patient does not produce fast-beating eye movements.
E. With warm water causes a slow eye deviation to the side of the irrigation.

65. Congenital oculomotor apraxia:
A. Is more common in girls than in boys.
B. Is associated with normal vertical saccades.
C. Is associated with horizontal head thrusting to fixate on a target.
D. May occur in children who have dysgenesis of the corpus callosum.
E. Does not have a well-defined pattern of inheritance.

66. Slow saccades may be seen in:
A. Wilson disease.
B. Huntington disease.
C. Myotonic dystrophy.
D. Whipple disease.
E. Myasthenia gravis.

67. Balint syndrome:
A. Is caused by bilateral parieto-occipital lesions.
B. Results in visual agnosia.
C. Results in simultagnosia.
D. Results in optic ataxia.
E. Results in ocular motor apraxia.

68. One-and-a-half syndrome:
- A. May be caused by demyelinating disease.
- B. Involves one medial longitudinal fasciculus and either the ipsilateral paramedian pontine reticular formation or abducens nerve nucleus.
- C. Is never caused by pontine tumors.
- D. Retains abduction in the contralateral eye.
- E. May be associated with facial weakness, if the facial nerve is involved.

69. Downgaze palsy may be caused by:
- A. Bilateral pontine lesion.
- B. Progressive supranuclear palsy.
- C. Whipple disease.
- D. Wilson disease.
- E. Tuberculosis.

70. Dorsal midbrain (Parinaud's) syndrome consists of:
- A. Pupillary light-near dissociation.
- B. Impaired divergence.
- C. Lid retraction.
- D. Convergence-retraction nystagmus.
- E. Upgaze paralysis.

71. Progressive supranuclear palsy (Steele-Richardson-Olszewski syndrome) consists of:
- A. Severe dementia.
- B. Muscle rigidity.
- C. Parkinsonism.
- D. Photophobia.
- E. Postural instability.

72. Tonic downward gaze deviations are associated with:
- A. Thalamic hemorrhage.
- B. Acute obstructive hydrocephalus.
- C. Hypoxic encephalopathy.
- D. Massive subarachnoid hemorrhage.
- E. Cerebellar hemorrhage.

73. Skew deviation:
- A. Is usually comitant.
- B. Occurs most commonly with peripheral neurologic lesions.
- C. Is frequently associated with globe torsion.
- D. Manifests with hypertropia on the involved side when the causative lesion is above the midbrain.
- E. May alternate on lateral gaze.

74. Ocular tilt reaction:
- A. Includes a skew deviation.
- B. Includes cyclotorsion of both eyes.

C. Includes head tilt to the side of the lower eye.
D. Can be caused by vestibular nerve lesions.
E. Is caused by a lesion of the contralateral intersitital nucleus of Cajal.

75. **Ocular motility signs of cerebellar disease include:**
    A. Opsoclonus.
    B. Saccadic dysmetria.
    C. Gaze-evoked nystagmus.
    D. Vertical nystagmus.
    E. Saccadic pursuit.

76. **Divergence paralysis may be associated with:**
    A. Miller-Fisher syndrome.
    B. Chiari malformation.
    C. Pontine tumors.
    D. Diazepam use.
    E. Niemann–Pick disease type C.

77. **Spasm of the near reflex:**
    A. Is characterized by intermittent convergence, miosis, and accommodation.
    B. Manifests with variable degrees of esotropia.
    C. Rarely presents with complaints of diplopia.
    D. Is usually non-organic.
    E. May be caused by head trauma.

78. **The left third cranial nerve contains fibers from the:**
    A. Left medial rectus subnucleus.
    B. Left superior rectus subnucleus.
    C. Left Edinger-Westphal nucleus.
    D. Left inferior rectus subnucleus.
    E. Caudal subnucleus to the levator palpebrae superioris.

79. **The fascicles of the third cranial nerve pass through the:**
    A. Red nucleus.
    B. Substantia nigra.
    C. Periaqueductal gray matter.
    D. Crus cerebri.
    E. Midbrain.

80. **An isolated third nerve nuclear lesion is:**
    A. Impossible if the patient has bilateral total third nerve palsies without ptosis.
    B. Possible if the patient has a unilateral third nerve palsy with contralateral superior rectus weakness and bilateral partial ptosis.
    C. Possible if the patient has bilateral medial rectus weakness.
    D. Possible if the patient has unilateral ptosis.
    E. Very rare.

81. **Fascicular third cranial nerve palsies:**
    A. Never spare the pupil.
    B. Can involve isolated extraocular muscles.
    C. Can involve only one division of the third nerve (superior or inferior).
    D. Are usually due to vascular etiologies.
    E. Are not associated with aberrant regeneration.

82. **Congenital third cranial nerve palsies:**
    A. Are commonly associated with aberrant regeneration.
    B. Are rare.
    C. Are associated with other neurologic abnormalities in many patients.
    D. Are not associated with cyclic oculomotor spasm.
    E. Usually occur because of lesions outside the midbrain.

83. **Cranial nerve IV:**
    A. Is the only cranial nerve to exit from the dorsal brainstem.
    B. Innervates the contralateral superior oblique muscle.
    C. Has the longest intracranial course.
    D. Palsy commonly results in horizontal diplopia.
    E. Palsies can be congenital or acquired.

84. **Lesions of the sixth cranial nerve:**
    A. Can cause the patient to turn develop a face turn toward the side of the palsy to obtain fusion.
    B. Do not affect the pupil.
    C. Are associated with an esotropia that is greater at near than at distance.
    D. Do not cause all abduction weaknesses.
    E. If nuclear, induce an ipsilateral gaze palsy.

85. **The sixth nerve nucleus:**
    A. Contains the cell bodies of two neuron types.
    B. Contains cell bodies that project to the lateral rectus muscle via the sixth cranial nerve.
    C. Contains cell bodies that project via the medial longitudinal fasciculus to the contralateral medial rectus nucleus.
    D. Is a gaze center.
    E. Is never associated with seventh nerve palsies.

86. **The third cranial nerve:**
    A. Passes between the posterior cerebral and superior cerebellar arteries.
    B. Runs alongside the posterior communicating artery.
    C. Runs below the fourth nerve in the cavernous sinus.
    D. Enters the orbit via the superior orbital fissure.
    E. Branches into two divisions in the anterior cavernous sinus.

87. **Parasympathetic fibers to the iris sphincter:**
    A. Travel along the nerve branch to the inferior oblique muscle.
    B. Synapse in the ciliary ganglion.

C. Travel in the long ciliary nerves.
D. Originate in the Edinger-Westphal nucleus.
E. Terminate in the iris and ciliary body.

88. The fourth cranial nerve:
    A. Runs between the posterior cerebral and superior cerebellar arteries.
    B. Runs along the lateral wall of the cavernous sinus below the first division of the trigeminal nerve.
    C. Has the longest intracranial course.
    D. Runs outside the annulus of Zinn.
    E. Crosses to the contralateral side after exiting the midbrain.

89. The sixth cranial nerve:
    A. Runs through the subarachnoid space along the surface of the clivus.
    B. Runs over the petrous apex of the temporal bone.
    C. Runs under the petroclinoid ligament.
    D. Runs medial to the internal carotid artery in the cavernous sinus.
    E. Enters the superior orbital fissure.

90. Traumatic sixth nerve palsies are associated with:
    A. Fractures of the petrous bone or clivus.
    B. Mastoid ecchymoses.
    C. A head turn toward the uninvolved eye.
    D. Esotropia.
    E. An ipsilateral abduction deficit.

91. A congenital superior oblique palsy:
    A. Is always associated with diplopia.
    B. Is usually associated with large vertical fusional amplitudes.
    C. Often demonstrate a head posture in early photographs.
    D. Is usually associated with full ocular motility.
    E. Is associated with objective evidence of globe torsion.

92. Aberrant regeneration of the third cranial nerve:
    A. May cause lid elevation on attempted adduction.
    B. May cause pupillary constriction on attempted adduction.
    C. May cause lid elevation on attempted upgaze.
    D. May cause globe retraction on attempted upgaze or downgaze.
    E. Is always due to an antecedent third nerve palsy.

93. Hydroxyamphetamine drops:
    A. Dilate the affected pupil when there is a preganglionic lesion causing Horner's syndrome.
    B. May falsely localize a postganglionic lesion producing Horner's syndrome as being preganglionic within 1 week of lesion onset by dilating the affected pupil.
    C. Should not be used within 3 weeks of cocaine drops.
    D. Help to localize the site of a Horner's syndrome lesion.
    E. Should be given 60 minutes to dilate the pupils before evaluating for an effect.

94. **Horner's syndrome in infants and children:**
    A. Is associated with complete ptosis.
    B. Is associated with contralateral hemifacial flush when the patient is crying or nursing.
    C. In a child with curly hair, produces limp hair on the affected side.
    D. Can be diagnosed with cocaine eye drops.
    E. May be associated with neuroblastoma.

95. **A tonic pupil associated with Adie's syndrome:**
    A. Occurs most commonly in young women.
    B. Will show segmental vermiform iris contractions in response to light.
    C. May have light-near dissociation.
    D. Ultimately will become the larger pupil.
    E. May demonstrate supersensitivity to cholinergic substances within the first week.

96. **Pupillary light-near dissociation may be caused by:**
    A. Pinealoma.
    B. Syphilis.
    C. Adie's syndrome.
    D. Cataract.
    E. Third nerve aberrant regeneration.

97. **Migraine:**
    A. Occurs before age of 10 years in 25% of migraine patients.
    B. Headache in patients who have common migraine begins unilaterally in 50% of patients.
    C. May be aborted during acute attacks with oral medication.
    D. Without aura is usually preceded by focal neurological deficits.
    E. Is commonly associated with nausea but rarely with vomiting.

98. **Ophthalmoplegic migraine:**
    A. Rarely spares the pupil.
    B. Usually involves the sixth cranial nerve.
    C. Is very rarely bilateral.
    D. Almost always involves the third cranial nerve.
    E. Usually begins in early childhood.

99. **Cluster headaches:**
    A. May be associated with Horner's syndrome.
    B. Rarely have nocturnal onset.
    C. Are more common in men than in women.
    D. Are usually unilateral and periorbital.
    E. Are very painful.

100. **Miller–Fisher syndrome:**
    A. Consists of ataxia, areflexia, and ophthalmoplegia.
    B. Is associated with hyperreflective deep tendon reflexes.
    C. Is associated with bilateral ptosis.
    D. Usually results in complete recovery.
    E. Is a variant of Guillain-Barre syndrome.

101. Carbon monoxide poisoning may be associated with:
   A. Homonymous hemianopia.
   B. Fluctuating visual acuity.
   C. Horner's syndrome.
   D. Metamorphopsia.
   E. Visual object agnosia.

102. Carotid artery occlusive disease is associated with:
   A. Ocular ischemic syndrome.
   B. Homonymous hemianopia.
   C. Facial numbness.
   D. Motor aphasia.
   E. Monocular blindness with contralateral hemiplegia.

103. Carotid-cavernous fistula may be associated with:
   A. Diplopia.
   B. Ocular ischemia.
   C. Exophthalmos.
   D. Enophthalmos.
   E. Venous stasis retinopathy.

ANSWERS

1. E. Short time to repetition (TR) is actually 200–700 ms. Long TR is 1500–3000 ms and very long TR is >6000 ms. Short time to echo (TE) is 20–35 ms. Long TE is 75-250 ms.

Table 11.1: General guidelines for the choice of neuroimaging techniques in neuro-ophthalmology.		
Area	Problem	Technique
Globe	Trauma	Noncontrast computed tomography
	Foreign body	Noncontrast computed tomography
	Calcification	Noncontrast computed tomography
	Retinoblastoma	Magnetic resonance imaging
	Melanoma	Magnetic resonance imaging
Orbit and optic nerve	Trauma	Noncontrast computed tomography
	Foreign body	Noncontrast computed tomography
	Hemorrhage	Noncontrast computed tomography
	Calcification/bony erosion	Noncontrast computed tomography
Area	Problem	Technique
	Thyroid ophthalmopathy	Fat-suppressed magnetic resonance imaging
	Optic nerve tumor	Gadolinium-enhanced, fat-suppressed magnetic resonance imaging

Contd...

Contd...

Chiasm and juxtasellar region	Aneurysm	Gadolinium-enhanced magnetic resonance imaging and magnetic resonance angiography or conventional angiography
	Aneurysm with acute hemorrhage	Contrast-enhanced computed tomography
	Calcification	Contrast-enhanced computed tomography
Retrochiasma region and posterior fossa	Acute hemorrhage	Noncontrast computed tomography

2. C. Vitreous actually yields a dark T1 and bright T2 image.
3. A. Gadolinium shortens T1 time to relaxation.
4. E. Magnetic resonance imaging is not contraindicated in patients with psychiatric disorders.
5. B. Magnetic resonance angiography is a form of noninvasive imaging that may miss aneurysms, plaques and ulcerations. It is generally considered less sensitive than conventional angiography but similar to computed tomographic angiography in efficacy. Magnetic resonance angiography tends to overdiagnose vascular stenosis and exhibits vessels smaller than noted in conventional angiography.
6. D. Conventional angiography is performed by placing a catheter intra-arterially. Complications including vasospasm, emboli and vessel dissection occur in 2.5% of cases.
7. E. Magnetic resonance imaging is preferred over computed tomography in the evaluation of uveal melanoma.
8. B. The optic nerve is about 8-10-mm long in the optic canal.
9. C. The ophthalmic artery runs inferior to the optic nerve in the optic canal. The circle of Zinn-Haller is formed by choroidal vessels, posterior ciliary arteries and the pial arteries, not the ophthalmic artery.
10. C. Optic neuropathies do not commonly produce metamorphopsia. This symptom is more typical of macular disease.

Table 11.2: Differentiation of optic nerve from macular disease by history.

Feature	Optic nerve	Macula
Onset	Variable	Variable
Course	Stable, progressive, or transient	Slow changes
Pain	Sometimes with eye movements	Rarely
Description of deficit	Dark or gray cloud	Metamorphopsia
Refractive error	Unchanged	Sometimes shift toward hyperopia

Neuro-ophthalmology

Table 11.3: Differentiation of optic nerve from macular disease by clinical examination		
Visual function	*Optic nerve*	*Macula*
Visual acuity	Variably reduced	Markedly reduced
Afferent pupillary defect	Present	Absent
Brightness sense	Very reduced	Slightly reduced
Color vision	Very reduced	Slightly reduced
Visual field	Variable	Normal or central scotoma

11. D. Macular disease can produce a central scotoma on Amsler grid testing.
12. A. Visual acuity with optic nerve hypoplasia is unpredictable and may remain intact.
13. C. Morning glory disc anomaly can be associated with serous retinal detachment.

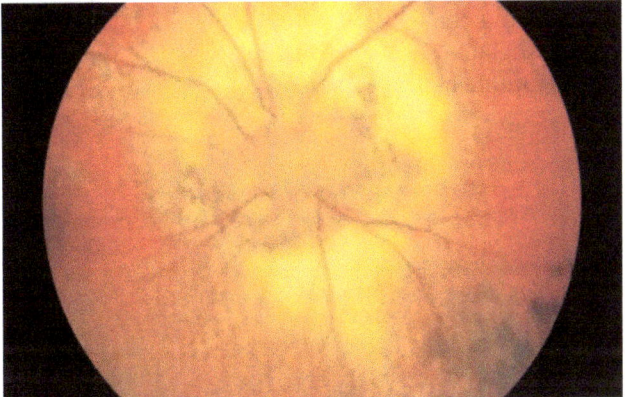

Fig. 11.1: Fundus photo of morning glory disc anomaly.

14. A. Transsphenoidal encephalocele is associated with morning glory disc anomaly but not optic disc coloboma.

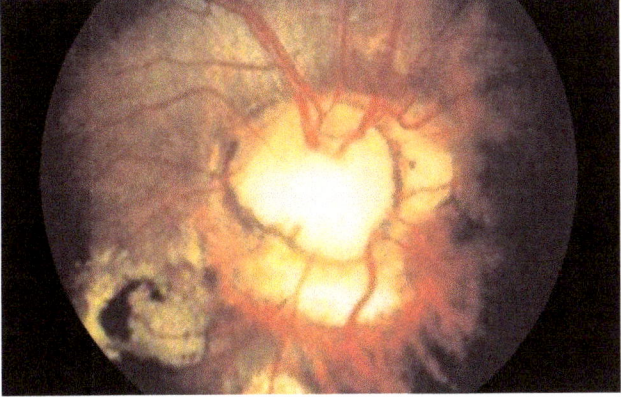

Fig. 11.2: Fundus photo of optic disc coloboma.

15. B. Optic pits can produce a visual field defect (paracentral or arcuate). They most commonly occur inferotemporally but can occur at any location in the optic disc.

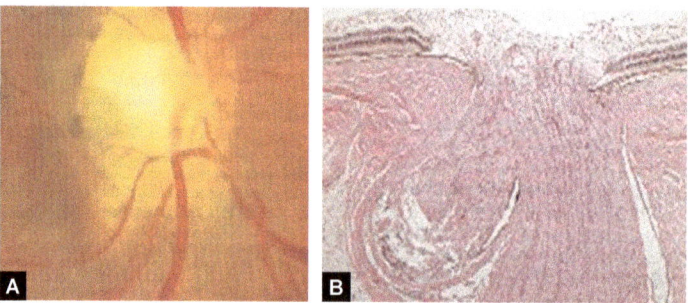

Figs. 11.3A and B: Fundus photo. (A) And histopathology; (B) Of an optic nerve pit.

16. D. Megalopapilla is a congenital, most commonly sporadic condition in which the optic nerve head appears larger, often simulating glaucomatous changes. It can be unilateral or bilateral. Megalopapilla is not associated with systemic conditions and therefore, does not require routine neuroimaging.

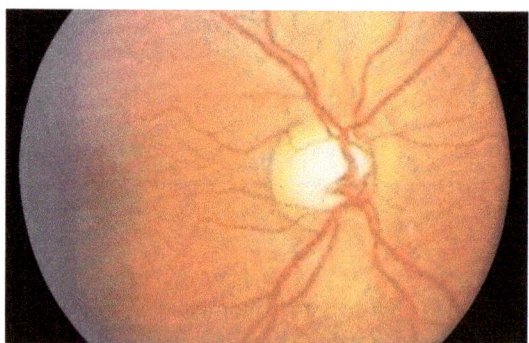

Fig. 11.4: Fundus photo of megalopapilla.

17. B. Congenital tilted disc syndrome is most often non-hereditary, though there have been reports of autosomal dominant inheritance.

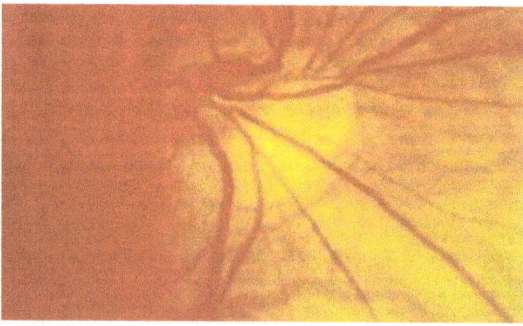

Fig. 11.5: Fundus photo of congenital tilted disc syndrome.

18. D. Ocular findings including chorioretinal lacunae are often found bilaterally in association with Aicardi syndrome.
19. C. Pseudotumor cerebri (Idiopathic intracranial hypertension) is idiopathic and therefore, the cause is unknown.
20. B. Axoplasmic transport is an oxygen dependent system that can be anterograde or retrograde. If anterograde, transport can occur at slow, intermediate, or rapid speeds.
21. E. Clinical signs of optic disc edema include vascular congestion with venous dilation, blurring of the optic disc margin, obliteration of the optic cup, anterior extension of the optic nerve head and choroidal folds.

Definition

Papilledema is optic disc edema (usually bilateral) that results from increased intracranial pressure.

Key Features

- Blurring of the optic disc margins.
- Anterior extension of the nerve head.
- Venous congestion of arcuate and peripapillary vessels.
- Hyperemia of the optic nerve head.

Associated Features

On fundus examination, several mechanical and vascular signs of optic disc edema occur. These include gross elevation of the optic nerve head, engorged and dusky veins, peripapillary splinter hemorrhages, and sometimes choroidal folds and retina striae.

22. D. Headaches associated with increased intracranial pressure are typically diffuse.
23. B. Acetazolamide, a carbonic anhydrase inhibitor is the first line treatment for idiopathic intracranial hypertension along with weight loss. Optic nerve sheath fenestration and ventriculoperitoneal shunt are surgical options that may be recommended in refractory cases.
24. D. Optic neuritis most often presents in young females with unilateral decreased vision, decreased color vision, afferent pupillary defect, pain around the eye and pain on extraocular movements. Pain often precedes visual symptoms. Optic neuritis develops over several days.
25. E. Neuroretinitis is characterized by optic disc edema and macular exudation in a stellate pattern. The most common cause is Bartonella henselae (associated with cat-scratch disease) but there are many other causes for neuroretinitis including sarcoidosis, tuberculosis, toxoplasmosis, syphilis and Lyme disease. Neuroretinitis is not associated with multiple sclerosis.

26. A. Parainfectious or postviral optic neuritis is most commonly seen in children 1-3 weeks after a viral infection. It may also occur following a vaccination. This type of optic neuritis may be unilateral or bilateral and may present with associated neuroretinitis. Optic disc edema may or may not occur. Meningoencephalitis is known to occur with this condition. Treatment is not necessary, though corticosteroids may shorten recovery time. Parainfectious optic neuritis is associated with an excellent visual prognosis.

27. E. Patients with optic neuritis are less likely to develop multiple sclerosis if disc swelling is present.

28. A. In the optic neuritis treatment trial, patients treated with intravenous corticosteroids followed by oral steroids recovered visual acuity 1-2 weeks faster than patients in the placebo arm and were less likely to develop multiple sclerosis at 2 years. However, there was no difference in the incidence of MS compared to patients that received a placebo at 3 years and there was no long-term difference in visual acuity. Patients who received oral steroids alone had no improvement in visual acuity over the placebo arm and were more likely to develop a subsequent episode of optic neuritis. Therefore, oral corticosteroids alone are not recommended in the treatment of optic neuritis.

29. D. Following an episode of optic neuritis, recovery of color vision and brightness is commonly incomplete.

30. D. Anterior ischemic optic neuropathy most commonly occurs in patients over the age of 50.

31. A. Arteritic anterior ischemic optic neuropathy results from short ciliary artery vasculitis.

32. C. Nonarteritic anterior ischemic optic neuropathy occurs equally in men and women.

33. D. Nonarteritic anterior ischemic optic neuropathy is associated with an improvement in visual acuity of at least 3 Snellen lines in 31% of patients according to the ischemic optic neuropathy decompression trial.

34. E. Joint pain is not a systemic feature associated with arteritic anterior ischemic optic neuropathy.

35. D. Erythrocyte sedimentation rate does not typically revert to a normal level after a single dose of corticosteroids but typically trends downward over the course of treatment.

36. C. Temporal artery biopsy can be performed up to 10 days after the initiation of corticosteroid treatment for arteritic anterior ischemic optic neuropathy without affecting biopsy results.

37. C. There has been no proven association between carotid occlusive disease and nonarteritic anterior ischemic optic neuropathy.

38. C. High-dose intravenous methylprednisone (1g/day) is most often recommended as initial treatment often followed by high-dose oral steroids. Daily aspirin may be used as an adjunctive therapy. Alternate-day corticosteroids would not be considered a sufficient treatment option.

39. D. There is a therapy that has been proven to be beneficial in the treatment of nonarteritic anterior ischemic optic neuropathy. The ischemic optic neuropathy decompression trial did not find any benefit to optic nerve sheath fenestration.
40. D. While diabetic papillopathy occurs in the setting of diabetic retinopathy in up to 80% of cases, it can also occur without any evidence of retinopathy.
41. A. Papillophlebitis is defined by monocular marked optic nerve edema and retinal venous congestion, most commonly occurring in young healthy patients.
42. A. Leber hereditary optic neuropathy is inherited through mitochondrial transmission.

Definition
Leber's hereditary optic neuropathy which arises from an inherited point mutation in mitochondrial DNA (most often 11778, less commonly 3460 or 14484), manifests in young adulthood, as a distinctive optic neuropathy.

Key Features
- Presents with hyperemia of optic disc, peripapillary telangiectasia and retinal vascular tortuosity.
- Results in relatively symmetric, significant visual impairment (usually 20/200 or worse).
- Loss of central visual acuity.
- Dyschromatopsia.
- Cecocentral visual field defects.
- Temporal optic disc pallor.
- Nerve fiber layer loss in the papillomacular bundle.

Associated Features
- Loss of hearing.
- Peripheral neuropathy.

43. E. Methanol ingestion can rapidly produce a severe toxic optic neuropathy.

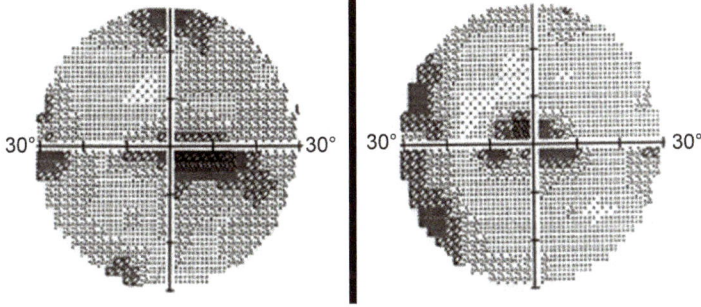

Fig. 11.6: Visual field with bilateral central scotoma secondary to toxic optic neuropathy.

44. D. A deficiency of folic acid can result in toxic optic neuropathy.
45. C. Gliomas of the optic pathway involve the optic nerve and/or chiasm. They can present with exophthalmos, vision loss, optic disc edema and optic disc pallor, and an APD. Magnetic resonance imaging (MRI) of gliomas reveal optic nerve enhancement with fusiform enlargement and kinking. For most patients, observation is the treatment of choice.
46. A. Optic nerve gliomas are associated with neurofibromatosis type 1.
47. E. Optic nerve sheath meningiomas arise from meningoepithelial cells, most often in middle-aged women. They are almost always benign and have a mortality rate of almost 0%. On MRI they produce a characteristic "tram track" sign. They are most commonly observed or treated with radiation therapy though surgical excision is an option if the tumor extends intracranially or in the setting of contralateral vision loss.
48. A. Traumatic optic neuropathy can result from direct or indirect trauma, though indirect trauma is a much more common cause. It always presents with an APD and vision loss. There is no proven treatment. Corticosteroids have been shown to have no benefit with regard to visual outcomes and have been suggested to increase mortality.
49. C. The optic chiasm contains macular fibers that cross in the posterior portion of the chiasm.
50. B. Pituitary adenomas comprise up to 15% of symptomatic intracranial tumors.
51. E. Suprasellar meningiomas are associated with neurofibromatosis-1.
52. D. Craniopharyngiomas more commonly affect the superior portion of the optic chiasm producing an inferior bitemporal visual field defect.
53. E. The most common visual field defect associated with chiasmal lesions is a bitemporal hemianopia. A junctional scotoma (central scotoma in one eye with temporal field loss in the other eye) is associated with lesions affecting the junction between the optic chiasm and optic nerve. An asymmetric or unilateral temporal visual field defect and a paracentral temporal visual field defect can also occur with chiasmal lesions.
54. A. Meningiomas are rarely malignant. The transitional type has concentrically arranged spindle cells that form whorls. Other types include syncytial tumors with intertwined cell membranes, fibroblastic tumors with elongated cells simulating fibroblasts and angioblastic tumors with prominent capillaries. They also commonly have psammoma bodies especially in association with whorls.
55. B. First line treatment for pituitary adenomas is typically medical. Prolactin secreting adenomas are often treated with bromocriptine or cabergoline (dopamine agonists), while growth hormone secreting tumors can also be treated with somatostatin analogs such as octreotide.

56. A. Surgical treatment of craniopharyngiomas may be via a transsphenoidal approach, craniotomy or subdiaphragmatic approach. Surgical excision is associated with a high recurrence rate, usually occurring within 2 years of resection. Cystic lesions are more difficult to treat and chemotherapeutic or radioactive agents may be placed within the cysts. After treatment, visual recovery occurs in only 50% of cases.
57. A. The lateral geniculate body contains axons from the contralateral eye that synapse in layers 1, 4 and 6. It also contains axons from the ipsilateral eye that synapse in layers 2, 3 and 5.
58. C. The primary visual cortex is also known as V1.
59. A. Non-organic vision loss includes malingering and hysteria.
60. B. Horizontal saccades are controlled by the paramedian pontine reticular formation, not the frontal lobe. Vertical saccades are controlled by the rostral interstitial nucleus.

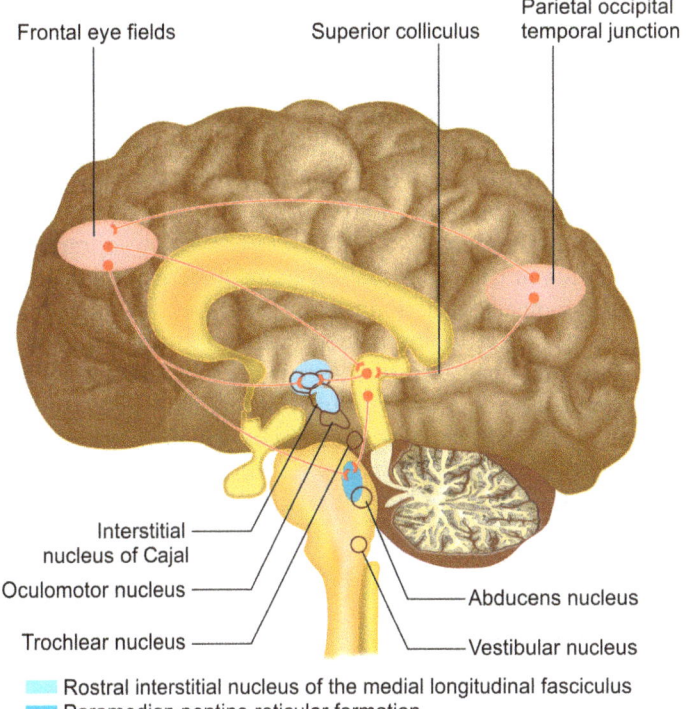

Fig. 11.7: Supranuclear center of eye movement.

61. B. Smooth pursuit eye movements track objects moving at <30° per second.
62. E. Vertical eye movements may be affected by various conditions including pineal tumors, brainstem tumors, pituitary adenomas, aneurysms, stroke, trauma and multiple sclerosis.
63. C. The oculocephalic or doll's eye reflex can overcome gaze palsies produced by supranuclear but not infranuclear lesions.

64. E. Vestibular caloric testing with cold water produces a slow eye deviation to the ipsilateral side with fast-beating eye movements to the contralateral side. The opposite occurs with warm water.
65. A. Congenital oculomotor apraxia is more common in boys than girls.
66. E. Myasthenia gravis is associated with faster than normal saccades.
67. B. Balint syndrome caused by bilateral parieto-occipital lesions results in the triad of simultanagnosia, ocular motor apraxia and optic ataxia. Simultanganosia is the inability to recognize the composite picture, while still being able to recognize each part of the picture separately. Optic ataxia is the inability to coordinate visual and motor systems.
68. C. One-and-a-half syndrome is commonly caused by stroke, demyelinating diseases such as multiple sclerosis and pontine abnormalities such as tumors. It presents with a horizontal gaze palsy and internuclear ophthalmoplegia. When the facial nerve is also involved, it is called eight-and-a-half syndrome.
69. A. Bilateral pontine lesions produce a horizontal gaze palsy with preservation of vertical gaze.
70. B. Dorsal midbrain syndrome may consist of impaired convergence (not divergence) as well as convergence retraction nystagmus, skew deviation, lid retraction, upgaze palsy and pupillary light-near dissociation. Causes of this syndrome include tumors of the pineal gland, multiple sclerosis and stroke.
71. A. Though forgetfulness is a feature of progressive supranuclear palsy, severe dementia is not usually a characteristic of the syndrome.
72. E. Tonic downgaze deviation is associated with thalamic hemorrhage, acute obstructive hydrocephalus, hypoxic encephalopathy or subarachnoid hemorrhage. It may also be associated with intraventricular hemorrhage in preterm infants. This presentation is not typically associated with cerebellar hemorrhage.
73. B. Skew deviation is a vertical deviation more commonly caused by central lesions than peripheral lesions. It may be comitant or incomitant. A skew deviation is one of the few supranuclear lesions that may cause diplopia. It may also result in abnormal globe torsion and it may alternate on lateral gaze. When a skew deviation alternates, it results in hypertropia of the eye that is abducting.
74. E. Ocular tilt reaction includes skew deviation, cyclotorsional abnormalities and head tilt. It is often caused by a lesion of the ipsilateral interstitial nucleus of Cajal.
75. A. Opsoclonus is not typically associated with cerebellar disease.
76. E. Secondary divergence insufficiency or paralysis has been associated with many causes including Miller-Fisher syndrome, Chiari malformation, pontine and midbrain tumors, diazepam use and abnormal intracranial pressure. While Neimann-Pick disease is associated with vertical gaze palsies, it is not typically associated with divergence insufficiency or paralysis.
77. C. Spasm of the near reflex usually presents with diplopia.

78. B. The superior rectus subnucleus crosses to innervate the contralateral superior rectus. Therefore, the left third cranial nerve contains fibers from the right superior rectus subnucleus.
79. C. The fascicles of cranial nerve III (CN III) pass through the midbrain. In the midbrain, they pass through the red nucleus and the crus cerebri. A lesion of the fasicular CN III at the red nucleus results in Benedikt's syndrome which is characterized by ataxia, tremor and possible loss of sensation. A lesion of the fasicular CN III at the crus cerebri results in Weber's syndrome which is characterized by contralateral hemiparesis. The fascicles also pass through the substantia nigra. While they are in close proximity to the periaqueductal gray matter, they do not pass through this structure.
80. D. Unilateral ptosis excludes the possibility of an isolated CN III nuclear lesion.
81. A. Fasicular third cranial nerve palsies may be pupil-sparing or they may involve the pupil. If involved, the degree of pupil involvement classically correlates to the degree of lid and motility abnormality. This type of palsy typically affects all CN III functions but may affect isolated extraocular muscles. They are most commonly caused by vascular etiologies, and the resultant ischemia is associated with varying degrees of recovery. Aberrant regeneration does not occur.
82. D. Congenital cranial nerve three palsies may be associated with cyclic oculomotor spasm. This condition is associated with alternating periods of a paretic phase (ptosis, pupil dilation and abduction) and a spastic phase (lid elevation, pupil constriction and adduction). Cyclic oculomotor spasm is not typically associated with acquired CN III lesions.
83. D. A lesion of the fourth cranial nerve produces a superior oblique palsy. This typically results in vertical diplopia. This diplopia will often worsen in downgaze, gaze to the contralateral side and ipsilateral head tilt.
84. C. CN VI palsies produce an esotropia that is worse at distance than near.
85. E. The nucleus of the sixth cranial nerve located in the pons is closely related to the facial nerve fasiculus, and therefore, often produces an ipsilateral peripheral facial nerve palsy.
86. C. The third cranial nerve runs superior to the fourth nerve along the lateral wall of the cavernous sinus.
87. C. Parasympathetic fibers to the iris sphincter muscle travel in the short ciliary nerves.
88. B. The fourth cranial nerve crosses to the contralateral side after exiting the midbrain. It runs between the posterior cerebral and superior cerebellar arteries before entering the cavernous sinus. Within the cavernous sinus, the fourth cranial nerve runs along the lateral wall below the third cranial nerve and above the first division of the trigeminal nerve. It then runs outside of the annulus of Zinn, entering the orbit via the superior orbital fissure.

89. D. The sixth cranial nerve runs lateral to the internal carotid artery and medial to CN III/IV/V1 in the cavernous sinus.
90. C. CN VI palsies may be caused by trauma. As with other causes of a CN VI palsy, a head turn toward the involved eye typically occurs to improve fusion.
91. A. A congenital superior oblique palsy does not typically manifest with diplopia, especially if it manifests early in childhood. However, a congenital superior oblique palsy that manifests later in life may present with intermittent vertical diplopia.
92. E. Aberrant regeneration of CN III is commonly caused by a CN III palsy. However, aberrant regeneration may also occur without preceding palsy.
93. C. Hydroxyamphetamine drops can be used in cases of Horner's syndrome to determine if the causative lesion is preganglionic or postganglionic. If the lesion is postganglionic, the affected pupil will dilate less than the normal pupil and the anisocoria will become exaggerated. If the causative lesion is preganglionic, the affected pupil will dilate more than the normal pupil and a reversal of anisocoria will occur. A lesion can be falsely identified as being preganglionic within 1 week of onset due to residual norepinephrine that remains in the damaged neurons in the iris. This test must be performed at least 3 days after cocaine has been administered, as cocaine prevents the uptake of hydroxyamphetimine.
94. A. Horner's syndrome is associated with an incomplete ptosis. In infants who develop an acquired Horner's syndrome, neuroblastoma must be considered.
95. D. Ultimately, the affected tonic pupil in Adie's syndrome will become the smaller pupil due to aberrant regeneration.
96. D. Light-near dissociation may occur with pinealoma, syphilis (Argyll-Robertson pupil) or Adie's syndrome secondary to aberrant regeneration.
97. D. Common migraines (or migraines without aura) are, by definition, not associated with focal neurological deficits.

Differentiation of headache types.
1.0 Migraine:

- Migraine without aura ("common migraine")
- *Migraine with aura:*
  - Migraine with typical aura
  - Migraine with prolonged aura (aura >60 minutes)
  - Familial hemiplegic migraine
  - Basilar migraine
  - Migraine aura without headache ("migraine equivalent", "migraine disorder")
- Ophthalmoplegic migraine
- Retinal migraine
- Childhood periodic syndromes (e.g. "abdominal migraine" and "vomiting attacks")
- Complications of migraine (including migrainous infarction)
- Migraine not fulfilling any of above criteria ("atypical migraine")

Neuro-ophthalmology

2.0 Tension-type headache:

- Episodic tension headache:
  - Episodic tension headache with disorder of pericranial muscles ("myofascial syndrome")
  - Episodic tension headache without disorder of pericranial muscles
- *Chronic tension-type headache:*
  - Chronic tension headache with disorder of pericranial muscles ("myofascial syndrome")
  - Chronic tension headache without disorder of pericranial muscles

3.0 Cluster-type headache:

- Typical cluster headache
- Chronic paroxysmal hemicrania
- Cluster headache-like disorders ("atypical cluster")

4.0 Miscellaneous headaches unassociated with structural, metabolic, or vascular disorders:

- Idiopathic stabbing pains ("ice pick headaches")

98. B. Ophthalmoplegic migraine almost always involves the third cranial nerve but sixth and/or fourth cranial nerve involvement is very rare. The pupil is almost always involved. This type of migraine is defined by a history of migraine with/without aura and ophthalmoplegia during a migraine episode. It is a diagnosis of exclusion and other causes of pupil-involving third cranial nerve palsy must be excluded via neuroimaging.

99. B. Cluster headaches are painful, unilateral and periorbital headaches occurring more commonly in med than women. This type of headache may be associated with tearing, conjunctival injection, rhinorrhea and Horner's syndrome. Episodes typically last 15 minutes to 3 hours and typically occur at least once per day with episodes characteristically occurring in clusters. Nocturnal episodes are common and may wake the patient from sleep.

100. B. Miller-Fisher syndrome is a variant of Guillain-Barré syndrome that is characterized by areflexia, ataxia and ophthalmoplegia. It is also associated with bilateral ptosis and absent deep tendon reflexes.

101. C. Carbon monoxide toxicity is associated with various visual field defects including homonymous hemianopia, fluctuating visual acuity, visual object agnosia, and metamorphopsia. The pupils are typically normal and Horner's syndrome does not typically occur.

102. C. Facial numbness is not typically associated with carotid artery occlusive disease.

103. D. Carotid-cavernous sinus (CC) fistulas are characterized by direct flow between the cavernous sinus and the carotid artery. They are high-flow and typically due to trauma. They present with arterialization of episcleral veins. They can also present with diplopia (secondary to decreased arterial blood supply to cranial nerves in the cavernous sinus), ocular ischemia, venous stasis retinopathy and exophthalmos which may be associated with a frozen globe. A bruit may be heard over the superior orbital vein.

CHAPTER 12

Strabismus

Stephanie J Weiss, Robert T Spector

QUESTIONS

Identify the INCORRECT answer for all questions (unless instructed otherwise).

1. **The extraocular muscles:**
    A. Develop in situ.
    B. Are innervated at 1 month of gestation.
    C. Develop from three separate foci, one for each innervating cranial nerve.
    D. Are of neural crest origin.
    E. Are in their final anatomic position by 6 months of gestation.

2. **Structures that pass through the annulus of Zinn include:**
    A. The nasociliary nerve.
    B. The oculomotor nerve.
    C. The trochlear nerve.
    D. The ophthalmic artery.
    E. The optic nerve.

3. **The Spiral of Tillaux describes the:**
    A. Medial rectus insertion 5.5 mm from the limbus.
    B. Inferior rectus insertion 6.5 mm from the limbus.
    C. Lateral rectus insertion 6.9 mm from the limbus.
    D. Superior rectus insertion 7.7 mm from the limbus.
    E. Superior oblique insertion 7.7 mm from the limbus.

4. **The oblique muscles:**
    A. Are directly supplied by the branches of the ophthalmic artery.
    B. Insert posterior to the equator.
    C. Insert near the vortex veins.
    D. Are supplied by the same blood vessels that supply the anterior segment of the eye.
    E. Insert on thicker sclera than the rectus muscles.

5. **The medial rectus muscle:**
   A. Is the only rectus muscle without fascial attachment to an oblique muscle.
   B. Can be damaged during endoscopic ethmoid sinus surgery.
   C. Has the longest tendon of any rectus muscle.
   D. Is the most common rectus muscle to be lost during strabismus surgery.
   E. Does not contribute to vertical movement.

6. **The lateral rectus muscle:**
   A. Is attached to the inferior oblique fascia.
   B. Maintains globe contact for a larger distance than all other rectus muscles.
   C. Primarily functions as an adductor.
   D. Contains only one anterior ciliary artery.
   E. Is innervated by the abducens nerve.

7. **The superior rectus muscle:**
   A. Forms an angle of 23° with the visual axis in the primary position.
   B. Is attached to the levator by fascial connections.
   C. Inserts farthest from the limbus of any rectus muscle.
   D. Elevates best when the globe is fully adducted.
   E. Is innervated by the superior division of the oculomotor nerve.

8. **The inferior rectus muscle:**
   A. Travels inferior to the inferior oblique muscle.
   B. Is attached to the fascia of the inferior oblique.
   C. If recessed, may lead to retraction of the lower lid.
   D. Is usually supplied by two anterior ciliary arteries.
   E. Is innervated by the inferior division of the oculomotor nerve.

9. **The superior oblique:**
   A. Tendon and muscle are approximately the same length.
   B. Forms an angle of 23° with the visual axis in primary position.
   C. Is connected to the superior rectus muscle by fascial attachments.
   D. Inserts near the optic nerve.
   E. Acts primarily to incyclotort the globe when in primary position.

10. **The inferior oblique:**
    A. Primarily acts to excyclotort the eye in primary position.
    B. Primarily acts to elevate the eye in adduction.
    C. Primarily acts to elevate the eye in abduction.
    D. Inserts near the lateral rectus.
    E. Inserts near the macula.

11. **Extraocular muscle innervation:**
    A. Of the rectus muscles occurs at the junction of the middle and posterior thirds.
    B. Of the inferior oblique muscle occurs temporal to the inferior rectus muscle.

C. Of the superior oblique muscle is always affected by retrobulbar anesthesia.
D. By the superior division of the oculomotor nerve includes the superior rectus and levator muscles only.
E. By the inferior division of the oculomotor nerve includes the medial rectus, inferior rectus, and inferior oblique muscles.

12. **Anterior ciliary arteries:**
    A. Accompany all extraocular muscles.
    B. Usually are distributed as one per lateral rectus muscle.
    C. Connect with the major arterial circle of the iris.
    D. Are permanently disrupted, if the muscle is detached from the globe.
    E. Supply most of the anterior segment circulation.

13. **Tenon's capsule:**
    A. Thickens at the equator of the globe and thins posteriorly.
    B. Begins 1 mm posterior to the limbus.
    C. Is a fibroelastic membrane with a smooth inner surface.
    D. Is penetrated by the rectus muscles about 10 mm posterior to the muscle insertions.
    E. Is easily repaired, if violated.

14. **The superior oblique trochlea:**
    A. Is attached to the frontal bone.
    B. Contains no cartilage.
    C. Contains a telescoping tendon in which the central fibers move farther than the peripheral ones.
    D. Alters the direction of the superior oblique muscle.
    E. Acts as the origin of the superior oblique tendon.

15. **Opticokinetic nystagmus techniques for evaluating visual acuity:**
    A. Measure visual acuity by means of a motor response.
    B. Have provided falsely normal responses in infants who are cortically blind.
    C. Usually overestimates visual acuity.
    D. Use square-wave gratings.
    E. Are difficult to standardize.

16. **Forced-choice preferential looking tests for evaluating visual acuity:**
    A. Demand that the infant be capable of making neck or eye movements.
    B. Are based on the preference of children to observe a homogenous stimulus over a pattern.
    C. Evaluate visual acuity by means of a motor response.
    D. Use square-wave gratings.
    E. Generally present the target only in a vertical orientation.

17. **Graded optotype tests include:**
    A. HOTV test.
    B. Sheridan–Gardiner test.
    C. Allen test.

D. Tumbling E chart test.
E. Checkerboard test.

18. Delayed visual maturation is:
A. Seen in infants up to three years of age.
B. Often seen in children who are developmentally delayed.
C. May have normal pupillary function.
D. Associated with a normal electroretinogram.
E. Not associated with nystagmus.

19. Corneal light reflex tests for use in measuring ocular alignment:
A. Do not take into account the angle kappa.
B. Do not require both eyes to be able to move to a given position.
C. Assume that each millimeter of light displacement is equal to 15° of decentration of the visual axis when performing a Hirschberg test.
D. Assume that the pupillary axis and optic axis coincide.
E. Are useful in infants.

20. Ophthalmic prisms:
A. Cannot be stacked base-to-base for accurate measurement of the deviation.
B. Are calibrated in the same way whether they are glass or plastic.
C. If plastic are held with the rear surface in the frontal plane.
D. Can be stacked with the bases 90° apart to measure horizontal and vertical deviations accurately.
E. Should be split between the two eyes to measure large deviations more accurately.

21. Cover tests:
A. Can identify and measure horizontal and vertical deviations.
B. Demand the fixing eye to move into the appropriate gaze position.
C. Ideally should be used with an accommodation-controlling target.
D. Can identify and measure torsional deviations.
E. Can separate phorias from tropias.

22. Forced duction testing:
A. Of rectus muscles requires care to avoid pushing the globe into the orbit.
B. Is "positive" in some patients who have muscle paresis.
C. Can often be performed in the office with cooperative adults.
D. Can help to separate restrictive from paretic causes of duction limitation.
E. Of oblique muscles requires care to avoid pushing the globe into the orbit.

23. Visual confusion:
A. Is defined as the simultaneous perception of two different visual stimuli by corresponding retinal elements.
B. Is the same as diplopia.
C. Is alleviated in children by anomalous retinal correspondence.

D. Occurs in adults who develop new onset of strabismus.
E. May be present and symptomatic in patients with visual acuity as low as 20/200.

24. **Suppression scotomas:**
    A. Remain visually significant when the strabismic eye fixates.
    B. Have different shapes in patients who have esotropia than in patients who have exotropia.
    C. Develop in children less than 9 years of age.
    D. Are absolute and facultative under binocular viewing conditions.
    E. Alleviate central diplopia.

25. **Monofixation syndrome:**
    A. Is associated with horizontal strabismus of 8 prism diopters or less.
    B. Occurs when patients have central fusion without peripheral fusion.
    C. May be associated with anisometropia.
    D. Usually has an absolute facultative scotoma.
    E. Generally associated with alignment stability.

26. **Monofixation syndrome is:**
    A. May be associated with a tropia and a superimposed phoria.
    B. Always associated with normal stereopsis.
    C. Associated with amblyopia in many cases.
    D. Seen in patients who have small vertical tropias.
    E. Associated with normal fusional vergence amplitudes.

27. **Panum fusional area:**
    A. Allows for fusion to occur in the absence of exact retinal correspondence.
    B. Straddles the horopter.
    C. Is circular in the fovea.
    D. Is the same size in the fovea as in the retinal periphery.
    E. Includes most objects that are stereoscopically appreciated.

28. **Stereopsis:**
    A. Requires binocular vision.
    B. Is not present at birth.
    C. May reach 10 seconds of arc.
    D. Is unrelated to interpupillary distance.
    E. Typically requires fusional abilities.

29. **Bagolini lenses:**
    A. Are plano lenses with finely ruled lines.
    B. Generate a Conoid of Sturm to a light target.
    C. Are placed in orthogonal orientation in a trial frame.
    D. Yield a single-line response in patients who have no binocular vision.
    E. Are difficult to use in small children.

30. **When evaluating for stereopsis:**
    A. The Titmus stereotest can detect stereopsis to a finer level than the Wirt stereotest.

B. Patients who do not have true stereopsis can sometimes succeed with the Titmus stereotest because of monocular clues.
C. Random dot stereotests may be useful as they contain few monocular clues.
D. Patients are shown a slightly different view of the same object for each eye.
E. Polarized glasses are often required.

31. **Congenital esotropia:**
    A. Presents before 6 months of age.
    B. Is rarely associated with amblyopia.
    C. Usually measures more than 35 prism diopters.
    D. Has no known racial predilection.
    E. Is the most common form of esotropia.

32. **Congenital esotropia is associated with:**
    A. Inferior oblique muscle overaction.
    B. Dissociated vertical deviation.
    C. Rotary nystagmus.
    D. Latent nystagmus.
    E. Superior oblique muscle overaction.

33. **Dissociated vertical deviation:**
    A. Manifests with an upward deviation of one eye.
    B. May coexist with inferior oblique overaction.
    C. May exist without coexistent horizontal strabismus.
    D. Is consistent with the Hering's law.
    E. Is usually asymmetric between the eyes.

34. **Reasonable expectations after medical and surgical treatment of congenital esotropia include:**
    A. Binocular vision.
    B. Equal visual acuity.
    C. Monofixation syndrome.
    D. Normal ductions and versions.
    E. Peripheral fusion.

35. **Accommodative esotropia:**
    A. May occur in myopes.
    B. Does not develop before 1 year of age.
    C. May be associated with A or V patterns.
    D. May have a normal accommodative convergence-to-accommodation ratio.
    E. May develop after successful treatment of congenital esotropia.

36. **Treatment options for accommodative esotropia include:**
    A. Miotic drops in infants and myopes.
    B. Correction of hyperopic refractive error.
    C. Bifocal glasses.

D. Surgical intervention.
E. Myopic overcorrection.

37. **Cyclic esotropia:**
    A. Is always acquired in childhood.
    B. May be related to trauma.
    C. Does not respond to anti-accommodative treatment measures.
    D. May be successfully treated via surgical intervention on days when the eyes are aligned.
    E. Most commonly obeys a cycle of 24 hours of alignment followed by 24 hours of esotropia.

38. **Mobius syndrome is associated with:**
    A. Exotropia.
    B. Mental retardation and polydactyly.
    C. Bilateral abduction deficit.
    D. Lower motor neuron seventh cranial nerve palsy.
    E. Atrophy of part of the tongue.

39. **Duane's syndrome:**
    A. Is bilateral in about 20% of cases.
    B. May be associated with Goldenhar syndrome.
    C. Type I rarely has more than 30 prism diopters of esotropia in primary position.
    D. Is caused by an absent third nerve nucleus.
    E. Has been described to occur with mirror image manifestations in identical twins.

40. **Duane's syndrome:**
    A. Represents congenital miswiring of the horizontal rectus muscles.
    B. Is often acquired.
    C. Does not resolve with time.
    D. Type III is the rarest form.
    E. Most commonly occurs as a Type I variant in the left eye of girls.

41. **Intermittent exotropia:**
    A. Is more common in premature children.
    B. Usually progresses in frequency.
    C. Is not associated with orbital anomalies.
    D. May lead to contraction of the lateral recti.
    E. Often causes the deviated eye to squint in bright sunlight.

42. **Nonsurgical treatment options for intermittent exotropia include:**
    A. Myopic spectacle overcorrection.
    B. Alternate eye occlusion.
    C. Fusional amplitude enhancement.
    D. Base-out prisms.
    E. Correction of amblyopia.

43. Surgical treatment of intermittent exotropia:
   A. Usually includes surgical manipulation of at least one lateral rectus muscle.
   B. Yields equivalent results whether symmetric lateral rectus muscle recessions or monocular recess/resect procedures are performed.
   C. Is indicated when frequency and amplitude of deviation are increasing.
   D. May be the initial form of treatment.
   E. May result in postoperative diplopia.

44. Primary inferior oblique muscle overaction:
   A. Is associated with excyclotorsion of the fundus.
   B. Is seen more commonly in intermittent exotropia than in congenital esotropia.
   C. May be unilateral.
   D. May be associated with a V-pattern strabismus.
   E. Does not provide a positive Parks-Bielschowsky three-step head-tilt test.

45. Over-elevation in adduction may be caused by:
   A. Tight lateral rectus muscles.
   B. Inferior oblique muscle overaction.
   C. A tight superior oblique tendon.
   D. Dissociated vertical deviation.
   E. The tethering effect in Duane's syndrome.

46. Primary superior oblique muscle overaction:
   A. Is associated with fundus excyclotorsion.
   B. May be associated with A-pattern strabismus.
   C. May be associated with hypertropia in primary position.
   D. Is associated with neurologic abnormalities.
   E. Is usually asymptomatic.

47. V-pattern esotropia:
   A. Is associated with esotropia worse in upgaze.
   B. Is associated with a chin-down head posture.
   C. May be associated with a superior oblique palsy.
   D. May be caused by inferior oblique overaction in some cases.
   E. Is more common than V-pattern exotropia.

48. A-pattern esotropia:
   A. Presents with esotropia worse in upgaze.
   B. Is associated with a chin-down head posture.
   C. May be associated with superior oblique muscle overaction.
   D. May be observed.
   E. Is often treated with superior oblique weakening procedures.

49. A-pattern exotropia:
   A. Is commonly associated with superior oblique muscle overaction.
   B. May be treated with downward translation of the lateral recti.

C. May be treated with procedures that weaken the superior oblique tendon.
   D. Always requires treatment.
   E. Is associated with a chin-down head posture.

50. **Aberrant regeneration of the third cranial nerve:**
    A. May result in lid elevation on attempted adduction.
    B. Commonly results in pupillary dilation on attempted adduction.
    C. May produce abnormal globe retraction.
    D. Is also known as oculomotor synkinesis.
    E. Is usually acquired.

51. **Congenital third nerve palsy:**
    A. Is typically associated with concurrent neurological abnormalities.
    B. Is rare.
    C. Usually causes hypotropia.
    D. Is usually unilateral.
    E. Usually causes loss of binocular function.

52. **Acquired third nerve palsy:**
    A. Is usually bilateral.
    B. In adults, is most often caused by vasculopathies.
    C. In children, is most commonly caused by trauma.
    D. In children, is rarely caused by vasculopathy.
    E. May be associated with torticollis.

53. **Anterior segment ischemia:**
    A. Usually occurs after surgical manipulation of 3 or more rectus muscles.
    B. Is more common in adults.
    C. Causes pain, corneal edema, and pupil abnormalities.
    D. Is usually associated with permanent visual loss.
    E. May be treated with topical or systemic steroids.

54. **Unilateral fourth nerve palsy:**
    A. Produces hypertropia and excyclotorsion of the affected eye.
    B. Often causes a head tilt to the same side as the paretic muscle.
    C. May be caused by closed head trauma.
    D. May be congenital.
    E. May be diagnosed using the Parks-Bielschowsky three-step head-tilt test.

55. **Sixth nerve palsies:**
    A. May be comitant when long-standing.
    B. Are associated with an ipsilateral head turn.
    C. May be congenital.
    D. Are associated with a larger deviation when the paretic eye is fixating.
    E. Is more commonly caused by neoplasm than trauma in children.

56. **Dissociated vertical deviation:**
    A. Involves upward deviation of either eye.
    B. The degree of deviation is always the same with each episode.

C. Is exacerbated by fatigue.
D. Is associated with congenital esotropia.
E. Typically presents between the ages of 2–3.

57. Surgical treatment options for dissociated vertical deviation include:
A. Superior rectus muscle recession.
B. Anterior translation of the inferior oblique muscle insertion.
C. Inferior rectus muscle resection.
D. Posterior fixation suture (Faden procedure).
E. Superior oblique tendon tuck.

58. Double elevator palsies:
A. Are usually associated with a normal Bell's phenomenon.
B. Are usually unilateral.
C. May be treated with Knapp procedure.
D. May be acquired.
E. May involve the levator palpebrae.

59. Brown's syndrome:
A. Is most common in the right eye of girls.
B. Is defined by restriction of elevation upon abduction.
C. May be associated with widening of the lid fissure in upgaze.
D. May be caused by trauma to the trochlea.
E. May have a familial association.

60. Treatment of Brown's syndrome:
A. Is required in all cases.
B. In acquired cases is often nonsurgical.
C. May involve corticosteroid injections.
D. May include superior oblique tenotomy.
E. May include silicone superior oblique tendon expanders.

61. Graves' ophthalmopathy:
A. Often causes extraocular muscle tendon enlargement.
B. Most commonly involves the inferior rectus muscles.
C. Causes restriction on forced duction testing.
D. Should be primarily treated by establishing a euthyroid state in most cases.
E. May be severe even when laboratory tests of thyroid function are normal.

62. Heavy eye syndrome:
A. Is associated with high myopia.
B. Is associated with fixed abduction of the involved eye.
C. May exhibit limited elevation of the affected eye.
D. May be treated surgically with loop myopexy.
E. Is progressive.

63. Anisometropic amblyopia:
A. Rarely occurs initially in children over 5–6 years of age.
B. Rarely occurs unless the anisometropia is present for at least 2 years.

C. Rarely occurs in patients with hyperopia.
D. May return upon cessation of treatment until about age of 10 years.
E. Occurs in patients with decreased visual acuity extending nasally and temporally in the visual field.

64. **Stimulus deprivation amblyopia:**
    A. May be caused by a lid lesion.
    B. Usually requires central lens opacity of at least 3 mm.
    C. May occur with full-time occlusion of one eye for more than 1 week per year of life.
    D. Rarely occurs after 2 years of age.
    E. May be bilateral.

65. **Strabismic amblyopia:**
    A. Will not usually develop after 6 years of age.
    B. May occur in patients with freely alternating strabismus.
    C. Is proportional to the degree of fixation preference.
    D. Occurs in patients who have a fixation preference.
    E. May be successfully treated in teenagers.

66. **Amblyopia may be associated with:**
    A. Amplification of the crowding phenomenon.
    B. Decreased contrast sensitivity.
    C. An afferent pupillary defect.
    D. Abnormal spatial visual processing.
    E. Increased saccadic amplitudes.

67. **Iatrogenic amblyopia:**
    A. Is often caused by patching during amblyopia treatment.
    B. Is usually reversible.
    C. Is associated with full-time patching.
    D. Typically occurs over months to years.
    E. Is more common in young children.

68. **Prisms may be effective for patients who have:**
    A. Abnormal head postures associated with congenital nystagmus.
    B. Purely torsional diplopia.
    C. Superior oblique palsy.
    D. Diplopia caused by sixth nerve palsy.
    E. Vertical strabismus.

69. **Botulinum toxin chemodenervation:**
    A. May be used as a treatment option for a sixth nerve palsy.
    B. Has a high success rate in treating exotropia.
    C. Is most successful in treating cases of overcorrection following strabismus surgery.
    D. Can result in temporary pupillary dilation.
    E. Is contraindicated in patients who have myasthenia gravis.

70. Globe perforation during strabismus surgery:
A. Rarely leads to retinal detachment.
B. Demands immediate retinal examination.
C. May not require immediate treatment.
D. Always requires treatment if the needle passes into the suprachoroidal space.
E. Occurs more commonly with cutting needles than with spatulated needles.

ANSWERS

1. D. The extraocular muscles are derived from mesoderm. All extraocular muscles develop in situ from three foci of cells, one for the third cranial nerve, one for the fourth cranial nerve and one for the sixth cranial nerve. They may be innervated by their cranial nerves as early as 1 month of gestation and they reach their final anatomic positions by 6 months of gestation.
2. C. The nasociliary nerve, oculomotor nerve, ophthalmic artery, optic nerve and abducens nerve all pass through the annulus of Zinn. The trochlear nerve does not pass through the annulus of Zinn.

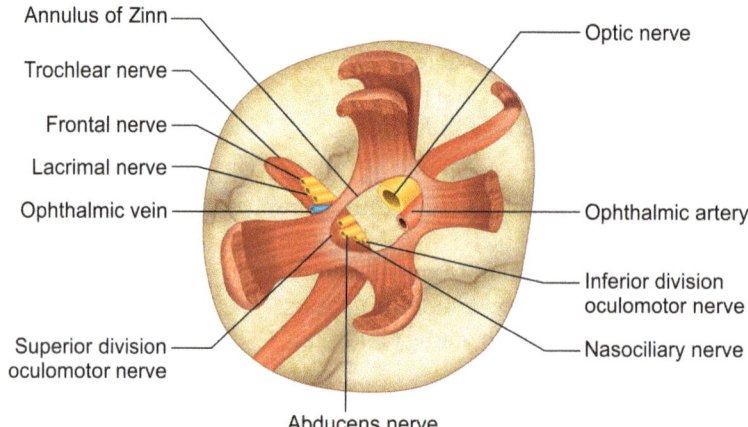

Fig. 12.1: Annulus of Zinn and surrounding structures.

3. E. The Spiral of Tillaux describes the relationship between the limbus and the insertion of the 4 rectus muscles. The medial rectus insertion is located 5.5 mm from the limbus. The inferior rectus insertion is located 6.5 mm from the limbus. The lateral rectus insertion is located 6.9 mm from the limbus. The superior rectus insertion is located 7.7 mm from the limbus. The superior and inferior oblique muscles are not included in the Spiral of Tillaux.
4. D. All of the extraocular muscles including the superior and inferior oblique muscles are directly supplied by the branches of the ophthalmic artery. The rectus muscles are supplied by one or two

anterior ciliary arteries which also supply the anterior segment of the eye. The blood vessels that supply the oblique muscles do not contribute to the blood supply for the anterior segment of the eye. The insertion of the oblique muscles in posterior to the equator, near the vortex veins. The sclera is thinnest posterior to the insertion of the rectus muscles. The sclera is, therefore, thicker at the site of oblique muscle insertions than at the rectus muscle insertions.

5. C. The lateral rectus, not the medial rectus, has the longest tendon of any rectus muscle. The superior oblique muscle has the longest tendon of any extraocular muscle.
6. C. The lateral rectus is a pure abductor. The medial rectus is a pure adductor.
7. D. The superior rectus elevates best when the globe is abducted 23°. In this position, the muscle becomes a pure elevator.
8. A. The inferior oblique muscle travels inferior to the inferior rectus muscle. Therefore, the inferior rectus muscle lies superior to the inferior oblique.
9. B. The superior oblique and inferior oblique muscles form an angle of 51° with the visual axis in primary position.
10. C. The primary action of the inferior oblique in primary gaze is excyclotorsion with secondary contributions to elevation and abduction. In adduction, the inferior oblique primarily acts to elevate the globe. However, in abduction, the inferior oblique primarily acts to excyclotort the globe.
11. C. The superior oblique muscle is innervated by the fourth cranial nerve which travels outside of the muscle cone. Therefore, the superior oblique is not usually affected by retrobulbar anesthesia. For reference, see the Table 12.1 on next page
12. A. The anterior ciliary arteries supply only the rectus muscles.

Table 12.2: Differential diagnosis of congenital esotropia.

Early-onset accommodative esotropia
Nystagmus blockage (compensation) syndrome
Möbius' syndrome
Duane's syndrome
Cyclic esotropia
Esotropia associated with visual loss in one eye, neurologic impairment, or increased intracranial pressure
Strabismus fixus and other fibrosis syndromes

13. E. Violating Tenon's capsule allows for fat to adhere to the globe and restrict movement of the globe. This action makes repair of Tenon's capsule difficult.
14. B. The trochlea is made of cartilage attached to the frontal bone. This structure acts as a pulley system by which the direction of the superior oblique is altered.

Table 12.1: Extraocular muscle characteristics.

Muscle	Origin	Insertion	Muscle length (mm)	Tendon length (mm)	Width of insertion (mm)	Direction of pull from 1° position (°)	Action: i. Primary ii. Secondary iii. Tertiary	Innervation (cranial nerve)
Medial rectus	Annulus of Zinn	5.5 mm behind nasal limbus	41	3.5	10.3	90	i. Adduction	Inferior III
Lateral rectus	Annulus of Zinn	6.9 mm behind temporal limbus	41	8	9.2	90	i. Abduction	VI
Superior rectus	Annulus of Zinn	7.7 mm behind superior limbus	42	5	10.6	23	i. Elevation ii. Incyclotorsion iii. Adduction	Superior III
Inferior rectus	Annulus of Zinn	6.5 mm behind inferior limbus	40	6	9.8	23	i. Depression ii. Excyclotorsion iii. Adduction	Inferior III
Superior oblique	Frontoethmoidal suture above annulus of Zinn	Posterior lateral, superior quadrant	32	26	10.3	51	i. Incyclotorsion ii. Depression iii. Abduction	IV
Inferior oblique	Posterior to lacrimal fossa	Posterior, lateral, inferior quadrant	35	1	9.6	51	i. Excyclotorsion ii. Elevation iii. Abduction	Inferior III

15. C. The use of optickokinetic nystagmus as a means for measuring visual acuity in infants may actually produce an underestimation in visual acuity in children who have a defect in the oculomotor system.
16. B. Forced-choice preferential looking is based on the assumption that children prefer to view a pattern over a homogenous stimulus. This test is useful for preverbal children and is easy to administer with limited equipment.
17. E. The checkerboard test is not an example of a graded optotype but is rather an example of a method of stimulus presentation utilized in visual evoked potential testing.
18. A. Delayed visual maturation may occur between the age of 6–12 months and is often seen in developmental delayed children. This syndrome is often associated with normally pupillary function, though a sluggish pupillary response may also be present. Electroretinogram is normal in these children, and they develop normal visual function later in life.
19. C. Corneal light reflex tests including the Hirshberg and Krimsky tests are useful in all patients including infants. The Hirshberg test compares the position of the corneal light reflex on the left and right eyes to determine an approximate deviation in ocular alignment. 1 mm of light displacement is equivalent to a 15 prism diopter deviation or 7° of decentration. The Krimsky test uses prisms to compare the corneal light reflex of the left and right eyes and quantify the degree of displacement.
20. B. Glass ophthalmic prisms are calibrated so that they must be held with the back surface perpendicular to the visual axis, while plastic prisms must be held with the back surface in the frontal plane.
21. D. Cover tests can identify and measure horizontal and/or vertical deviations. While they can identify some torsional deviations, it is not possible to measure torsional deviations via cover tests.
22. E. Forced duction testing of the oblique muscles requires the globe to be depressed into the orbit prior to manipulation of the globe in order to properly isolate the oblique tendon or muscle.
23. B. Visual confusion is different than diplopia. Visual confusion occurs when different visual stimuli are simultaneously perceived by corresponding retinal elements in each eye. Diplopia is the perception of a single object by different retinal elements in each eye.
24. A. Suppression scotomas develop in children younger than 9 years of age to alleviate diplopia. This type of scotoma is absolute and facultative under binocular conditions when the affected eye is misaligned. However, under monocular conditions when the strabismic eye is fixating, the scotoma disappears entirely.
25. B. By definition, monofixation syndrome occurs when patients have peripheral fusion without central fusion. There is typically an absolute, facultative, central scotoma. Monofixtion syndrome also typically presents with a small tropia (up to 8 prism diopters of esotropia or exotropia or up to 2 prism diopters of hypertropia or

hypotropia) with possible superimposed phoria. Often, normal fusional vergence amplitudes are present. This syndrome may be caused by anisometropia or following surgical correction of congenital strabismus. Amblyopia commonly develops.

26. B. While some stereopsis may be present in patients with monofixation syndrome, normal stereopsis is never present.
27. D. Panum fusional area increases in size in the retinal periphery.
28. D. Stereopsis is a form of depth perception that relies on binocular vision and usually fusion. Stereoacuity evaluates the disparity between two images (typically horizontal) that permits perception of depth. Stereoacuity is most sensitive in the fovea and decreases in the retinal periphery. It also increases with increasing object distance and is directly proportional to interpupillary distance.
29. B. Bagolini lenses are plano lenses with fine lines across the lenses. They are placed in front of both eyes in an orthogonal orientation and the patient is typically asked to view a light target in the distance. In patients with binocularity, an X-shaped figure is perceived. Non-binocular patients will see only one line.
30. A. When evaluating for stereopsis, the Titmus stereotest can detect 3,000 to 40 seconds of arc. The Wirt stereotest can detect stereopsis as fine as 14 seconds of arc.

Congenital Esotropia

Definition

Inward deviation of the visual axes that develops before 6 months of age.

Key Features

- Esotropia greater than 35 Δ.
- Cross-fixation.
- No binocular vision.
- Typical refractive error between +1.50 and +3.00.
- Initially, similar deviation at distance and near fixation.

Associated Features

- Inferior oblique overaction.
- Dissociated vertical deviation.
- Latent horizontal and manifest rotary nystagmus.
- Amblyopia in 25–40% of patients.

Accommodative Esotropia

Definition

Inward deviation of the visual axes caused by high hyperopia, a high accommodative convergence-to-accommodation ratio, or both.

Key Features

- Initially, intermittent acquired esotropia.
- Esotropia larger at near than distance fixation.

Associated Features

- High accommodative convergence-to-accommodation ratio
- Age of onset usually between 18 months and 3 years.

31. B. Congenital esotropia is the most common form of esotropia and has been reported in 1% of the population. There is no known racial predilection associated with this form of esotropia. Congenital esotropia is defined by at least 35 prism diopters of esotropia. While patients may cross-fixate which would help to prevent amblyopia, 25–40% of patients will still develop amblyopia.

Duane's Syndrome

Definition

Congenital absence of the medial or lateral rectus muscles, or both, often associated with strabismus.

Key Feature

Retraction of the affected globe(s) on attempted adduction.

Associated Features

- Ptosis on attempted adduction.
- Elevation or depression of the globe on attempted adduction.
- Limitation of abduction, adduction, or both.
- Esotropia or exotropia in some patients that is usually acquired and rarely larger than 30 Δ.

32. E. Superior oblique overaction is not associated with congenital esotropia. Inferior oblique overaction and dissociated vertical deviation have been found to occur in up to 75% of cases. Nystagmus is also commonly present in patients with congenital esotropia. Latent nystagmus is most commonly associated with congenital esotropia, while rotatory nystagmus has also been reported in rare cases.

33. D. Dissociated vertical deviation is defined by an upward deviation of one eye while the other eye fixates on a target. Because one eye drifts upward with a corrective saccade downward while the other eye remains stable and fixated on a target, dissociated vertical deviation disobeys Hering's Law. This deviation can occur in either eye, but the deviation is typically asymmetric. It is associated with horizontal strabismus in many cases including congenital esotropia.

34. A. Following treatment of congenital esotropia, good visual acuity can be expected in both eyes. While monofixation syndrome and peripheral fusion will often develop, binocular vision does not usually develop following treatment.
35. B. Accomodative esotropia typically occurs in patients with moderate to high hyperopia who manifest with a greater deviation upon near than distance fixation. While high hyperopia is typical, it is also possible to develop accommodative esotropia in patients with myopia. The accommodative convergence-to-accommodation ratio may be high or normal. The onset is typically between 18 months and 3 years of age with onset possible at any time from 6 months of age to 7 years of age.
36. E. Treatment of accommodative esotropia largely consists of correction of hyperopia and miotic drops such as ecothiophate iodide 0.125%. Bifocal glasses are also often used. Surgical intervention may be indicated but is typically aimed at correcting only the non-accomodative component of esotropia. Patients should not undergo surgery without first correcting refractive error. Myopic overcorrection is not a treatment option for accommodative esotropia.
37. A. Cyclic esotropia presents with alternating 24 hour periods of intact ocular alignment followed by 24 hour periods of large angle esotropia. This typically develops in children age 3–4 but can also develop later in life. While the cause of this form of esotropia is unclear, it has been associated with trauma, infection, neurosurgical intervention and strabismus surgery. While cyclic esotropia does not respond well to anti-accomodative measures, surgical intervention has a high success rate whether it is performed when ocular alignment is intact or esotropia is present.
38. A. Mobius syndrome presents with bilateral abduction deficits and possible esotropia. It is associated with upper motor neuron seventh nerve palsies more commonly than lower motor neuron seventh nerve palsies. Twelfth nerve palsies are also associated with Mobius syndrome and often present with atrophy of the tongue.
39. D. Duane's syndrome is a congenital condition caused by an absent sixth nerve nucleus. This leads to anomalous innervation of the medial and lateral rectus muscles which causes glove retraction to occur on attempted adduction. Duane's syndrome is bilateral in approximately 20% of cases. 30% of cases have systemic associations including Goldenhar syndrome. Cases of Duane's syndrome have been reported identical twins with mirror image manifestations.
40. B. Duane's syndrome is a congenital condition that, by definition, is not acquired. There are 2 types of Duane's syndrome. Type I is the most

common and accounts for 85% of cases. This type is most common in the left eyes of girls and presents with severe limitations in abduction in addition to globe retraction on attempted adduction. Type II accounts for approximately 14% of cases and presents with limited abduction and exotropia. Type III occurs in 1% of cases and presents with limited abduction and adduction with esotropia or exotropia.

41. C. Intermittent exotropia is defined as an intermittently present outward deviation of the visual axes in one or both eyes. This type of deviation has been associated with mechanical and orbital abnormalities that induce a restrictive deviation. Intermittent exotropia is more common in patients born prematurely and patients with a family history of strabismus. One early sign of intermittent exotropia is squinting of the deviated eye especially in bright lights. Over time, the frequency of deviation commonly increases. This often results in contraction of the lateral recti which in turn increases the degree of deviation.

42. D. The mainstay of nonsurgical treatment for intermittent exotropia is correction or overcorrection of myopia. This can improve accommodative convergence. Correction of other refractive errors to improve visual acuity has also been suggested. Other less successful but still utilized nonsurgical treatment options include patching of alternating eyes, enhancement of fusional amplitudes, base-in prisms, and correction of amblyopia.

43. D. Surgical treatment of intermittent exotropia should never be attempted without first attempting nonsurgical techniques including myopic correction. Surgical intervention is indicated when exotropia decompensates and becomes constant, when the frequency and amplitude of deviation occur and when symptoms increase. Bilateral lateral rectus recession or unilateral medial rectus resection with lateral rectus recession are the most commonly employed surgical techniques and yield approximately similar outcomes in most reports. Bilateral medial rectus resection is less common but may also be employed.

44. B. Primary inferior oblique overaction is most commonly associated with congenital esotropia and has been reported in up to 72% of patients with congenital esotropia. Inferior oblique overaction occurs less commonly in association with congenital exotropia.

45. C. While a tight lateral rectus muscle can result in over-elevation in adduction, a tight superior oblique muscle is not associated in over-elevation in adduction.

46. A. Primary superior oblique overaction produces an incyclotorsion of the fundus as opposed to primary inferior oblique overaction which produces excyclotorsion.

47. A. V-pattern esotropia is often caused by inferior oblique overaction which produces an esotropia that is worse in downgaze. This often causes a chin-down posture to develop.
48. B. A-pattern esotropia is defined as an esotropia that is worse in upgaze. This presentation often results in a chin-up head posture to minimize deviation. It is typically caused by superior oblique overaction. Small deviations can be observed but larger or symptomatic deviations associated with an abnormal head posture are often treated with superior oblique weakening procedures. Superior oblique weakening procedures include recession and silicone tendon expanders.
49. D. A-pattern exotropia may be observed if the degree of deviation and incomitance is minimal and an abnormal head posture does not develop. If an abnormal head posture (typically chin-down) develops or if the degree of incomitance is greater than 10 prism diopters, several surgical options exist. If superior oblique overaction is not present, translation of the lateral rectus muscles downward may be employed. If superior oblique overaction is present, superior oblique weakening procedures may be performed.
50. B. Aberrant regeneration of the third cranial nerve also known as oculomotor synkinesis develops when axons regenerate improperly. This can lead to globe retraction, lid elevation and/or pupillary constriction (not dilation) upon attempted adduction and/or downgaze.
51. A. Congenital third nerve palsies are rare usually unilateral and typically result in loss of binocular fusion. They are typically idiopathic and are not associated with concurrent neurological abnormalities. Congenital third nerve palsies typically present with exotropia, hypotropia and ptosis. The pupil may or may not be involved.
52. A. Acquired third nerve palsies are usually unilateral, though they rarely occur bilaterally. They present with exotropia, hypotropia and/or ptosis. In older individuals, diplopia may develop. Torticollis may also develop which is caused by a head turn to the contralateral side in an effort to minimize diplopia. In children, acquired third nerve palsies are most commonly caused by trauma and are almost never associated with vascular lesions. In adults, when a cause is determined, the most common cause is vasculopathic.
53. D. Anterior segment ischemia typically occurs when 3 or more rectus muscles are operated on, causing disruption of multiple anterior ciliary arteries. This presents with uveitis, pain, corneal edema and pupillary abnormalities. Treatment usually consists of topical or systemic steroids. This complication of strabismus surgery is more

common in adults with vascular disease that predisposes the patient to vascular compromise. However, this can also occur in children.
54. B. A unilateral fourth nerve palsy typically results in a head tilt to the contralateral side.
55. E. Sixth nerve palsies may be congenital or acquired, and result in pure esotropia as the lateral rectus is the only affected muscle. In children, a sixth nerve palsy is more commonly associated with trauma than neoplasm. It is essential that all children with a sixth nerve palsy undergo neurological imaging to rule out neoplasm or hemorrhage associated with trauma. Patients may develop an ipsilateral head turn early in the course of the palsy. This often resolves with long-standing paresis secondary to the development of a comitant esotropia as the antagonist muscle contracts.
56. B. Dissociated vertical deviation (DVD) is characterized by an upward drifting of one eye as the other eye fixates on a target and remains stable. This will occur in either eye. The degree of deviation varies with each episode and is commonly asymmetric with one eye tending to deviate more than the other. Episodes of deviation can occur during periods of good fixation but episodes are exacerbated by episodes of fatigue or inattention. There is an association with DVD and congenital esotropia though DVD does not typically present until age 2–3.
57. E. Treatment options for DVD include recession of the superior rectus muscles, resection of the inferior rectus muscles, anterior displacement of the inferior oblique and the Faden procedure (posterior fixation suture). Superior oblique tendon tuck is not used to treat DVD.
58. A. Double elevator palsy is defined by a paresis of the superior rectus and inferior oblique (muscles involved in upgaze). This paresis leads to hypotropia of the involved eye. Bell's phenomenon is usually absent in patients with a double elevator palsy. Treatment of this deviation most commonly involves transposition of the medial and lateral rectus tendons to the insertion of the superior rectus. This procedure is known as Knapp procedure. The levator palpebrae may also be involved, and lid surgery may also be indicated in these cases. Double elevator palsies may be congenital or acquired. Evaluation of acquired cases requires neuroimaging to rule out brain lesions.
59. B. Brown's syndrome affects the tendon of the superior oblique muscle. This results in impaired upgaze that is worse in adduction (not abduction). This is also associated with widening of the lid fissure in upgaze. The tendon dysfunction may be congenital or may be acquired. There have been reports suggesting a familial association as well. Reports have suggested that Brown's syndrome occurs more commonly in girls and in right eyes. While most commonly unilateral,

bilateral cases have also been reported. Acquired cases have been associated with trauma or inflammation. The dysfunction may be located in the trochlear region.

60. A. Brown's syndrome is not necessary if the symptoms are intermittent. Treatment is advocated in cases of significant visual symptoms, abnormal head position and/or strabismus. In acquired cases, early treatment should be restricted to conservative and medical management as the degree of restriction may change or resolve over the course of the disease. In early cases, steroid injections may help with inflammation and prisms may help with diplopia. For cases of longstanding restriction, surgical procedures to reduce restriction and free the superior oblique tendon are suggested. This may include a superior oblique tenotomy or a silicone superior oblique tendon expander.

61. A. Graves' ophthalmopathy is an autoimmune inflammatory condition that causes enlargement of the extraocular muscles with sparing of the tendons. While a hyperthyroid state may increase the risk of developing Graves' ophthalmopathy, this presentation can occur even after the patient has been euthyroid for years. This is a restrictive ophthalmopathy and, therefore, forced duction testing will reveal restriction. Ocular manifestations include lid lag, lid retraction, exophthalmos, ocular surface disease, strabismus and compressive optic neuropathy. Conservative treatment options include prisms for diplopia caused by strabismus and frequent lubrication for surface disease induced by the exophthalmos. Systemic steroids may be indicated to help with active inflammation. Surgical treatment may also be necessary to treat strabismus and/or compressive optic neuropathy. If orbital decompression is necessary to prevent compressive optic neuropathy, this procedure should be performed prior to correction of strabismus. Otherwise, additional correction of strabismus may be required following decompression.

62. B. Heavy eye syndrome presents with hypotropia, limited elevation and fixed adduction (not abduction) in an eye with high myopia. This is a progressive disorder that may be treated surgically with loop myopexy.

63. C. Anisometropic amblyopia may occur in patients with asymmetric hyperopia or myopia.

64. D. Stimulus deprivation amblyopia occurs as a result of occlusion of the visual axis. This can be caused by anything that blocks the visual axis including lid lesions, corneal opacities or lens opacities. Typically, lens opacities must be at least 3 mm in diameter to be visually significant. Even relatively short periods of deprivation can cause amblyopia (1 week per age of life). Like anisometropic amblyopia, stimulus

deprivation amblyopia typically occurs up to age 5–6 years. Amblyopia may occur bilaterally in cases of bilateral occlusion of the visual axis.

65. B. Strabismic amblyopia occurs only in patients with a fixation preference. Patients who freely alternate will not develop amblyopia as both eyes are used equally and will therefore develop normally. The degree of amblyopia is directly proportional to the degree of fixation preference because the eye that is not preferred will progressively develop loss of foveal visual acuity. Strabismic amblyopia typically occurs up to age 5–6 years but may recur up to age 9–10 years if treatment cessation occurs. Successful treatment has been reported in patients into their teenage years.

66. E. Amblyopia is associated with decreased contrast sensitivity, abnormal spatial visual processing and amplification of the crowding phenomenon. A mild afferent pupillary defect can occur in severe cases of amblyopia. Amblyopia is associated with decreased (not increased) saccadic amplitudes.

67. D. Iatrogenic amblyopia usually occurs as a result of full-time patching of the "good" eye as part of amblyopia treatment. It is more common in young children who have rapidly developing visual systems. As a result, it typically develops rapidly and would not take years to develop.

68. B. Prisms are most useful in the treatment of small degrees of purely horizontal or vertical strabismus with diplopia. This includes diplopia induced by a sixth nerve palsy. Patients with congenital nystagmus who develop an abnormal head posture to accommodate a null point may also benefit from prism correction. Patients with superior oblique palsies may benefit from prisms but the induced excyclotorsion will limit their usefulness. Patients wiith purely torsional deviations would not benefit from prism as prism correction cannot address torsional misalignments.

69. B. Botulinum toxin chemodenervation has limited value in treating cases of exotropia with success rates of only 13% of cases.

70. D. Globe perforation during strabismus surgery poses a risk for retinal detachment but this is rare due to the formed vitreous in the young patients typically undergoing strabismus surgery. If the needle passes only into the suprachoroidal space, no treatment is indicated and retinal detachment typically will not occur. If the needle penetrates the retina, the risk for retinal detachment increases. All cases of suspected retinal detachment should undergo thorough retinal evaluation.

Milton Keynes UK
Ingram Content Group UK Ltd.
UKHW050739090724
445259UK00003B/18

9 789352 706105